Caring for children born small for gestational age

Development of this book was supported by funding from Sandoz

Caring for children born small for gestational age

Editor in chief
Siegfried Zabransky

Contributors

Miguel Alejandre Alcázar
Sarah Appel
Nordie Bilbao
Jörg Dötsch
Thomas Eggermann
A Kubilay Ertan
Anke Ertan
Fabian Fahlbusch
Martijn JJ Finken
Thomas Harder
Fritz Haverkamp
Axel Hübler
Berthold Huppertz
Prakash M Kabbur
Barbara Kaesmann-Kellner
Ruth Kuschewski
David D Martin
Eva Nüsken

Kai-Dietrich Nüsken
Dirk Manfred Olbertz
Nisha Parikh
Andreas Plagemann
Peter K Plinkert
Thomas Reinehr
Niels Rochow
Eva Rother
Paul Saenger
Ralf Schild
Roland Schweizer
Sebastian Straube
Ellen Struwe
Regina Trollmann
Anja Tzschoppe
Manfred Voigt
Patricia Vuguin
Philipp S van de Weyer

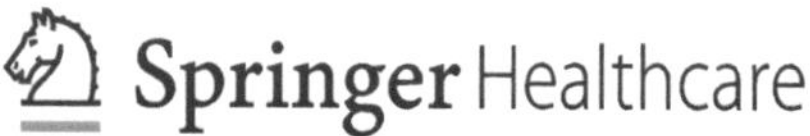

Published by Springer Healthcare Ltd, 236 Gray's Inn Road, London, WC1X 8HB, UK.

www.springerhealthcare.com

British Library Cataloguing-in-Publication Data.

A catalogue record for this book is available from the British Library.

ISBN 978-1-908517-85-2

Although every effort has been made to ensure that drug doses and other information are presented accurately in this publication, the ultimate responsibility rests with the prescribing physician. Neither the publisher nor the authors can be held responsible for errors or for any consequences arising from the use of the information contained herein. Any product mentioned in this publication should be used in accordance with the prescribing information prepared by the manufacturers. No claims or endorsements are made for any drug or compound at present under clinical investigation.

Project editor: Katrina Dorn
Designer: Joe Harvey
Artworker: Sissan Mollerfors
Production: Marina Maher
Printed in Great Britain by Latimer Trend and Co. Ltd.

Contents

SECTION ONE
Normal intrauterine development of the fetus

1 Fetal development 1

Siegfried Zabransky

2 Intrauterine aspects 11

Kai-Dietrich Nüsken

3 Maternal nutrition 25

Siegfried Zabransky

SECTION TWO
Interference with intrauterine fetal development

15 Growth hormone treatment 191

Roland Schweizer and David D Martin

16 Renal function 209

Jörg Dötsch

Author biography

Professor Dr. Med. Siegfried Zabransky studied human medicine at the University Erlangen-Nuernberg/Bavaria and University Innsbruck/Austria and received his PhD (Dr Med) from the University of Erlangen. He underwent his clinical training at the Hospital Eichstätt/Bavaria and at the children's hospital at the University of Erlangen-Nuernberg in surgery, gynecology, internal medicine, pediatrics. Professor Zabransky was house office at the University of Erlangen-Nuernberg, the Institute of Nuclear Medicine Free University Berlin and the children's hospital at the University Free University, Kaiserin Auguste Victoria Haus, where he became an assistant professor. Professor Zabransky served as assistant medical director and head of section of pediatric endocrinology and diabetology at the University of Saarland in Homberg until 2002, where he provided support to approximately 50 doctoral candidates. He was also head of the screening laboratory and poison control center of Saarland. His research interests include work done in hormones at the University of Goettingen (under Professor Dr.A.von zur Mühlen) and University of Munich (under Professor Scriba), and in the children's hospital of the University of Pittsburgh (in the research laboratory of Professor Foley). Additional research interests include newborn screening for endocrine and metabolic diseases, thyroid diseases in children, growth (inter alia growth study with evaluation of new growth charts for children; functional tests), puberty, and other general topics of pediatric endocrinology. He has over 100 publications, including 5 books. He is currently Head of Institute for Pediatric Endocrinology and Preventive Medicine (IPEP), Head of Medizinischer - Verlag Siegfried Zabransky, and works as a consultant. From 2003, he has organized the annual proceedings of interdisciplinary SGA workshops and serves as editor-in-chief (www.sga-syndrom.de).

zabransky.siegfried@web.de

Preface

During the last few years, many scientific articles related to several aspects of children born small for gestational age (SGA) or exposed to intrauterine growth restriction (IUGR) have been published by endocrinologists and other medical experts. The intention of this book is to summarize the most important topics about SGA/IUGR from a practical point of view.

The target audience for this book is gynecologists, obstetricians, midwives, neonatologists, pediatricians, endocrinologists, neurologists, psychiatrists, and nutritionists, as well as general practitioners and family practice physicians.

The estimated frequency of children born SGA and/or IUGR varies from 3–10% of all live births. Being born SGA and exposure to IUGR are contributors to the morbidity and mortality of newborns, particularly in underdeveloped areas of Asia and Africa where undernutrition and malnutrition are the frequent causes of disturbances to fetal growth. In so-called 'developed countries' with relatively higher living standards, avoidable causes of fetal growth restriction, such as alcohol consumption and smoking, can prevent normal fetal development.

Depending on when growth disturbances begin and the causes, there are numerous acute consequences and long-term effects of being born SGA. Initially, gynecologists, obstetricians, and neonatologists are involved but, later in childhood and during puberty, pediatricians, (especially pediatric endocrinologists and neurologists) may also have a role in providing patient care. In adulthood, metabolic syndrome and cardiovascular diseases are considered the most serious long-term effects and require continued medical care. Thus, despite being a condition that may begin before birth, it can be a lifelong condition that requires medical care across several specialities.

This book summarizes normal fetal development and interferences of fetal growth, as well as acute and long-term consequences. Prevention and pre-natal and post-natal care are described and considerations for future research are also discussed.

Most of the authors are members of a German working group, SGA-Syndrome (www.sga-syndrom.de). Initiated by Siegfried Zabransky, the group was formed in 2003 and holds annual workshops that focus primarily on topics such as SGA, IUGR, and fetal programming.

Acknowledgements

I thank my son, Dr. Markus Zabransky, who stimulated the conception of this book, and Sandoz International for funding of this project.

I also thank Katrina Dorn from Springer Healthcare for her valuable editorial support.

Finally, I wish to thank all of the contributors for their involvement.

Siegfried Zabransky, Homburg, 2013.

The development of this book was supported by Sandoz.

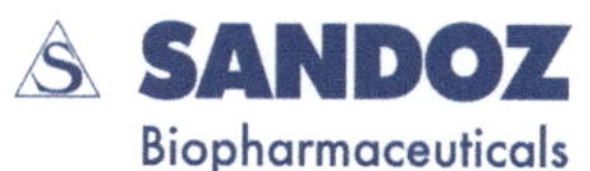

Normal intrauterine development of the fetus

Chapter 1

Fetal development

Siegfried Zabransky

Prenatal development

Conception signifies the fusion of a female (ovum) and a male (sperm) gamete, usually in the ampulla of the uterine tube. The result of this process is the production of a zygote, or fertilized ovum, which migrates down the fallopian tube to reach the uterus. The phases following conception include:

- implantation;
- placentation;
- embryonic period;
- fetal period.

Implantation

Implantation of the zygote into the wall of the uterus takes place approximately 9 days (ranging from 6–12 days) after ovulation. The blastocyst is created, which is composed of an inner cell mass called an embryoblast (made up of embryonic stem cells that will go on to form all of the body structures), an outer layer of cells and a trophoblast (which becomes the placenta) [1]. Insulin-like growth factor 1 (IGF-1) regulates the differentiation of cytotrophoblasts into syncytiotrophoblasts, which secrete progesterone and promote uterine lining integrity and extravillous cell formation [2–5].

S. Zabransky (ed.), *Caring for Children Born Small for Gestational Age*,
DOI: 10.1007/978-1-908517-90-6_1, © Springer Healthcare 2013

Placentation

Development of the placenta (or placentation) starts with the invasion of the syncytiotrophoblasts into the maternal endometrium and the reconfiguring of uterine spiral blood vessels to ensure blood supply to the blastocyte. This results in blood perfusion to the placenta because of the decreased resistance of these vessels. Placentation is regulated by local oxygen supply as well as immunological and growth factors (eg, IGF-1 and IGF-2), which act as endocrine, autocrine, and paracrine regulators [6]. The placentation process typically occurs 7–8 days after fertilization.

Embryonic period

The embryonic period lasts 56 days (8 weeks from fertilization). During this time, 90% of the body's organ systems are established [7] and the embryo divides into three distinct layers. Due to the rapid pace of differentiation, the embryo is very vulnerable during this phase and within the first 8 weeks the incidence of deformities that lead to miscarriages is approximately 10% (decreasing to 1% by the end of the embryonic period), while the frequency of neural tube defects is 2.5% (later decreasing to 0.1%) [8]. After the eighth week, the fetus starts to show recognizable human features, although the head is still relatively large in appearance.

Fetal period

During the fetal period (which lasts from the ninth week until birth), the organs that began to form during the embryonic period continue to grow and begin to differentiate during a process called organogenesis. During this period, major organs such as the brain, lungs, and liver grow isometrically in relation to the fetal body, while smaller organs like the thymus and spleen grow three to five times faster. The largest increase of length occurs during the second trimester, while weight tends to increase during the third trimester [9].

Gestational age

Gestational age is calculated from the first day of the last menstruation to the day of delivery. On average, it is 12–14 days longer than the conceptional age (with an error of calculation +/− 5 days), which refers to the time elapsed between the day of conception and the day of delivery. Gestational age is more commonly used to estimate the expected date of delivery because many women can recall when their last menstrual period began but may not be able to pinpoint when conception occurred. Thus, a full-term pregnancy is defined when the fetus has a conceptional age of 38 weeks or a gestational age of 40 weeks.

Measuring fetal growth

Ultrasound examination makes it possible to obtain information about implantation, placental position and morphology, volume of amniotic fluid, presence of a multiple pregnancy, fetal position and morphology, vitality of the embryo/fetus, sex, gestational age, and fetal growth (for comparison with standard growth curves).

As early as 4.5 weeks gestational age, a gestational sac can be identified, which grows approximately 1 mm per day [10,11]. Until approximately 20 weeks gestational age, fetal length is measured from the crown of the head to the rump; after 20 weeks, it is measured from crown to heel. Several other parameters, especially in combination, allow estimation of fetal proportion, length, and weight development (Table 1.1). Fetal weight can be estimated by polynomial equations combining biparietal diameter, femur length, and abdominal circumference [12,13] (Table 1.1). Below is a list of auxological parameters that can be measured by ultrasound examination:

- biparietal diameter;
- head circumference;
- occipitofrontal diameter;
- femur length;
- humerus length;
- abdominal circumference;
- crown–rump length.

It should be noted that standards for birth weight and length may be very different in several countries and regions, depending on different ethnographic factors and nutritional conditions, as well as different health care systems. Additionally, a child born as part of a multiple birth is more likely to have a lower birth weight than a singleton [17] (Table 1.2).

Length and weight development of the fetus

Gestational age (weeks)	Length (inches)	Weight (oz)	Length (cm)	Mass (g)
	(Crown to rump)		(Crown to rump)	
8	0.630	0.040	1.60	1
12	2.130	0.490	5.40	14
15	3.980	2.470	10.1	70
16	4.570	3.530	11.6	100
	(Crown to heel)*		(Crown to heel)*	
20	6.460	10.58	16.4	300
24	11.81	17.32	30.0	600
28	14.80	35.45	37.6	1005
32	16.69	60.04	42.4	1702
35	18.19	84.06	46.2	2383
35	19.13	100.8	48.6	2859
38	19.61	108.7	49.8	3083
40	20.16	122.1	51.2	3462
42	20.28	130.0	51.5	3685

Table 1.1 Length and weight development of the fetus. *After 20 weeks, fetal size is measured from crown to heel. Data adapted from Doubilet et al 1997, Hadlock et al 1992, and Usher et al 1969 [14–16].

Frequency of low and very low birth weight in children born as singletons or a part of a multiple birth

Birth weight (g)	Singletons	Twins	Triplets
<2500	6.1%	52.2%	91.5%
<1500	1.1%	10.1%	31.9%

Table 1.2 Frequency of low and very low birth weight in children born as singletons or a part of a multiple birth. Adapted from Alexander et al [17].

Regulation of fetal growth

Normal fetal growth is regulated by the intrauterine and placental environment, the fetal genome, and several maternal (eg, hormonal, nutritional) and environmental factors. Especially in utero, the environment determined by maternal and placental function is important for fetal growth [18]. This is true not only for the development of the organs but also for metabolic processes where genetic factors play an important role (eg, diabetes). Throughout pregnancy, the placenta is crucial for transport and exchange of nutrients, trace elements, vitamins, and oxygen from the mother.

The estimated influence of the maternal genome on the birth weight of the children is 20%, while environmental factors account for 60%; other factors account for the remaining 20% [19]. The genetic influence is almost entirely maternal in origin, with low paternal genetic correlation [20,21]. As such, maternal height is an important determinant of birth size and reflects an association between height, uterine size, and blood flow. However, the genetic correlation in birth weight is rather low, and non-genetic maternal environmental influences appear to be more important [18]. For example, Brooks et al showed that the intrauterine milieu is more important for determining birth weight than purely genetic factors [22]. In 62 cases of ovum donation, donor weight, donor birth weight, and the birth weight of the donor's children were not significantly correlated. Furthermore, in animal studies, it has been shown that fetuses with the same genotype (eg, identical twins) will be different sizes if grown in different uteruses, depending on the breed and maternal size [23]. Normal fetal growth in late gestation is constrained by uteroplacental factors.

Placental regulation of fetal growth

Maintaining an adequate supply of nutrients to the fetus depends on sufficient uteroplacental perfusion (via maternal blood supply), placental weight and surface, and placental active transport capacity for amino acids, lipids, and glucose [18]. The predominant binding protein in placental tissue is IGF-binding protein 3 (IGFBP3) and it is expressed in high levels by trophoblasts and fibroblasts of the villous stroma [24].

Especially during the early phase of pregnancy, the placenta develops its own metabolic activities in order to supply the embryo with glycogen, cholesterol, and fatty acids [25,26]. There are selective processes for nutrient transport. The placenta also acts as an excretory organ for carbon dioxide, urea, uric acid, bilirubin, and other substances that could harm the fetus. Additionally, the placenta is regarded as an endocrine organ because it not only has regulatory effects on embryo and fetal survival but on maternal metabolism as well. Placental hormones include progesterone, estrogen, placental adrenocorticotrophic hormone, human chorionic gonadotropin, and gonadotropin-releasing hormone, among others [25].

Hormonal regulation of fetal growth

Hormones and growth factors are essential for fetal growth and promoting the utilization of available substrates [27]. Growth hormone (GH) is detectable in cells of the anterior lobe of the fetal hypophysis from the sixth gestational week and active secretion starts from 8th gestational week. In fetal circulation, GH is evident from the twelfth gestational week. In the middle of the gestation (ie, week 20), GH levels in the plasma reach very high values (approximately 100 ng/mL) [28], only to decrease later in the pregnancy, which is most likely a result of gradual activation of IGF-1-mediated feedback on a hypophyseal level [29].

Although high circulating-GH concentrations are detectable during the second half of the pregnancy, GH is not necessarily important for fetal growth regulation. For example, children born with anencephaly are born with an absence of GH but still may have a normal body length at birth. Additionally, children with congenital GH deficiency caused by gene defects or a defect of the hypothalamo–hyphyseal axis can also be average length at birth [30]. Possibly, during the fetal period, GH may have a greater influence on metabolism and body composition than body length. Interestingly, in children born small for gestational age (SGA), GH concentrations in cord blood are elevated when compared with eutrophic and hypertrophic children [31].

IGF is produced in all fetal tissues and during later fetal development, fetal IGF-1 serum levels correlate with fetal body weight [32]. Fetal growth is regulated by fetal insulin and IGF-2 and IGF-1, whereas GH and thyroid hormones play a secondary role. This is in contrast to the postnatal growth regulation, which is dominated by GH and IGF-1. The postnatal growth-promoting effect of GH is mediated by IGF-1, and IGF-1 secretion depends on stimulation by GH. Regulation of hypothalamo-hypophyseal hormones (GHRH) and external stimuli (eg, hypoglycemia) is intact at birth. The typical pattern of the spontaneous GH secretion with low values during the day and sleep-associated secretion at night develops during the first 6 weeks after birth [28].

Whereas IGF-2 is the primary growth factor of embryonic growth, IGF-1 (which is produced in the liver and other tissues) is the dominant fetal growth regulator in late gestation, as well as postnatally [33].

IGF-2 is evident in the fetal circulation during the first trimester and its concentration increases up to the birth (whereas GH levels decrease). Prenatally, IGF-II is regulated independently from GH [31].

Fetal insulin is most likely to be the primary growth-promoting factor in prenatal life, which is predominantly regulated by fetal glucose availability [34]. The somatogenic actions of insulin are mediated through IGF release [35,36], whereas its direct effects are on adipogenesis [37]. Thus, IGF synthesis is mainly regulated through nutrient supply (and thus, deficiency) [30,38–40].

Glucocorticoids also affect fetal growth and maturation [41]. The barrier enzyme 11 *b*-hydroxysteroid type 2, localized in the placenta, protects the fetus from maternal glucocorticoids. However, maternal undernutrition downregulates this enzyme and, as a result, the fetus can be exposed to increasing levels of glucocorticoids, which can intensify fetal growth restriction. Additionally, extended exposure to maternal glucocorticoids may induce intrauterine growth restriction (IUGR) [41]. Human glucocorticoid receptors and GH receptor proteins are evident from the fifteenth gestational week in fetal chondrocytes, osteoblasts, fibroblasts, and the epidermis [42].

References

1   Wilcox AJ, Baird DD, Weinberg CR. Time of implantation of the conceptus and loss of pregnancy. *N Eng J Med*. 1999;340:1796-1799.
2   Bhaumick B, George D, Bala RM. Potentiation of epidermal growth factor induced differentiation of cultured human placental cells by insulin-like growth factor I. *J Clin Endocrinol Metab*. 1992;74:1005-1011.
3   Milio LA, Hu J, Douglas GC. Binding of insulin-like growth factor I to human trophoblast cells during differentiation in vitro. *Placenta*. 1994:15:641-651.
4   Lacey H, Haigh T, Westwood M, Aplin JD. Mesenchymally-derived insulin-like growth factor I provides a paracrine stimulus for trophoblast migration. *BMC Dev Biol*. 2002;2:5.
5   Aplin JD, Lacey H, Haigh T, Jones CJ, Chen CP, Westwood M. Growth factor -extracellular matrix synergy in the control of trophoblast invasion. *Biochem Soc Trans*. 2000;28:199-202.
6   Roberts CT, Owens JA, Sferuzzi-Perri AN. Distinct actions of insulin-like growth factors on placental development and fetal growth: lessons from mice and guinea pigs. *Placenta*. 2008;29:42-47.
7   O'Rahilly R, Müller F. Developmental stages in human embryos: revised and new measurements. *Cells Tissues Organs*. 2010;192:73-84.
8   Shiota K. Teratothanasia: prenatal loss of abnormal cenceptuses and the prevalence of various malformations during human gestation. *Defects Orig Artic Ser*. 1993;29:189-199.
9   Mullis PE, Tonella P. Regulation of fetal growth: consequences and impact of being born small. *Best Pract Res Clin Endocrinol Metab*. 2008;22:173-190.

10 Nyberg DA, Mack LA, Lasing FC, Patten RM. Distinguishing normal from abnormal gestational sac growth in early pregnancy. *J Ultrasound Med.* 1987;6:23-27.

11 Robinson HP, Fleming JE. A critical evaluation of sonar "crown-rump length" measurements. *Br J Obstet Gynaecol.* 1975;82:702-710.

12 Shepard MJ, Richards VA, Berkowitz RI, Warsof SL, Hobbins JC. An evaluation of two equations for predicting fetal weight by ultrasound. *Am J Obstet Gynecol.* 1982;142:47-54.

13 Hadlock FP, Harrist RB, Sharman RS, Deter RL, Park SK. Estimation of fetal weight with the use of head, body, and femur measurements: a prospective study. *Am J Obstet Gynecol.* 1985;151:333-337.

14 Doubilet PM, Benson CB, Nadel AS, et al. Improved birth weight table for neonates developed from gestations dated by early ultrasonography. *J Ultrasound Med.* 1997;16:241.

15 Hadlock FP, Shah YP, Kanon DJ, et al. Fetal crown rump length: reevaluation of relation to menstrual age with high resolution real-time US. *Radiology.*1992;182:501.

16 Usher R, McLean F. Intrauterine growth of live-born Caucasian infants at sea level: standards obtained from measurements in 7 dimensions of infants born between 25 and 44 weeks of gestation. *Pediatrics.* 1969;74.901-910.

17 Alexander GR, Kogan M, Martin J, et al. What are the fetal growth patterns of singletons, twins, and triplets in the United States? *Clin Obstet Gynecol.* 1998;41:115-125.

18 Gluckman PD, Pinal CS. Regulation of fetal growth by the somatotrophic axis. *J Nutr.* 2003;133:1741-1746.

19 Milner RDG. Prenatal growth control. In: Gluckman PD, Heymann MA, eds. *Perinatal and pediatric pathophysiology: a clinical perspective.* London, UK: Hodder and Stoughton; 1993:163-169.

20 Polani PE. Chromosomal and other genetic influences on birth weight variation. In: Elliott K, Knight J, eds. *Ciba Foundation Symposium 27 - Size at Birth.* Chichester, UK: John Wiley and Sons; 2008:127-159.

21 Robson EB. The genetics of birth weight. In: Faulkner F, Tanner JM, eds. *Human Growth: Principles and Prenatal Growth.* New York: Plenum Press; 1978:285-297.

22 Brooks AA, Johnson MR, Steer PJ, et al. Birth weight: nature or nurture? *Early Hum Develop.* 1995;42:29-35.

23 Walton A, Hammond J. The maternal effects on growth and conformation in Shire horse-Shetland pony crosses. *Proc Royal Soc Lond.* 1938; 125:311-335.

24 Forbes K, Westwood M. The IGF axis and placental function. *Horm Res.* 2008;69:129-137.

25 Petraglia F, Florio P, Nappi C, Genazzini AR. Peptide signaling in human placenta and membranes: autocrine, paracrine, and endocrine mechanisms. *Endocr Rev.* 1996;2:156-186.

26 Moore KL, Persaud TVN. *Embryologie, Lehrbuch und Atlas der Entwicklungsgeschichte des Menschen.* New York, NY: Auflage, Schattauer Verlag Stuttgart; 1996:128-140.

27 Evain-Brion D. Hormonal regulation of fetal growth. *Horm Res.* 1994;42:207-214.

28 Wollmann Hartmut A. Die Wachstumshormonregulation vom Fetus zum Kindesalter. In: Wollmann HA, Ranke MB, eds. *Perinatale Endokrinologie.* Mannheim, Germany: Palatium Verlag (J&J edition); 2002:11-20.

29 Gluckman PD. The role of pituitary hormones, growth factors and insulin in the regulation of fetal growth. In: Clarke JR, ed. *Oxford reviews of reproductive biology 8.* Oxford, UK: Clarendon Press; 1986:1-60.

30 Gluckman PD, Gunn AJ, Wray A, et al. Congenital idiopathic growth hormone deficiency associated with prenatal and early postnatal growth failure. The International Board of the Kabi Pharmacia International Growth Study. *J Pediatr.* 1992;121:920-923.

31 De Zegher F, Kimpen J, Raus J, Vanderschueren-Lodeweyckx M. Hypersomatotropism in dysmature infant at term and preterm birth. *Biol Neonate.* 1990;58:188-191.

32 Gluckman PD. Thendocrine regulation of fetal growth in late gestation. The role of insulin-like growth factors. *J Clin Endocrinol Metab.* 1995;4:1047-1050.

33 D'Ercole AJ, Applewhite GT, Underwood LE. Evidence that somatomedin is synthesized by multiple tissues in the fetus. *Dev Biol*. 1980;75:315-328.

34 Oliver MH, Harding JE, Breier BH, Gluckman PD. Fetal insulin-like growth factor (IGF)-I and IGF-II are regulated differently by glucose or insulin in the sheep fetus. *Reprod Fertil Dev*. 1996;8:167-172.

35 Fowden AL. The role of insulin in prenatal growth. *J Dev Physiol*. 1989;12:173-182.

36 Fowden AL, Hughes P, Comline RS. The effects of insulin on the growth rate of the sheep fetus during late gestation. *Q J Exp Physiol*. 1989;74:703-714.

37 Cheek DB, Brayton JB, Scott RE. Overnutrition, overgrowth and hormones (with special reference to the infant born of the diabetic mother). *Adv Exp Med Biol*. 1974;49:47-72.

38 Gluckmann PD, Grumbach MM, Kaplan SL. The neuroendocrine regulation and function of growth hormone and prolactin in mammalian fetus. *Endocr Rev*. 1981;2:363-395.

39 Klempt M, Bingham B, Breier BH, Baumbach WR, Gluckman PD. Tissue distribution and ontogeny of growth hormone receptor messenger ribonucleic acid and ligand binding to hepatic tissue in the midgestation sheep fetus. *Endocrinology*. 1993;132:1071-1077.

40 Breier BH, Ambler GR, Sauerwein H, Surus A, Gluckman, PD. The induction of hepatic somatotrophic receptors after birth in sheep is dependent on parturition associated mechanisms. *J Endocrinol*. 1994;141:101-108.

41 Seckl JR. Glucocorticoids, feto-placental 11beta-hydroxysteroid dehydrogenase type 2, and the early life origins of adult disease. *Steroids*. 1997;62:89-94.

42 Werther GH, Haynes K, Waters MJ. Growth hormone receptors are expressed on human fetal mesenchymal tissues – identification of messenger ribonucleic acid and GH-binding protein. *J Clin Endocrinol Metab*. 1993;76:1638-1646.

Development of this book was supported by funding from Sandoz

Chapter 2

Intrauterine aspects

Kai-Dietrich Nüsken

Fetoplacental unit

The fetoplacental unit is a part of the materno-fetoplacental unit and normal fetal growth and development is achieved when there is adequate interaction between all parts. The placenta serves as an exchange interface between mother and fetus and this chapter will focus on fetoplacental processes, including bidirectional transport, communication, and interaction between the fetus and the placenta.

The placenta strongly influences the fetal phenotype because it regulates the maternal-placental-fetal transport of nutrients and oxygen. The placenta therefore has a high metabolic activity to meet its own as well as fetal demands. The most important role of the placenta is the delivery of nutrients, oxygen, placental hormones, signaling molecules, and cytokines to the fetus. To compliment this, the fetus delivers hormones, signaling molecules, cytokines, and waste to the placenta, which influences placental morphology and function.

Fetal nutrition

Normal fetal nutrition depends on the adequate supply of macronutrients (eg, carbohydrates, fat, proteins/amino acids), micronutrients (eg, trace elements, vitamins), and electrolytes from the placenta to the fetus, and the adequate elimination of fetal metabolic end products. Preconditions for adequate fetal growth include sufficient maternal nutrient availability,

S. Zabransky (ed.), *Caring for Children Born Small for Gestational Age*, DOI: 10.1007/978-1-908517-90-6_2, © Springer Healthcare 2013

adequate trophoblast invasion, placental growth, and increasing utero-placental and fetoplacental blood flow [discussed further in Chapter 8]. Nutrient supply to the fetus is mediated in part by simple diffusion, facilitated diffusion and active transport. Endocytosis and exocytosis also play a role. Thus, placental nutrient supply to the fetus can be influenced by a number of different mechanisms: modulation of food availability by hormonal modification of maternal eating behavior and metabolism, adaptation of placental blood flow, adjustment of placental metabolism and growth, and activation of transport processes [1–3].

Transport of nutrients
Glucose
Glucose is essential for fetal growth. Almost all fetal circulating glucose is provided via facilitated diffusion transporters in the placenta [3]. The most important placental glucose transporter is glucose transporter 1 (GLUT1), which is found in the microvillus and basal membranes of the syncytiotrophoblast, as well as in endothelial cells. As GLUT1 is abundantly present in the microvillus membrane, but not in the basal membrane, basal GLUT1 may be rate-limiting for transplacental glucose transfer. Glucose transporter 3 (GLUT3) may enhance glucose uptake in fetal placental arteries [4] and is also found in stromal cells [5]. Both GLUT1 and GLUT3 are insulin-independent. Glucose transporter 4 (GLUT4), the insulin dependent isoform, is found in placental stromal cells but does not seem to influence maternal-fetal glucose transport.

In perfusion studies under physiological conditions, transplacental glucose flux was insulin-independent and only limited by nutrient availability (eg, maternal-fetal glucose gradient and uteroplacental blood flow). GLUT1 expression and activity were relatively constant at physiological extracellular concentrations (20–220 mg/dL) in vitro, but decreased at high concentrations (>360 mg/dL) [3,6]. At these high glucose concentrations, GLUT1-mediated transport of glucose is saturable. Notably, glucose is subject to significant placental metabolism. The placenta stores glucose in the form of glycogen and releases it mainly in the form of lactate [3], which is used for energy production by the fetus and may also function as an energy store [6].

Amino acids

Amino acids are important energy substrates and are the basic elements of proteins, which play key roles in metabolic pathways, tissue formation, and hormonal signaling. Alterations in amino acid supply, even when limited to a single (essential) amino acid, may have wide-ranging effects on fetal development. Therefore, amino acid transporter systems have been the subject of numerous studies and reviews that have focused on placental location, functioning, and complex characteristics of the transporters [7,8].

Transplacental amino acid supply depends on transport across the microvillus and basal syncytiotrophoblast, as well as the metabolism within the syncytiotrophoblast [9]. In a normal pregnancy, the concentration of amino acids is higher in fetal plasma than maternal plasma, suggesting active transport. Because the relationship between umbilical venous and maternal plasma amino acid concentrations is not the same for all amino acids [9], selective active transfer of specific amino acids is suggested.

In the microvillus membrane, there are two main classes of amino acid transporters:

- accumulative transporters belonging to the system A family;
- the X_{AG}^- system and amino acid exchangers [7,10].

Both classes work together in the microvillus membrane to supply an adequate amount of amino acids to the basal membrane. Within the syncytiotrophoblast, amino acids may be considerably metabolized [11]. However, there are limited data available pertaining to amino acid metabolism in the human placenta. Glutamate, which is a major neurotransmitter, may be metabolized to glutamine in the human syncytiotrophoblast [11], which may protect the fetus from neurotoxic glutamate concentrations.

Transporters in the basal membrane appear to regulate the amount and type of amino acids transferred to the fetus. A number of transporters localized in the basal membrane have been identified, including amino acid exchangers, accumulative transporters, sodium-dependent exchangers, and facilitated diffusion channels. However, the specific transporters involved in the regulatory process still need to be identified [7].

Lipids

The transplacental supply of lipids is complex and only partially understood. Some authors estimate that approximately half of fetal body fat at term is due to fetal lipogenetic activity, whereas the other half is due to maternal–fetal transfer [3]. Fatty acids provide an important energy source and are the main source of fetal fat accumulation, 90% of which occurs during the last 10 weeks of pregnancy [12]. Moreover, long-chain polyunsaturated fatty acids and cholesterol are essential for fetal development as they form part of cell membranes and functional molecules. An insufficient supply may result in complications such as impaired neuronal development, blood clotting disorders, and vascular damage [13].

Maternal hyperlipidemia during pregnancy can cause a concentration gradient between mother and fetus and in this setting free fatty acids are able to pass the placenta by simple diffusion. However, only 1% of fatty acids are free and, therefore, the majority of circulating fatty acids can only pass the placenta after processing or by transport mechanisms. Hydrolysis of triglycerides (derived from lipoproteins) by lipoprotein lipase and subsequent uptake of fatty acids (by either diffusion or placental plasma membrane fatty acid binding proteins [FABPs] and transporters present in the syncytiotrophoblast) is an important source of lipids. Apart from diffusion, binding proteins and transporters considerably affect fatty acid transport. Fatty acid translocase, plasma membrane FABP, fatty acid transport protein, and intracellular FABPs are all involved [14]. Triglycerides are also taken up as low-density lipoproteins (LDL) or very-low-density lipoprotein by receptor-mediated endocytosis [3,12]. Transport of cholesterol may occur by uptake of LDL via the LDL-receptor by endocytosis [15].

Placental nutrient sensing and efficiency

The placenta is able to detect the nutritional status of the mother and the nutritional demands of the fetus, and reacts to both via regulation of placental function (eg, fetoplacental nutrient transport by modification of transporter abundance and activity), and with modification of placental morphology (eg, placental surface area and vascularization). Signals of maternal and fetal nutritional status relate to the concentrations of circulating nutrients, insulin-like growth factor (IGF), insulin, glucocorticoids, and leptin (Figure 2.1) [2]. Maternal partial pressure of oxygen also influences transplacental nutrient transport because the placenta metabolically adapts to hypoxia [2].

With respect to placental weight, placental efficiency is especially important and is often expressed as fetal weight (in grams [g]) divided by placental weight (g_{fw}/g_{pw}) [2]. Placental efficiency can be increased in case of adverse environmental conditions to support the fetus in achieving its genetically determined growth potential [2]. For example, in rats fed an isocaloric, 8% low-protein diet (compared to 18–20% protein

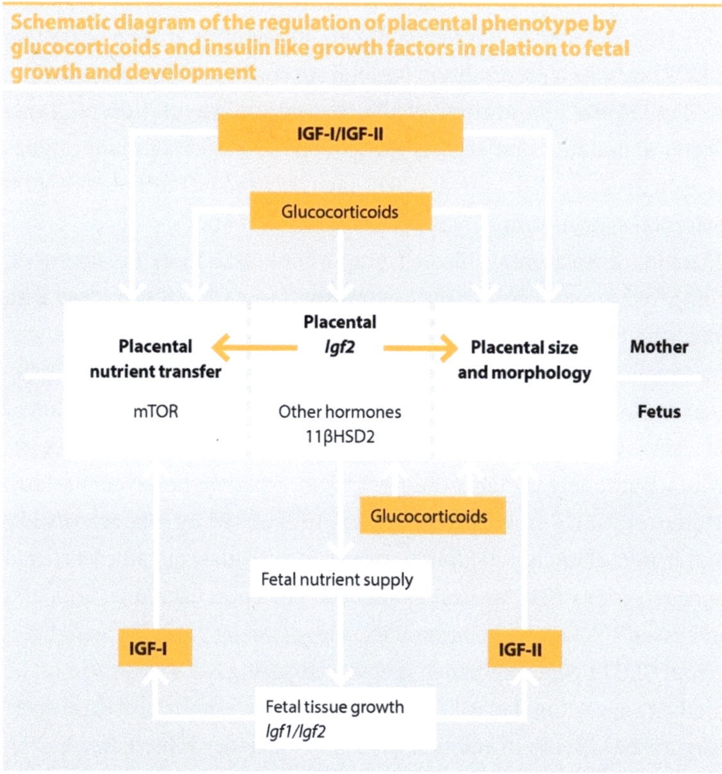

Figure 2.1 Schematic diagram of the regulation of placental phenotype by glucocorticoids and insulin like growth factors in relation to fetal growth and development. Orange boxes, circulating hormones; white boxes, regulated processes. Gene expression is shown in italics. IGF, insulin like growth factor; 11βHSD2, 11β-hydroxysteroid-dehydrogenase type 2; mTOR, mammalian target of rapamycin. Reprinted with permission from Fowden et al [2].

in a normal diet), placental efficiency increased by about 10% because there was a greater reduction of placental weight than fetal weight [16]. This is because the placenta supplies as much substrate as possible to the fetus [16]. Accordingly, in humans, small placentas are most often more efficient than heavy placentas [17].

Decreased placental efficiency indicates a suboptimal placental-fetal nutrient transfer, possibly due to placental insufficiency. Decreased placental efficiency is often associated with restricted oxygen availability [2,3,18]. In rats with uteroplacental insufficiency induced by bilateral ligation of the uterine arteries, placental efficiency decreased by approximately 20% because fetal weight, but not placental weight, was reduced [19]. However, under hypoxic conditions, intrauterine growth restriction (IUGR) may be a precondition for fetal survival by saving oxygen [2].

Functional adaptations of the placenta by regulation of transporter abundance and activity have been the subject of many studies [2,8,18,20,21,25,29]. In fetal IUGR, samples from full-term or pre-term placental syncytiotrophoblasts and basal membranes showed no differences in transplacental glucose transport or in GLUT1 expression when compared to controls [8]. Glucose transport in six IUGR placentae with abnormalities in umbilical arterial Doppler measurements also showed no alteration. However, decreased GLUT1 expression and glucose transport in IUGR pregnancies have been observed [20]. The expression of placental GLUT1 transporters is downregulated in maternal diabetes, which putatively protects the fetus from excess hyperglycemia [20]. Moreover, GLUT transporters are downregulated by glucocorticoids, and maternal undernutrition is associated with elevated glucocorticoid concentrations [21], as well as reduced placental exchange area and increased thickness of placental exchange barrier [22]. Increased placental GLUT1 gene expression is observed during IGF-I treatment of the mother, suggesting that IGF-1 promotes transplacental glucose transport (Figure 2.1) [2,23]. In addition, placental efficiency is increased during maternal IGF-I treatment in guinea pigs [24].

Because amino acids also are important energy substrates for the fetus, impaired transplacental amino acid transport is associated with IUGR [25,26]. In full-term IUGR neonates (as diagnosed by Doppler velocimetry), system A amino acid transporter activity across the microvillus membrane is significantly reduced compared to neonates born average for gestational age [25]. In twins with discordant birth weight, fetal concentrations of total essential, nonessential, and branched chain amino acids were significantly lower in twins with IUGR compared with twins born average for gestational age or in concordant twin pairs [27]. Roos et al. suggested that the placental mammalian target of rapamycin (mTOR) pathway might be a key candidate linking nutrient availability to fetal growth [28]. In a study on cultured primary trophoblasts, the investigators found that inhibition of the mTOR pathway significantly reduced the activity of system A, system L, and taurine amino acid transporters [29]. However, rapamycin treatment did not significantly decrease the protein expression of any of the transporter isoforms. Thus, mTOR signaling seems to regulate the activity of placental amino acid transporters without altering the amount of protein expression (Figure 2.1) [2,29].

In guinea pig model, maternal IGF-1 treatment increased amino acid transport and the expression of the amino acid transporter SLC38A2 gene [24]. Fetal IGF-1 treatment in sheep has been shown to reduce the placental clearance of amino acids from the fetal circulation [30]. Placenta-specific knock-out of IGF-2 in mice reduces placental growth, but increases placental efficiency, the ratio of transported amino acids/ placental weight, and the placental expression of the amino acid transporters SLC38A4 and SLC2A1 [31]. Glucocorticoids may also affect placental amino acid transport (Figure 2.1) [2].

Focusing on fatty acid transport, perfusion studies in placentae without pathology showed a constant transport capacity across a 2.5-fold range in placental weight [32]. The authors of the study concluded that, especially in small fetuses, a very high amount of transport capacity has to be lost to limit fetal growth [32]. However, the lipid profile of IUGR fetuses is unclear. Fetuses that are SGA may be hypertriglyceridemic [33], which supports the notion that triglyceride transfer does not limit fetal weight gain or growth. However, there is also evidence that lipoprotein lipase activity is impaired in IUGR placenta at term [13], which may result in reduced transplacental supply of free fatty acids.

Morphological adaptations of the placenta include modification of placental surface area, thickness of diffusion barrier, vascularization, and uteroplacental blood flow. Efficient placentas are usually small [34]. In mice, efficient placentae show a clearly increased ratio of surface area:placental weight [35]. The thickness of the diffusion barrier is increased in inefficient placentas of guinea pigs during malnutrition [20]. Adequate placental vascularization and utero-placental blood flow is a precondition for fetal growth and development. Whether or not increased vascular endothelial growth factor (VEGF) expression and angiogenesis contribute to modification of placental efficiency is still controversial and appears to depend on the species [2].

Oxygenation of the fetoplacental unit

An adequate, balanced supply of oxygen is vital for survival and the development of the fetoplacental unit. Both over- and undersupply of oxygen may have adverse effects and induce pathologies, including placental insufficiency and IUGR. The oxygenation of the fetoplacental unit has recently been reviewed [36,37]. See Chapter 9 for a more in-depth discussion of placental anatomy and perfusion.

Oxygen tension

In the first trimester, the endovascular trophoblast forms plugs that occlude the spiral arteries. Therefore, the intervillus space is filled with plasma and the nutrition of the fetus is histiotrophic (by endometrial glands). The mean intervillus oxygen tension during the first 10 weeks of pregnancy is about 20 mmHg (~3%). A low oxygen environment during this developmental stage is important to protect the fetoplacental unit from oxidative stress, as sufficient antioxidative properties are not available [38].

Between the tenth and twelfth week of pregnancy, the spiral arteries are further transformed and the plugs disappear. Maternal blood is able to enter the intervillus space, and the nutrition of the fetus is now hemotrophic. The mean intervillus oxygen tension rises to about 60 mmHg (~9%). At this time, the fetoplacental unit is able to provide sufficient antioxidative mechanisms. For sufficient exchange of nutrients and gases, as well as for integrity of the villus trophoblast, funnel-shaped spiral arteries are important as they allow a high perfusion of the intervillus space at a low flow rate. Throughout the ongoing pregnancy, uteroplacental perfusion is increased by dilatation of the uterine arteries, which is a necessary adaptation to and precondition for exponential growth of the fetus. The mean intervillus oxygen tension during this time decreases slightly from about 60 mmHg to about 50 mmHg (Figure 2.2) [36,39].

Relation of oxygenation to fetal growth

In early pregnancy, increased placental blood flow leads to increased oxygen tension, which, in turn, induces placental oxidative stress, impaired invasion, reduced vascularization, and can lead to reduced blood flow and pathologies, including IUGR, later in pregnancy [40]. In the second and third trimesters, the fetoplacental unit is at risk from acute or chronic hypoxia rather than from oxidative stress. Impaired oxygenation of the fetus may be pre-placental (eg, maternal anemia, high altitude pregnancy), uteroplacental (eg, shallow invasion, impaired spiral artery conversion), or post-placental (eg, disturbed perfusion of the fetal side of the placenta). As the placenta is not able to provide

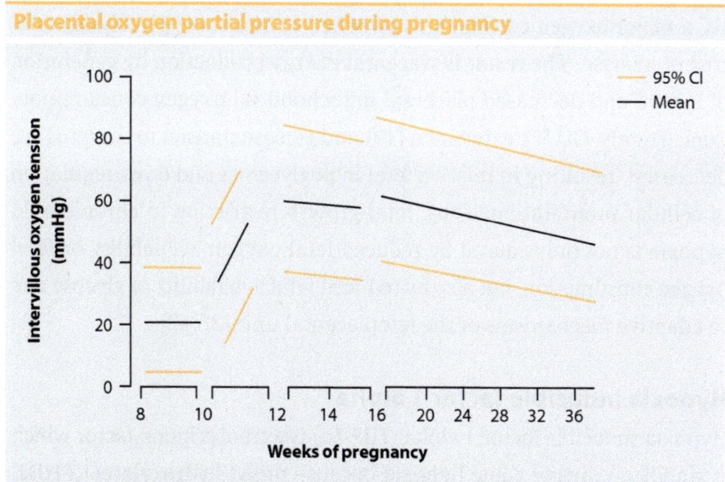

Figure 2.2 Placental oxygen partial pressure during pregnancy. The mean (black lines) and 95% confidence intervals of oxygen partial pressure (orange lines) throughout gestation in the intervillous space in the human. CI, confidence interval. Reprinted with permission from Zamudio [39].

more than 60 mmHg partial pressure of oxygen, even an adequately supplied fetus is in a chronic state of borderline hypoxemia. Both fetal partial oxygen pressure in umbilical cord blood and placental efficiency (birth weight:placental weight ratio) are related to weight at birth [41]. Newborns with IUGR show decreased partial oxygen pressure in umbilical arterial and venous blood and decreased placental efficiency. By contrast, infants born large for gestational age have increased partial pressure of oxygen [41].

However, the fetoplacental unit has efficient mechanisms to counteract fetal hypoxemia. Results observed in high-altitude pregnancies show that both the placenta and the fetus are involved in the adaptations [36,42]. An important placental mechanism to save oxygen is the reduction of its own high oxygen consumption via metabolic adaptation. In high-altitude pregnancies there is a 33% reduction in maternal oxygen partial pressure and a 25% reduction in uteroplacental blood flow, but only a 10% reduction in umbilical venous oxygen partial pressure and no reduction of fetal oxygen consumption [36]. Interestingly, while birth weight is reduced by 10%, placental weight shows no reduction [36]. The placenta therefore is less efficient during chronic hypoxia [36,42]. During this time, the placenta extracts more glucose from the maternal blood because aerobic glycolysis, a major oxygen consumer, is switched to anaerobic glycolysis at the cost of glucose. The result is placental energy production by generation of lactate and decreased placental mitochondrial oxygen consumption. Concurrently, GLUT1 expression [19] and glucose transfer to the fetus are decreased, resulting in relative fetal hypoglycemia and downregulation of cellular proliferation. Thus, fetal growth restriction in chronic mild hypoxia is not only caused by reduced fetal oxygen availability or fetal oxygen consumption, but also by reduced fetal availability of glucose due to adaptive mechanisms of the fetoplacental unit [36,42].

Hypoxia inducible factor 1 alpha

Hypoxia-inducible factor 1 alpha (HIF-1α) is a transcription factor which is stabilized during acute hypoxia because prolyl hydroxylases (PHD1, PHD2, PHD3), which regulate HIF activity, are inhibited by hypoxia. After forming a heterodimer with HIF-1β (an aryl hydrocarbon receptor nuclear translocator), HIF-1α translocates into the cellular nucleus and promotes the transcription of multiple genes. During chronic hypoxia, stabilization of HIF-1α decreases again in several tissues and HIF-2α may be more important for the regulation of gene expression [43]. Nevertheless, HIF-1α protein expression is increased in placental tissue in pregnancies at a high altitude where there is mild chronic hypoxia. Maternal circulating VEGF and erythropoietin, both of which are HIF-regulated, also are elevated in high altitude pregnancies [44].

Additionally, several hypoxia-independent mechanisms of HIF-1α induction are known, among them cytokines (interleukin-1β, tumor necrosis factor α), growth factors (IGF-II, transforming growth factor 1β), and hormones (angiotensin II) [45,46]. In conclusion, HIF-1α-mediated mechanisms may be crucial for both the hypoxic response and regulative processes during normoxia in the fetoplacental unit during all three trimesters of pregnancy.

References

1 Murphy VE, Smith R, Giles WB, Clifton VL. Endocrine regulation of human fetal growth: the role of the mother, placenta, and fetus. *Endocr Rev*. 2006;27:141-169.
2 Fowden AL, Sferruzzi-Perri AN, Coan PM, Constancia M, Burton GJ. Placental efficiency and adaptation: endocrine regulation. *J Physiol*. 2009;587:3459-3472.
3 Desoye G, Gauster M, Wadsack C. Placental transport in pregnancy pathologies. *Am J Clin Nutr*. 2011;94:1896S-1902S.
4 Illsley NP. Glucose transporters in the human placenta. *Placenta*. 2000;21:14-22.
5 Hahn D, Blaschitz A, Korgun ET, et al. From maternal glucose to fetal glycogen: expression of key regulators in the human placenta. *Mol Hum Reprod*. 2001;7:1173-1178.
6 Gluckman PD, Pinal CS. Maternal-placental-fetal interactions in the endocrine regulation of fetal growth: role of somatotrophic axes. *Endocrine*. 2002;19:81-89.
7 Cleal JK, Lewis RM. The mechanisms and regulation of placental amino acid transport to the human foetus. *J Neuroendocrinol*. 2008;20:419-426.
8 Jansson T. Amino acid transporters in the human placenta. *Pediatr Res*. 2001;49:141-147.
9 Cetin I, de Santis MS, Taricco E, et al. Maternal and fetal amino acid concentrations in normal pregnancies and in pregnancies with gestational diabetes mellitus. *Am J Obstet Gynecol*. 2005;192:610-617.
10 Bröer S. Adaptation of plasma membrane amino acid transport mechanisms to physiological demands. *Pflügers Arch*. 2002;444:457-466.
11 Chung M, Teng C, Timmerman M, Meschia G, Battaglia FC. Production and utilization of amino acids by ovine placenta in vivo. *Am J Physiol*. 1998;274:E13-E22.
12 Haggarty P. Placental regulation of fatty acid delivery and its effect on fetal growth - a review. *Placenta*. 2002;23:S28-S38.
13 Magnusson AL, Waterman IJ, Wennergren M, Jansson T, Powell TL. Triglyceride hydrolase activities and expression of fatty acid binding proteins in the human placenta in pregnancies complicated by intrauterine growth restriction and diabetes. *J Clin Endocrinol Metab*. 2004;89:4607-4614.

14 Duttaroy AK. Transport of fatty acids across the human placenta: a review. *Prog Lipid Res.* 2009;48:52-61.

15 Schmid KE, Davidson WS, Myatt L, Woollett LA. Transport of cholesterol across a BeWo cell monolayer: implications for net transport of sterol from maternal to fetal circulation. *J Lipid Res.* 2003;44:1909-1918.

16 Fernandez-Twinn DS, Ozanne SE, Ekizoglou S, Doherty C, James L, Gusterson B, Hales CN. The maternal endocrine environment in the low-protein model of intra-uterine growth restriction. *Br J Nutr.* 2003;90:815-822.

17 Salafia CM, Zhang J, Miller RK, Charles AK, Shrout P, Sun W. Placental growth patterns affect birth weight for given placental weight. *Birth Defects Res A Clin Mol Teratol.* 2007;79:281-288.

18 Zamudio S, Baumann MU, Illsley NP. Effects of chronic hypoxia in vivo on the expression of human placental glucose transporters. *Placenta.* 2006;27:49-55.

19 Reid GJ, Lane RH, Flozak AS, Simmons RA. Placental expression of glucose transporter proteins 1 and 3 in growth-restricted fetal rats. *Am J Obstet Gynecol.* 1999;180:1017-1023.

20 Hahn T, Barth S, Weiss U, Mosgoeller W, Desoye G. Sustained hyperglycemia in vitro down-regulates the GLUT1 glucose transport system of cultured human term placental trophoblast: a mechanism to protect fetal development? *FASEB J.* 1998;12:1221-1231.

21 Hahn T, Barth S, Graf R, et al. Placental glucose transporter expression is regulated by glucocorticoids. *J Clin Endocrinol Metab.* 1999;84:1445-1452.

22 Roberts CT, Sohlstrom A, Kind KL, et al. Maternal food restriction reduces the exchange surface area and increases the barrier thickness of the placenta in the guinea-pig. *Placenta.* 2001;22:177-185.

23 Currie MJ, Bassett NS, Gluckman PD. Ovine glucose transporter-1 and -3: cDNA partial sequences and developmental gene expression in the placenta. *Placenta.* 1997;18:393-401.

24 Sferruzzi-Perri AN, Owens JA, Pringle KG, Robinson JS, Roberts CT. Maternal insulin-like growth factors-I and -II act via different pathways to promote fetal growth. *Endocrinology.* 2006;147:3344-3355.

25 Glazier JD, Cetin I, Perugino G, et al. Association between the activity of the system A amino acid transporter in the microvillous plasma membrane of the human placenta and severity of fetal compromise in intrauterine growth restriction. *Pediatr Res.* 1997;42:514-519.

26 Jansson T, Scholtbach V, Powell TL. Placental transport of leucine and lysine is reduced in intrauterine growth restriction. *Pediatr Res.* 1998;44:532-537.

27 Bajoria R, Sooranna SR, Ward S, Hancock M. Placenta as a link between amino acids, insulin-IGF axis, and low birth weight: evidence from twin studies. *J Clin Endocrinol Metab.* 2002;87:308-315.

28 Roos S, Powell TL, Jansson T. Placental mTOR links maternal nutrient availability to fetal growth. *Biochem Soc Trans.* 2009;37:295-298.

29 Roos S, Lagerlöf O, Wennergren M, Powell TL, Jansson T. Regulation of amino acid transporters by glucose and growth factors in cultured primary human trophoblast cells is mediated by mTOR signaling. *Am J Physiol Cell Physiol.* 2009;297:C723-731.

30 Bloomfield FH, van Zijl PL, Bauer MK, Harding JE. A chronic low dose infusion of insulin-like growth factor I alters placental function but does not affect fetal growth. *Reprod Fertil Dev.* 2002;14:393-400.

31 Sibley CP, Turner MA, Cetin I, et al. Placental phenotypes of intrauterine growth. *Pediatr Res.* 2005;58:827-832.

32 Haggarty P, Allstaff S, Hoad G, Ashton J, Abramovich DR. Placental nutrient transfer capacity and fetal growth. *Placenta.* 2002;23:86-92.

33 Biale Y. Lipolytic activity in the placentas of chronically deprived fetuses. *Acta Obstet Gynecol Scand.* 1985;64:111-114.

34 Salafia CM, Zhang J, Miller RK, Charles AK, Shrout P, Sun W. Placental growth patterns affect birth weight for given placental weight. *Birth Defects Res A Clin Mol Teratol.* 2007;79:281-288.

35 Coan PM, Angiolini E, Sandovici I, Burton GJ, Constância M, Fowden AL. Adaptations in placental nutrient transfer capacity to meet fetal growth demands depend on placental size in mice. *J Physiol.* 2008;586:4567-4576.

36 Schneider H. Oxygenation of the placental-fetal unit in humans. *Respir Physiol Neurobiol.* 2011;178:51-58.

37 Burton GJ, Woods AW, Jauniaux E, Kingdom JC. Rheological and physiological consequences of conversion of the maternal spiral arteries for uteroplacental blood flow during human pregnancy. *Placenta.* 2009;30:473-482.

38 Burton GJ, Hempstock J, Jauniaux E. Oxygen, early embryonic metabolism and free radical-mediated embryopathies. *Reprod Biomed Online.* 2003;6:84-96.

39 Zamudio S. Hypoxia and the placenta. In: Kay HH, Nelson DM, Wang Y, eds. *The placenta. From development to disease.* Oxford, UK: Blackwell Publishing; 2011:43-49.

40 Genbacev O, Zhou Y, Ludlow JW, Fisher SJ. Regulation of human placental development by oxygen tension. *Science.* 1997;277:1669-1672.

41 Lackman F, Capewell V, Gagnon R, Richardson B. Fetal umbilical cord oxygen values and birth to placental weight ratio in relation to size at birth. *Am J Obstet Gynecol.* 2001;185:674-682.

42 Illsley NP, Caniggia I, Zamudio S. Placental metabolic reprogramming: do changes in the mix of energy-generating substrates modulate fetal growth? *Int J Dev Biol.* 2010;54:409-419.

43 Löfstedt T, Fredlund E, Holmquist-Mengelbier L, Pietras A, Ovenberger M, Poellinger L, Påhlman S. Hypoxia inducible factor-2 alpha in cancer. *Cell Cycle.* 2007;6:919-926.

44 Zamudio S, Wu Y, Ietta F, Rolfo A, Cross A, Wheeler T, Post M, Illsley NP, Caniggia I. Human placental hypoxia-inducible factor-1alpha expression correlates with clinical outcomes in chronic hypoxia in vivo. *Am J Pathol.* 2007;170:2171-2179.

45 Pringle KG, Kind KL, Sferruzzi-Perri AN, Thompson JG, Roberts CT. Beyond oxygen: complex regulation and activity of hypoxia inducible factors in pregnancy. *Hum Reprod Update.* 2010;16:415-431.

46 Patel J, Landers K, Mortimer RH, Richard K. Regulation of hypoxia inducible factors (HIF) in hypoxia and normoxia during placental development. *Placenta.* 2010;31:951-957.

Development of this book was supported by funding from Sandoz

Chapter 3

Maternal nutrition
Siegfried Zabransky

Introduction

For normal growth development, a fetus needs an adequate quantity and quality of nutrition from the mother via the placenta. In order to lessen the risk of fetal growth restriction and being born small for gestational age (SGA) – and the long-term consequences of these conditions – it is crucial that malnutrition during pregnancy is prevented. As the lifestyle of the mother greatly influences fetal development, promoting and supporting maternal nutrition should be a point of focus for disease prevention programs. Any nutritional advice must take into consideration the needs of both the mother and the fetus.

Caloric requirements

From the second trimester onward, an increased energy supply of approximately 250–300 kcal/day above the normal daily caloric requirement is necessary for normal physical development of the fetus [1]. Thus, once pregnancy enters the second trimester, the average daily total caloric requirement is approximately 1800–2500 kcal/day [2–5].

Weight gain

The recommended weight gain during pregnancy depends on the mother's weight before conception. An appropriate gain in weight can influence the duration of pregnancy and birth weight of the baby (Table 3.1) [5].

S. Zabransky (ed.), *Caring for Children Born Small for Gestational Age*,
DOI: 10.1007/978-1-908517-90-6_3, © Springer Healthcare 2013

Gain in weight depending on weight of mother before pregnancy		
Body mass index before pregnancy	**Total recommended weight gain (kg)**	**Recommended weekly gain in weight from 12th week onwards (kg)**
Normal (18.5–24.9)	11.5–16.0	0.4
Underweight (>18.5)	12.5–18.0	0.5
Overweight (29.9–39.9)	7.0–11.5	0.3
Obese (>40.0)	6.0	0.2

Table 3.1 Gain in weight depending on weight of mother before pregnancy. Adapted with permission from Rasmussen [6].

Composition of nutrients

The recommended proportion of dietary nutrients is similar in all women, including those who are pregnant: approximately 55% from carbohydrates, 10–15% from protein, and 30–35% from fat [7].

Carbohydrates

Carbohydrates are considered the most important type of 'fuel' for supporting muscle and brain activity. Monosaccharides (eg, glucose, fructose) and disaccharides (eg, lactose, sucrose) are needed to cover acute physical needs and can induce an elevation of blood sugar very rapidly. During pregnancy, complex carbohydrates are the preferred source of carbohydrates in the diet as they are metabolized slowly and blood sugar elevation is more moderate. Additionally, they often provide improved satiety, which is important for appetite and weight control.

Examples of foods that contain complex carbohydrates include certain cereals, brown rice, pulses, and wholemeal products. Foods containing simple carbohydrates (eg, products containing white flour) are more likely to contain monosaccharides and are less favorable by comparison. When consuming complex carbohydrates, mothers should insure a sufficient liquid intake (approximately 2 liters per day), which is necessary to 'soak up' dietary fiber and prevent constipation.

Protein

Although the suggested protein intake for young women is approximately 50 g/day, pregnant women are advised to consume more than the general recommended amount. Upon entering the fourth gestational month, the protein requirement increases as a result of increased fetal growth, which translates to an increased daily intake of protein (1.3 g/day per kg of body weight) [1]. Good sources of protein include low-fat dairy products, eggs, fish, lean meat, and poultry.

Protein requirements do not decrease immediately after giving birth; in fact, breastfeeding mothers need an additional 1 g of protein to produce 100 mL of breast milk [8].

Fatty acids

Long-chain and multiple unsaturated omega-3 and omega-6 fatty acids are known as essential fatty acids and are necessary for healthy development and growth. Specifically, they are required for stability and function of cell membranes and development of the brain and central nervous system. Deficiency of essential fatty acids may induce growth restriction, disturbances of water and electrolyte metabolism, and development of skin disorders. Fish such as herring, mackerel, tuna, and salmon are very good sources of essential fatty acids. Margarine also contains polyunsaturated fatty acids.

Animal-based fats should be reduced in favor of vegetarian fats (eg, sunflower oil, olive oil) because they have lower levels of cholesterol and have a higher content of essential unsaturated fatty acids. Food sourced from animals tends to contain more saturated fatty acids and cholesterol, and thus, when consumed in excess, may increase the risk of cardiovascular diseases [9]. However, in addition to quantity, the relation of saturated to unsaturated fatty acids is also important [9,10].

Vitamins and trace elements

Iodine

Iodine is an essential trace element that is able to pass from the maternal blood stream to the fetus through the placenta. Thus, iodine deficiency during pregnancy also leads to iodine deficiency of the fetus. During pregnancy, the mother's daily iodine requirement increases and supplementation becomes necessary as the recommended amount cannot generally be met through food intake alone. The consequences of fetal iodine deficiency include developmental interferences due to hypothyroidism.

Supplementation with 200 µg iodine daily during pregnancy and during the breastfeeding period is recommended, along with an increased intake of iodine-rich food such as fish and milk [11].

Vitamin A

Vitamin A (or retinol) is important for cholesterol synthesis, biochemical transformations in the biosynthesis of steroids (eg, gonadal steroids), night vision, healthy skin, and normal immune system functioning. Vitamin A, via retinol, all-*trans* and 9-*cis* retinoic acid metabolites, regulates several genes, that are responsible for embryonal development processes, cell division, and differentiation of cells. It also acts a growth factor. Excessive dietary intake of vitamin A has been associated with teratogenicity in humans [12,13].

Vitamin A is primarily found in animal-derived foods, especially liver. Other sources of vitamin A include dairy products, egg yolk, and fish. However, vegetarian provitamin A carotenoid may satisfy vitamin A needs as humans are able to transform carotin to retinol. Carotin is found in food that contains beta-carotene, alpha-carotene, and beta-cryptoxanthin, including certain vegetables (eg, carrots) and fruit (eg, cantaloupe). The recommended daily intake of vitamin A is 700 µg for women, which increases to 770 µg during pregnancy.

Vitamin A deficiency is a serious problem and is prevalent worldwide. According to the World Health Organization (WHO), approximately 5–10 million children develop eye problems (eg, xerophthalmia, dry eye) due to vitamin A deficiency per year, of which nearly half a million go blind [14]. In developed countries, vitamin A supplementation is generally not necessary if the pregnant woman has an adequate diet. However, daily intake should not exceed 6000 IU, with the exception of patients with diseases that can result in vitamin A deficiency (eg, limited intestinal absorption). Especially during the first trimester, pregnant women should abstain from eating vitamin A-enriched food due to a possible induction of malformations of the neural system [15]. Inadvertent or accidental intake of vitamin A doses that exceed 25,000 IU/day is not an indication for an abortion but does require individual risk evaluation and ultrasonographic examination [16].

Vitamin D

With the help of vitamin D precursors, ultraviolet light is converted in the skin to vitamin D (cholecalciferol/vitamin D_3), which is metabolized in the liver to form $25(OH)D_3$. The biologically active form of vitamin D, $1,25(OH)_2D_3$ (or calcitriol), is synthesized in the kidneys). The normal concentration range of vitamin D ($25(OH)D_3$) in blood serum is 70–110 nmol/L. Patients with vitamin D serum levels <50 nmol/L are considered to be vitamin D deficient. The Endocrine Society practice guidelines recommend 1500–2000 IU daily vitamin D supplementation during pregnancy and breastfeeding [17,18].

For most of the European population, sunlight exposure is insufficient to satisfy the suggested vitamin D requirement through endogenous production. Therefore, in these populations, supplementation of vitamin D is necessary. Risk groups for vitamin D deficiency include children, pregnant woman, and breastfeeding mothers, as well as elderly persons. Vitamin D enables maintenance of normocalcemia by promotion of enteral reabsorption, release of calcium from the bones, and inhibition of renal calcium excretion. There is a positive feedback loop between calcium serum level and parathyroid secretion. Vitamin D also influences neuromuscular coordination, normal skeletal development, and bone stability. A fetus develops most of its organ systems and the collagen matrix for the skeleton during the first and second trimesters, with calcification beginning during the third trimester. Therefore, as pregnancy progresses, maternal and fetal demand for calcium increases. The fetus is wholly dependent on the mother for vitamin D that passes from the placenta into the blood stream of the fetus [17,19,20].

Preeclampsia and caesarean section occur more often in pregnant women that are vitamin D deficient [21,22]. Studies in several countries have demonstrated the positive effects of vitamin D supplementation on the rate of preterm infant and gestational complications such as hypertonia, gestational diabetes mellitus, preeclampsia, and vaginal infections [21,22].

Folate

Folate (folic acid) is required for normal fetal development and growth. The recommended daily intake of folate for women of childbearing age is 400 µg. Optimal folate intake helps to prevent neural tube defects and is generally achieved with daily supplements of folate 4 weeks before conception until the end of the 12th gestational week. Woman that have had previous pregnancies with neural tube defects are recommended to take 4 mg folate daily during the same period of time [23]. Folate supplementation may also prevent other malformations such as cleft lip and palate [24]. Folate-enriched foods include dark leafy vegetables, legumes, some types of fruit (eg, strawberries), wholemeal products, eggs, meat, fish, and poultry.

Iron

Maternal iron requirements increase as a result of greater maternal blood volume and fetal requirement [25]. Despite physiologic changes to enhance iron absorption during pregnancy, many women still go on to develop iron-deficiency anemia during pregnancy. The WHO estimates that the worldwide prevalence of anemia among pregnant women is 42%; the prevalence of anemia is much higher in less developed nations compared with industrialized nations [26]. In Western Europe, the prevalence of iron-deficient anemia in pregnant women is estimated to be >20% (decreasing to 10% post partum) [27]. Definitions for anemia in pregnant and non-pregnant women are provided in Figure 3.1.

All levels of anemia require iron supplementation. A ferritin serum level ≤30 µg/L is an indication for iron supplementation, even without anemia. A reliable assessment of ferritin serum level may be difficult to obtain as it is an acute-phase protein and may be elevated in conditions

Defining anemia

The WHO definition of anemia in pregnancy is:

- <11.0 g/dL Hb during the first and third trimester;
- <10.5 g/dL during the second trimester;
- <10.0 g/dL Hb postpartum

WHO definition of anemia in non-pregnant women:

- 10 g/dL: grade 1 (mild);
- 7–10 g/dL: grade 2 (moderate);
- >7 g/dL: grade 3 (severe)

Figure 3.1 Defining anemia. Hb, hemoglobin; WHO, World Health Organization. Data taken from WHO [27].

with acute inflammatory processes. Therefore, C-reactive protein (CRP) levels should be analyzed as well.

The most common reason for iron-deficient anemia is an unbalanced hypocaloric or a predominantly vegetarian, plant-based diet. Although supplementation is generally not necessary for women with a balanced diet, regular blood tests are recommended to monitor Hb, hemocrit, ferritin, CRP, and differential blood count levels. Iron supplementation is only recommended in cases with proven anemia, as a fetus with an iron deficiency may be at higher risk of being growth-restricted [28]. The recommended daily requirement in pregnancy is 30 mg and 20 mg during the breastfeeding period [29,30]. Good sources of iron include fortified whole grains, lean meat, beans, seafood, nuts, dried fruit, and dark leafy vegetables. Vitamin C increases the absorption of iron when taken at the same time.

Vegetarian diet

A vegan (total omission of eating animal protein), vegetarian (plant-based diet that may include the consumption of dairy products or eggs), or a nutritionally unbalanced diet during pregnancy may lead to a greater risk of vitamin deficiency (especially vitamin A, B12, and D), as well as trace elements such as iodine. The Healthy Start Young Family Network recommends vitamin supplementation with a vegetarian diet [31].

Hygienic precautions

Hygienic precautions should be followed, as many otherwise healthy foods are at risk of being contaminated with toxoplasma, listeria, hepatitis, and salmonella pathogens. Thus, it is very important to wash hands before and after meal preparation, and before eating, and to wash fruit and vegetables thoroughly. Additionally, raw meat may be contaminated with the pathogen *Toxoplasma gondii*, which is transferred especially by cat excrement. Therefore, all pregnant women should be careful when contacting cats and avoid eating or handling raw animal products.

An example can be seen with listeriosis, an infection that can occur when a person eats food that has been contaminated with listeria monocytogenes bacteria. Listeria monocytogenes are found in animals (eg, cats, cattle), as well as in soil and contaminated water. Raw meat, dairy products, fruit, vegetables, and other foods may be infected with the bacteria. People at increased risk of listeriosis include developing fetuses, newborn babies, and pregnant women. The bacteria may cause a gastrointestinal illness, blood infection, or even meningitis. Infection during pregnancy can lead to a miscarriage or still birth, as the bacteria is able to cross the placenta and infect the fetus. Listeria monocytogenes is very resistant and can only be killed by cooking or frying at a high temperature, sterilization, and pasteurization.

Caffeine consumption should be limited to a maximum of 300 mg per day [32].

References

1   Pitkin RM. Nutritional influences during pregnancy. *Med Clin North Am*. 1977;61:3-15.

2   Biesalski H-K. *Ernährungsmedizin* [Nutritional medicine]. Stuttgart: Thieme; 2004.

3   Deutsche Gesellschaft für Ernährung, Österreichische Gesellschaft für Ernährung, Schweizerische Gesellschaft für Ernährungsforschung, Schweizerische Vereinigung für Ernährung. *Referenzwerte für die Nährstoffzufuhr*. Frankfurt: Umschau/Baus; 2008.

4   European responsible nutrition alliance (ERNA). Facts about vitamins, minerals and other food components with health effects. ERNA website. www.erna.org. Accessed February 20, 2013.

5   Ute K, Rösch R. *Ernährungsberatung in schwangerschaft und stillzeit* (German). Hippokrates: Stuttgart; 2008.

6   Rasmussen KM, Yaktine AL. *Weight gain during pregnancy: reexamining the guidelines*. Washington DC: National Academies Press; 2009.

7   Food and Nutrition Board, Institute of Medicine, National Academies. Dietary Reference Intakes for Energy, Carbohydrate, Fiber, Fat, Fatty Acids, Cholesterol, Protein, and Amino Acids (2002/2005). National Academies website. www.nap.edu/catalog.php?record_id=10490. Accessed February 20, 2013.

8   Institute of Medicine (IOM). *Institute of Medicine Subcommittee on Lactation: nutrition during lactation*. Washington DC: National Academy Press; 1991.

9   Hunter JE. n-3 fatty acids from vegetable oils. *Am J Clin Nutr*. 1990;51:809-814.

10 Odeleye OE, Watson RR. Health implication of the n-3 fatty acids. *Am J Clin Nutr*. 1991;53:177-178.

11 Heseker H. [Functions, physiology, metabolism, recommendations and supply in Germany] (German). *Ernährungs-Umschau*. 2000;47:243-245.

12 Hathcock JN, Hattan DG, Jenkins MY, et al. Evaluation of vitamin A toxicity. *Am J Clin Nutr*. 1990;52:183-202.

13 Lammer ET, Chen DT, Hoar RM, et al. Retinoic acid embryopathy. *N Eng J Med*. 1985;313:837-841.

14 Miller RK, Hendrickx AG, Hummler H, Wiegand UW. Periconceptional vitamin A use: how much is teratogen? *Reprod Toxicol*. 1998;12:75-88.

15 Wiegand UW, Hartmann S, Hummler H. Safety of vitamin A: recent results. *Int J Vitam Nutr Res*. 1998;68:411-416.

16 Azaïs-Braesco V, Pascal G. Vitamin A in pregnancy: requirements and safety limits. *Am J Clin Nutr*. 2000;71(5 suppl):1325S-1333S.

17 Holik MF, Binkley NC, Bischoff-Ferrari HA, et al. Evaluation, treatment and prevention of vitamin D deficiency, an Endocrine Society clinical practice guideline. *J Clin Endocrinol Metab*. 2011;96:1-20.

18 Institute of Medicine (IOM). *Dietary reference intakes of calcium and vitamin D*. IOM website. www.iom.edu/Reports/2010/Dietary-Reference-Intakes-for-Calcium-and-Vitamin-D.aspx. Accessed February 20, 2013.

19 Holik MF. Vitamin D deficiency. *N Engl J Med*. 2007;357:266-281.

20 Lewis S, Lucas RM, Halliday J, Ponsonby AL. Vitamin D deficiency and pregnancy: from preconception to birth. *Mol Nutr Food Res*. 2010;54:1092-1102.

21 Bodnar LM, Catov JM, Simhan HN, Holick MF, Powers RW, Roberts JM. Maternal vitamin D deficiency increases the risk of preeclampsia. *J Clin Endocrinol Metab*. 2007;92:3517-3522.

22 Merewood A, Mehta SD, Chen TC, Bauchner H, Holik MF. Association between vitamin D deficiency and primary caesarean section. *J Clin Endocrinol Metab*. 2009;94:940-945.

23 US Preventive Services Task Force. Folic acid for the prevention of neural tube defects: US Preventive Services Task Force recommendation statement. *Ann Intern Med*. 2009;150:626-631.

24 Wilcox AJ, Lie RT, Solvoll K, et al. Folic acid supplements and the risk of facial clefts: a national population-based control study. *BMJ*. 2007;334:46.

25 Drake VJ. Micronutrient needs during pregnancy and lactation. Oregon State University – Linus Paul Institute;2011. www.lpi.oregonstate.edu/infocenter/lifestages/pregnancyandlactation/index.html#iron. Accessed February 20, 2013.

26 McLean E, Cogswell M, Egli I, Wojdyla D, de Benoist B. Worldwide prevalence of anaemia, WHO Vitamin and Mineral Nutrition Information System, 1993-2005. *Public Health Nutr*. 2009;12:444-454.

27 World Health Organization (WHO). Iron deficiency anemia: assessment, prevention and control. Geneva, Switzerland: WHO; 2011. www.who.int/nutrition/publication/en/ida_assessment_prevention_control.pdf. Accessed February 20, 2013.

28 Pavord S, Myers B, Robinson S, Allard S, Strong J, Oppenheimer C; British Committee for Standards in Haematology. UK guidelines on the management of iron deficiency in pregnancy. *Br J Haematol*. 2012;156:588-600.

29 Heseker H. [Functions, physiology, metabolism, recommendations and supply in Germany] (German). *Ernährungs-Umschau*. 2000;47:243-245.

30 Kiss H, Konnaris C. [Guideline, Austrian Society for Gynecology and Obstetrics] (German). *Speculum*. 2011;29:19-21.

31 Koletzko B, Bauer CP, Bung P, et al. [Nutrition in pregnancy - practice recommendations of the network, Healthy Start - Young Family Network] (German). *Dtsch Med Wochenschr*. 2012;137:1366-1372.

32 Kuczkowski KM. Caffeine in pregnancy. *Arch Gynecol Obstet*. 2009;280:695-698.

Development of this book was supported by funding from Sandoz

Chapter 4

Prenatal care, surveillance, and risk assessment

Anke Ertan, A Kubilay Ertan

Introduction

The aim of prenatal surveillance and care is to monitor and minimize health risks to the mother and to ensure the birth of a healthy baby by anticipating problems and implementing necessary interventions to minimize morbidity. Several components are involved to achieve this goal and this chapter will have an emphasis on the prenatal care and surveillance given to pregnant women in Germany.

During the initial clinical visit after a pregnancy has been confirmed, a general case history is assessed from blood and urine samples and patients are tested for several conditions, including sexually transmitted diseases (eg, HIV), iron levels, blood type, antibodies (eg, rubella), antigens (eg, hepatitis B), and other infections. Throughout the pregnancy, blood pressure, weight, iron levels, and urine samples need to be regularly monitored and analyzed. Prenatal care also includes control of uterine fundal height, fetal heart rate, and if necessary, the length of the cervix.

The gynecologist/obstetrician, midwife, nurse practitioner, perinatologists, or general practitioner (primary care during pregnancy varies between countries) should inform the pregnant women about lifestyle, nutrition, supplements, and offer an evaluation for genetic risk factors. In many countries (eg, US, UK, Scandinavia), it is more common for prenatal care to be performed by midwives, general practitioners, or

S. Zabransky (ed.), *Caring for Children Born Small for Gestational Age*, 35
DOI: 10.1007/978-1-908517-90-6_4, © Springer Healthcare 2013

a combination of the two. Patients should also be informed about the risk of adverse effects due to drugs, tobacco, or alcohol consumption during pregnancy. A Pap smear examination should be given if one has not been performed in the previous 6 months.

Evaluation of risk factors

The first step in the evaluation of risk factors during pregnancy is to obtain the medical history of the parents and their families. This includes taking into consideration all of the conditions listed in Figure 4.1.

Estimation of gestational age

To determine the due date, the crown–rump length of the embryo during the first trimester is the most reliable measurement (confidence interval +/– 6 days, compared to +/– 8 days for the biparietal diameter measurement and +/– 10 days for the gestational sac diameter) [2]. If there was not an ultrasound performed in the first trimester, the transverse

Risk factors during pregnancy

1. General family health history:

- diabetes;
- hypertension;
- genetic disorders;
- predisposition for thrombosis;
- allergies;
- skeletal deformations;
- medications currently being taken;
- previous operations or medical procedures;
- exposure to teratogens/drugs

2. History of problems during previous pregnancies:

- habitual abortion;
- previous still-birth or neonatal death;
- previous preterm infant;
- previous delivery of an infant born small or large for gestational age
  - multiparity;
  - previous infant with Rh isoimmunization/Rh disease;
  - previous infant with known or suspected genetic disorders or congenital anomaly

3. History of reproductive tract disorders:

- myoma;
- cervical lesions;
- uterine anomalies [1]

Figure 4.1 Risk factors during pregnancy.

cerebellar diameter corresponds to the pregnancy week until 22 weeks gestation [2,3].

Ultrasound screening

Pregnant women should ideally be screened 2–3 times during pregnancy and should be transferred to a specialist in case of any abnormalities or suggestive signs such as abnormal amniotic fluid volume, fetal growth deviations or disproportion, body surface abnormalities, atypical four-chamber view, arrhythmia, or single umbilical artery.

Ultrasound screening is organized differently all over the world. For example, the German Society for Ultrasound in Medicine (DEGUM) has established a three-level system [4]:

- *Level I*: screenings carried out by qualified gynecologists who have a good knowledge of normal fetal anatomy.
- *Level II*: screenings with a specialist that has several years of experience in detection of fetal anomalies.
- *Level III*: screening with specialists that are active in scientific research in prenatal centers and fetal treatment.

According to the DEGUM prenatal care guidelines, three ultrasound examinations should be performed at weeks 8–12, weeks 18–22, and weeks 28–32 gestational age [4]. However, in the UK, the National Institute for Health and Clinical Excellence (NICE) recommends two ultrasound examinations: a first trimester screening, and a second scan between weeks 18 and 20 [5]. In the US, the Mayo Clinic suggests that an ultrasound is performed in the first trimester to confirm and date the pregnancy and another is done in the second trimester (between weeks 18 and 20) to visualize the fetal anatomy [6,7]. In Scandinavian countries, two or three ultrasound scans are recommended and usually performed by a midwife [8]. In this chapter, we will primarily discuss the ultrasound procedure followed in Germany.

First ultrasound screening

The goal of the first screening (performed between weeks 8–12 of pregnancy) is to detect an intact intrauterine pregnancy, determine gestational age, check for multiple pregnancies, and detect any abnormalities of embryonic development [4]. If multiple pregnancies are found, chorionicity and amionicity should be recorded.

In order to definitively diagnose intrauterine growth restriction (IUGR) later in the pregnancy, the determination of gestational age is very important at this stage, as the range of variation of biometric parameters is known to be smallest during the first trimester. The crown–rump length and the biparietal diameter can be used at this stage to evaluate the due date [9].

Nuchal translucency scan

The measurement of the nuchal transluceny (NT) and the assessment of the free β-human chorionic gonadotropin (β-hCG) and pregnancy-associated plasma protein-A (PAPP-A) in maternal serum at 11–14 weeks has become a recognized and well-established risk calculation method [10]. It is generally performed towards the end of the first trimester and assesses the thickness of soft tissues via the nape of the neck. This procedure is recommended in high-risk pregnancies and in older women, as they are at greater risk of carrying a fetus with chromosomal defects [11].

The NT diameter, the levels of β-hCG and PAPP-A, maternal age, and the presence and the length of the fetal nasal bone are the main data used to determine suggestive signs in the diagnosis of chromosomal abnormalities, especially Trisomy 21 (Down's syndrome). The detection rate is over 90%, for a positive screening rate of 5% [10,12].

Second ultrasound screening

In many countries, the second ultrasound screening is performed sometime during weeks 18–22 to assess fetal development, search for fetal anomalies, identify abnormal amniotic fluid volumes and structures, and determine the location of the placenta. Four biometric parameters should be recorded at this stage: biparietal diameter, head circumference, abdominal circumference, and femur length. If any suggestive signs of abnormal fetal growth are found, the patient should be referred to a specialist.

Third ultrasound screening

The main objective of the third ultrasound screening (performed during weeks 29–32) is to monitor fetal growth, search for additional abnormalities, and determine fetal position.

Chorionic villus sampling/amniocentesis

Both chorionic villus sampling and amniocentesis are used for prenatal diagnosis of genetic diseases, including Trisomy 21, 18, and 13, and various metabolic diseases. Chorionic villus sampling is often performed if an early diagnosis is required (8–11 weeks gestational age; carrying a 2–5% risk for abortion), whereas the amniocentesis is performed at weeks 15–17 (1% or 2% risk for abortion) for later diagnosis in cases of sonoanatomic anomalies or fetuses at high risk for genetic disorders (ie, high risk determined as a result of NT measurement) [13].

Prenatal assessment of fetal weight

A standard component of prenatal care is monitoring fetal growth. The most commonly used biometric data (biparietal diameter, head circumference, abdominal circumference, and femur length) are incorporated into a formula to calculate estimated fetal weight. There are numerous formulas that can be used to interpret the data. For example, the most popular formulas used in Germany are the modified Hadlock I/II/III/IV, Hansmann or Merz formulae.

Nevertheless, there is no consensus on a formula to calculate the exact weight of the fetus in all cases, which is shown by the diversity of the formulae and revisions that are continually proposed [1]. Especially for fetuses above or below the normal range, the mean and the standard deviation of error of estimated fetal weight appears to be greater than 10% and can lead to an underestimation of large and an overestimation of small fetuses [14]. However, sonographic weight estimation is still the best method for identifying fetuses whose birth weight is likely to be below the tenth percentile for gestational age [15].

Determining presence of fetal growth restriction

Customized growth curves help sonographers to identify deviations from the normal percentiles or a stagnation of fetal growth. Additionally, body proportions such as the head circumference/abdominal circumference (AC) or femur length/AC ratio are proposed for evaluating fetuses with asymmetric fetal growth [16,17].

As soon as suboptimal growth occurs and is detected, the primary caregiver needs to determine its cause and severity. The most important task at this stage is to distinguish a constitutionally small fetus from a growth-restricted fetus. A fetal survey is often necessary, as major congenital anomalies are frequently associated with abnormal weight gain of the fetus.

Approximately 10% of fetal growth restriction is accompanied by congenital anomalies [18], including omphalocele, diaphragmatic hernia, skeletal dysplasia, and congenital heart defects. Consequently, fetal karyotyping should be suggested to the parents in case of structural anomalies, early or severe fetal growth restriction (ie, below the third percentile), or polyhydramnios. If the fetus or the mother show any suggestive signs for viral infection (eg, cytomegalovirus, parvovirus), maternal serum should be examined for evidence of seroconversion [19].

Doppler velocimetry

In compromised fetal growth, Doppler ultrasound is a noninvasive technique used to evaluate growth-restricted fetuses at high risk by providing information about the uteroplacental, fetoplacental, and fetal blood circulation. Chronically increased resistance in the placental blood circulation leads to chronic fetal hypoxia, often resulting in growth restriction and altered fetal hemodynamics. The histopathological findings in the placenta correlate with the Doppler findings in the uterine and umbilical arteries [20].

Fetal growth restriction is associated with diminished flow and abnormal Doppler waveforms in maternal and fetal blood vessels. The perinatal mortality in pregnancies complicated by fetal growth restriction can be reduced by the assessment of Doppler flow with appropriate intervention [15]. An abnormal waveform in the uterine artery is associated in fetal growth restriction with early delivery, reduced birth weight, oligohy-dramnios, neonatal admission to the intensive care unit, and a prolonged hospital stay [21]. A recent meta-analysis showed that the use of uterine artery Doppler and follow-up intervention reduces perinatal mortality by up to 38% and improves perinatal outcome [22].

Although the sensitivity of the systolic/diastolic ratio or pulsatility index of the umbilical artery was shown to be smaller than the estima-tion of the fetal weight in detecting risks associated with fetal growth restriction, the specificity and positive predictive value turned out to be higher [23]. Consequently, the sonographic estimation of fetal weight below the tenth percentile, in combination with abnormal umbilical artery Doppler velocimetry, is highly predictive of fetal growth restric-tion and is the best tool to identify those at risk of an adverse outcome [15]. Measurements of additional fetal arteries or veins also give reliable information about perfusion and indicate the centralization or decompen-sation in a chronically hypoxic and/or malnourished fetus [22]. Perhaps, in the near future, 3D ultrasonography can improve the accuracy of fetal weight estimation by using 3D volumetric measurements.

Screening for diseases

In order to screen for gestational diabetes, a glucose test is often given between weeks 24–26. The recommended cut-offs for the diagnosis of gestational diabetes are [24]:

- fasting glucose level: >92 mg/dL (5.1 mmol/L);
- glucose 1 hour after test: >180 mg/dL (10.0 mmol/L);
- glucose 2 hours after test: >153 mg/dL (8.5 mmol/L).

In cases of other detected infections, evidence of seroconversion for cytomegalovirus, rubella, varicella, or maternal diseases affecting the pregnancy (eg, diabetes), the patient is referred to a specialist and/or a specialized hospital for perinatology.

Prenatal care in Germany: the Mutterpass

Since the introduction of the MutterPass (or 'mother passport') in Germany 45 years ago, perinatal mortality has decreased from 34 per 1000 births in the 1960s to 4.69 per 1000 in 2004 [25].

The Mutterpass has been accompanied by technical improvements to ultrasound examinations in order to identify at-risk growth-restricted fetuses and encourage closer cooperation between pediatricians providing perinatal care.

The introduction of the Mutterpass has played a positive role because Germany is one of the only European countries with such a program and now has a low perinatal mortality rate (Figure 4.2) [27]. This medical system reduces the risk of missing important risk factors and enables every obstetrician to screen each patient in a systematic manner. Highly qualified obstetricians that specialized in sonographic diagnosis (ie, three-level ultrasound concept) have also helped to reduce the numbers of missed malformations and increased monitoring of high risk pregnancies [4].

Additionally, in Germany, every pregnant woman is protected by law (Mutterschutzgesetz; law for maternity protection) [26]. It defines the rights and obligations during pregnancy, the possibility of an employment ban, and the strains to account for in the different periods of pregnancy. If there is likely to be a risk to the unborn child or the mother due to the mother's given occupation, a gynecologist is able to pronounce an employment ban for the rest of the pregnancy or to request a reduction of

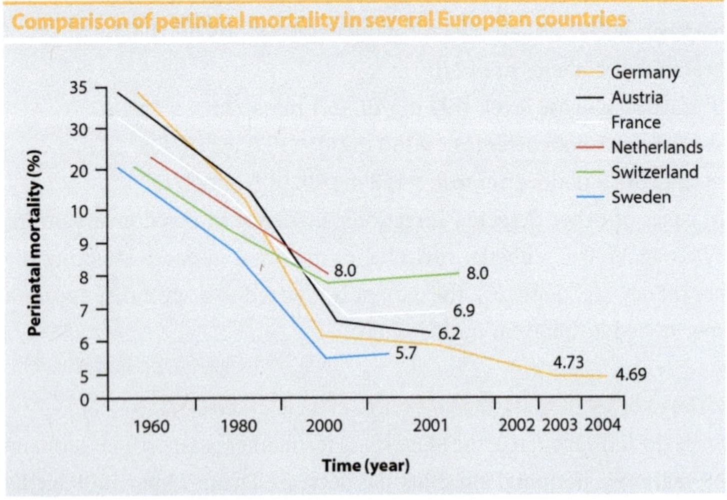

Figure 4.2 Comparison of perinatal mortality in several European countries. [27].

working time 6 weeks before birth and 8 weeks after delivery (or 12 weeks in a multiple pregnancy). In this type of situation, an employer is legally obliged to release the mother from work.

References

1   DeChernay AH, Pernoll M. *Current obstetric gynecologic diagnosis and treatment. 8th edn*. New York: McGraw Hill Professional; 1994.

2   Merz E. Fetal weight estimation. In: Merz E, ed. *Ultrasound in Obstetrics and Gynecology, Volume 1: Obstetrics*. New York, NY: Thieme; 2002:163-165.

3   Reece EA, Goldstein I, Pilu G, Hobbins JC. Fetal cerebellar growth unaffected by uterine growth retardation: a new paper for prenatal diagnose. *Am J Obstet Gynecol*. 1987;157;632.

4   Deutsche Gesellscaft für Ultraschall in der Medizin e.V (DEGUM). [*Section Gynecology and Obstetrics*]. DEGUM website. www.degum.de/Gynaekologie_Geburtshilfe.263.0.html. Accessed February 20, 2013.

5   National Institute for Health and Clinical Excellence (NICE). Antenatal care: routine care for the healthy pregnant woman. Clinical guides CG62 (2008). NICE website. www.nice.org.uk/CG62. Accessed February 20, 2013.

6   Hill LM, Breckle R, Gehrking WC. Prenatal detection of congenital malformations by ultrasonography. Mayo Clinic experience. *Am J Obstet Gynecol*. 1985;151:44-50.

7   Harms RW. Mayo clinic guide to a healthy pregnancy. New York, NY: William Morrow and Company; 2004.

8   World Health Organization (WHO). Training in diagnostic ultrasound: essentials, principals and standards. WHO website. www. whqlibdoc.who.int/trs/WHO_TRS_875.pdf. Accessed February 20, 2013.

9   Rempen, A. Vaginale sonographie im ersten trimenon. II. quantitative parameter. *Z.Geburth. u. Perinat*. 1991;195:163-171.

10 Pandya PP, Snijders RJM, Johnson SP, Brizot M, Nicolaides KH. Screening for fetal trisomies by maternal age and fetal nuchal transclucency thickness at 10–14 weeks of gestation. *Br J Obestet Gynecol*. 1995;102:957-962.

11 Sheppard C, Platt LD. Nuchal translucency and first trimester risk assessment: a systematic review. *Ultrasound Q*. 2007;23:107-116.

12 Nicolaides K, Shawwa L, Brizot M, Snijders R. Ultrasonographically detectable markers of fetal chromosomal defects. *Ultasound Obstet Gynecol*. 1993;3:56-59.

13 Merz E. Invasive prenatal diagnosis. In: Eichhorn, ed. *Ultrasound in Obstetrics and Gynecology, Volume 1: Obstetrics*. New York: Thieme; 2002:530-538.

14 MacKenzie AP, Stephenson CD, Funai EF. *Prenatal sonographic assessment of fetal weight*. UpToDate Clinical Reference Library. Wolters Kluwer Health website. www.uptodate.com/contents/prenatal-sonographic-assessment-of-fetal-weight. Accessed February 20, 2013.

15 Divon MY. *Diagnosis of fetal growth restriction*. UpToDate Clinical Reference Library. Wolters Kluwer Health website. www.uptodate.com/contents/diagnosis-of-fetal-growth-restriction. Accessed February 20, 2013.

16 Campbell S. Ultrasound measurement of fetal head to abdomen circumference ration in the assessment of growth retardation. *Br J Obstet Gynaecol*. 1977;155:1197.

17 Hadlock FP, Deter RL, Harrist RB, et al. A date-independent predictor of uterine growth retardation: femur length/abdominal circumference ratios. *Am J Roentgenol*. 1983;141:979.

18 Mendez H. Introduction to the study of pre- and postnatal growth in humans: a review. *Am J Med Genet*. 1985;20:63.

19 Resnik, R. *Fetal growth restriction: evaluation and management*. UpToDate Clinical Reference Library. Wolters Kluwer Health website. www.uptodate.com/contents/fetal-growth-restriction-evaluation-and-management. Accessed February 20, 2013.

20 Fok RY, Pavlova Z, Benirschke K. The correlation of arterial lesions with umbilical artery Doppler velocimetry in the placenta of small-for-date pegnancies. *Obstet Gynecol*. 1990;75:578-583.

21 Trudinger BJ, Cook CM. Umbilical and uterine artery flow velocity waveforms in pregnancy associated with major fetal abnormality. *Br J Obstet Gynaecol*. 1985;92:666-670.

22 Ertan K, Tanriverdi A. Doppler sonography in obstetrics. In: Kurjak A, Chervenak FA, eds. *Donald School Textbook of Ultrasound in Obstetrics and Gynecology*. New Delhi: Jaypee; 2011:499-520.

23 Ott WJ. Comparison of dynamic image and pulsed Doppler sonography for the diagnosis of uterine growth retardation. *J Clin Ultrasound*. 1990;18:3-7.

24 de Sereday MS, Damiano MM, González CD, Bennett PH. Diagnostic criteria for gestational diabetes in relation to pregnancy outcome. *J Diabetes Complications*. 2003;17:115-119.

25 World Health Organization (WHO). Neonatal and Perinatal Mortality, Country, Regional and Global Estimates 2004. WHO website. www. whqlibdoc.who.int/publications/2007/9789241596145_eng.pdf. Accessed February 20, 2013.

26 Bundesministerium für Familie, Senioren, Frauen und Jugend. *Mutterschutzgesetz - Leitfaden zum Mutterschutz*. www.bmfsfj.de/BMFSFJ/Service/themen-lotse,did=3156.html. Accessed February 20, 2013.

27 Berufsverband der Frauenärzte e.V. [Professional Association of Gynaecologists eV] (BVD). BVD website. www.bvf.de. Accessed February 20, 2013.

Development of this book was supported by funding from Sandoz

Chapter 5

Birth weight percentiles: an international comparison

Niels Rochow, Manfred Voigt, Dirk Manfred Olbertz, Sebastian Straube

Somatic development of neonates

Somatic development at birth is associated with a number of postnatal and life-long health outcomes [1]. In clinical practice, percentile curves of birth weight, length, and head circumference are calculated according to gestational age and, along with growth indices derived from these parameters, are used to estimate neonatal somatic development. These percentiles allow an estimation of, for example, the birth weight of a particular neonate compared to other neonates of the same sex who were born after the same duration of pregnancy. A birth weight in the 50th percentile means that 50% of neonates of the same sex and gestational age were smaller (lighter) than the child in question. A birth weight on the 10th or 90th percentile means that 10% or 90% of comparable children were smaller (lighter), respectively.

By convention, neonates are considered appropriate for gestational age (AGA) if they are between the 10th and 90th percentiles, small for gestational age (SGA) if they are smaller than the 10th percentile, and large for gestational age (LGA) if they in the 90th percentile, with regard to the anthropometric parameter or index in question. Importantly, the birth weight percentile curves describe somatic development at birth; they are not, strictly, intrauterine growth charts. Generally, percentile

S. Zabransky (ed.), *Caring for Children Born Small for Gestational Age*,
DOI: 10.1007/978-1-908517-90-6_5, © Springer Healthcare 2013

values are calculated with regard to the week of gestation and the percentile curves illustrated in this chapter were all calculated in this manner. However, week-specific percentiles may suffer from the disadvantage of being less accurate than day-specific ones. When using tabulated percentiles, weekly average values overestimate the SGA rate at the beginning of the week and underestimate the SGA rate at the end of the week, and conversely for the LGA rate [2].

Factors influencing birth weight

Anthropometric measurements of the newborn are affected by genetic factors and the intrauterine milieu. Birth weight is influenced mainly by maternal constitution, diseases, nutrition, and lifestyle (Figure 5.1).

Differences in birth weight percentiles between countries

Ethnic background and geographic origin can affect birth weight percentiles. For example, we have previously shown that the 10th, 50th, and 90th birth weight percentiles of neonates born in Germany to mothers originating from Asia were below those of neonates born in Germany

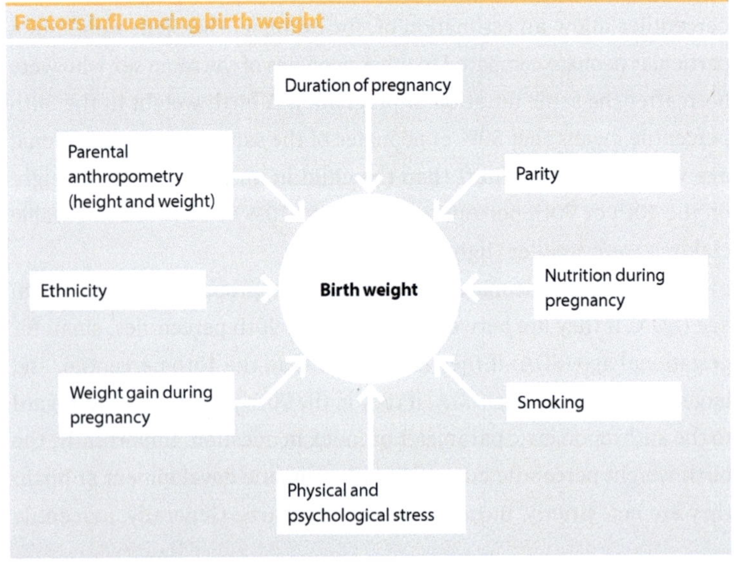

Figure 5.1 Factors influencing birth weight.

to mothers from Germany [3]. We also compared data from Taiwanese neonates [4] with the data from the German perinatal survey, finding that the Taiwanese percentiles were below those of neonates born in Germany to mothers from Asia [3]. These robust observations are likely due to a combination of genetic, nutritional, and lifestyle differences.

In this chapter, we will compare percentiles of birth weight for gestational age from a number of countries. Table 5.1 details the sources of the percentiles discussed with information on the times of data collection and the size of the cohorts.

From these sources, we found that considerable between-country differences exist. Percentile curves are illustrated in Figure 5.2 and Figure 5.3.

Table 5.2 shows the 10th and 90th percentiles at 40 completed weeks of gestation in tabulated form. Among our examples of international birth weight percentiles, there are differences for the 10th percentile of up to 215 g for girls and 235 g for boys. For the 90th percentiles, the largest differences in cut-off values were 393 g for girls and 424 g for boys. Because of these large differences, using the wrong set of curves can be problematic. For example, if percentile curves with cut-off values that are too high are used, AGA newborns may be wrongly classified as SGA, and LGA newborns as AGA, and so on. Based on such misclassifications, inappropriate healthcare management may be initiated.

International birth weight percentile charts

Country	Neonatal cohort (years)	Sample size (n)	Reference
Austria	1999–2004	454,155	Mayer et al [5]
Canada	1994–1996	676,605	Kramer et al [6]
Germany	1995–2000	2.3 million	Voigt et al [7]
Hungary	1990–1996	799,688	Joubert [8]
Israel	1991–2005	82,066	Davidson et al [9]
Kuwait	1998–2000	36,493	Alshimmiri et al [10]
Norway	1967–1998	>1.8 million	Skjaerven et al [10]
Spain	1999–2002	9,362	Carrascosa Lezcano et al [11]
Taiwan	1998–2002	1,298,389	Hsieh et al [4]
USA	1998–2006	257,855	Olsen et al [13]

Table 5.1 International birth weight percentile charts. Data taken from [4–13].

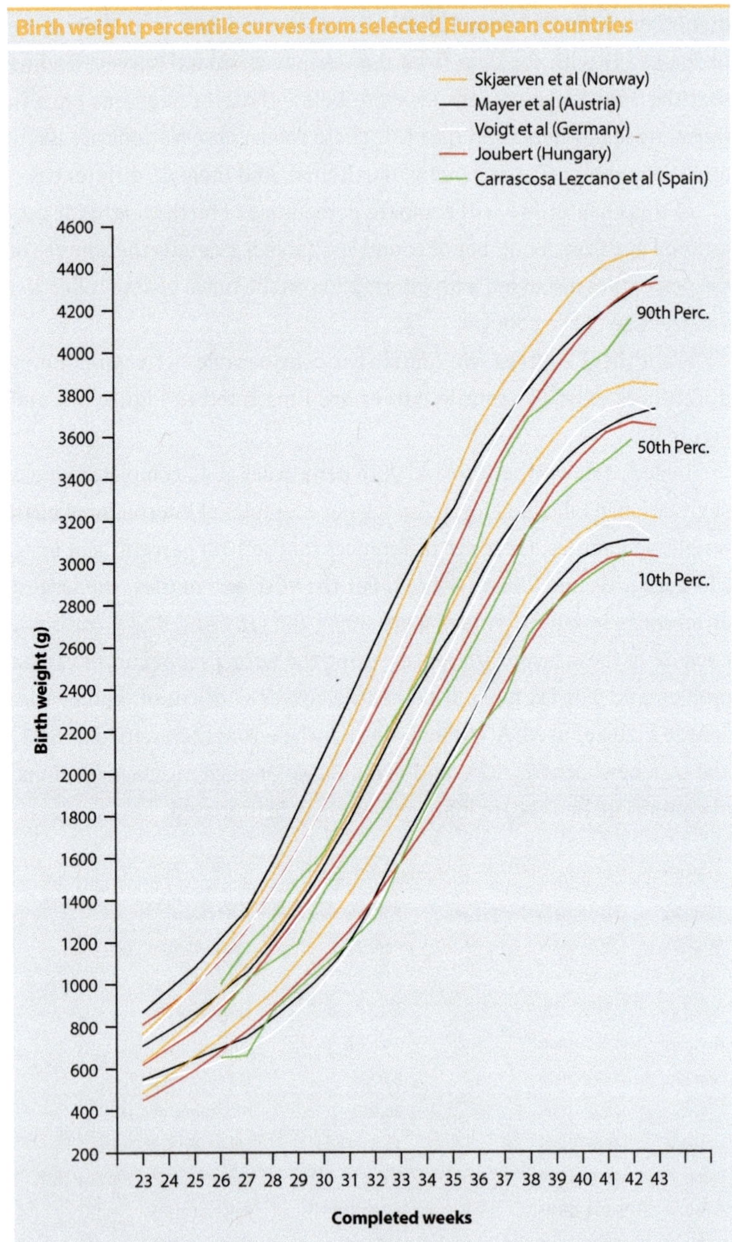

Figure 5.2 Birth weight percentile curves from selected European countries. Data taken from [5,7,8,11–12].

Birth weight percentile curves from Germany and selected non-European countries

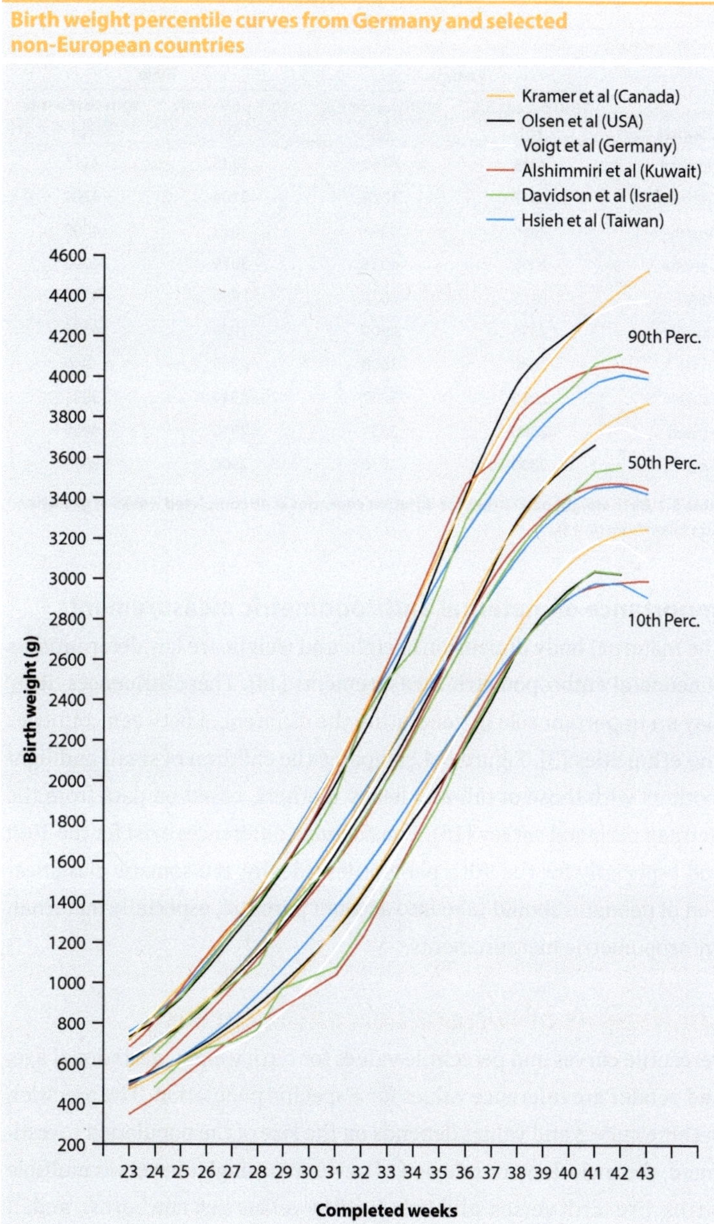

Figure 5.3 Birth weight percentile curves from Germany and selected non-European countries. Data taken from [4,6,7,9,10,13].

Birth weight percentiles for different countries at 40 completed weeks of gestation

Country	Female		Male	
	10th percentile (g)	90th percentile (g)	10th percentile (g)	90th percentile (g)
Norway	3015	4140	3135	4315
Germany	2977	4024	3104	4204
Austria	2956	3994	3013	4099
Canada	2955	4034	3079	4200
USA	2855	4070	2950	4232
Hungary	2835	3900	2925	4075
Israel	2830	3808	2935	3940
Taiwan	2816	3747	2914	3891
Kuwait	2800	3858	2910	4005
Spain	2800	3770	2900	3910

Table 5.2 Birth weight percentiles for different countries at 40 completed weeks of gestation. Data taken from [4–13].

Importance of maternal anthropometric measurements

The maternal body dimensions height and weight are key determinants of neonatal anthropometric measurements [14]. These influences likely play an important role in generating the differences between countries and ethnicities [3]. Figure 5.4 compares the children of small and light mothers with those of tall and heavy mothers, based on data from the German perinatal survey [15]. Considerable differences exist for the 10th and especially for the 90th percentiles. Ideally, the somatic classification of neonates should take into account parental, especially maternal, anthropometric measurements.

Limitations of current percentile curves

Percentile curves and percentile values for birth weight, gestational age, and gender are reference values for a specific population. The precision of these curves and values depends on the size of the population investigated, the inclusion or exclusion of newborns (singleton versus multiple births, live birth versus stillbirth, healthy versus sick newborns), and, if applicable, curve-smoothing procedures.

Differences in the 10th and 90th birth weight percentile curves between neonates of women with different heights and weights

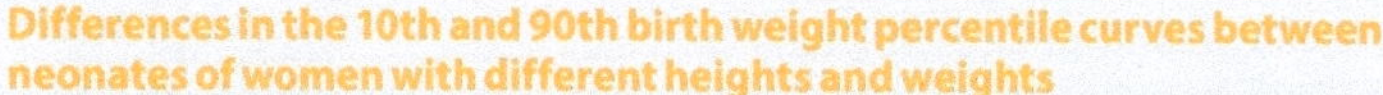

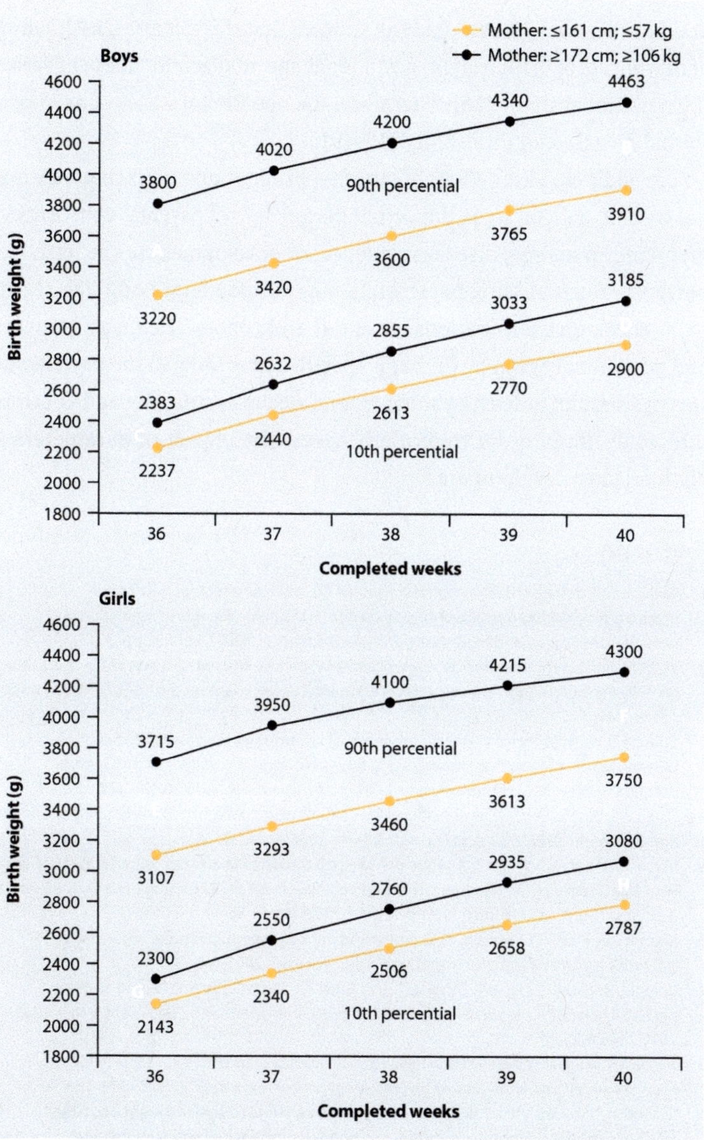

Figure 5.4 Differences in the 10th and 90th birth weight percentile curves between neonates of women with different heights and weights. A, diff.: 580 g; B, diff.: 53 g; C, diff.: 146 g; D, diff.: 285 g; E, diff.: 608 g; F, diff. 550 g; G, diff.: 157 g; H, diff.: 293 g. Modified with permission from Voigt et al 2011 [15].

Furthermore, the percentile curves or values for birth weight cannot be used to assess the nutritional status of the infant (amount of body fat and fat-free mass). A recent study showed that the somatic classification of newborns for birth weight, gestational age, and gender does not reflect the nutritional status [16]. Therefore, the nutritional status of newborns should be assessed differently [17–19].

An additional limitations of current perinatal surveys is that they may not contain data on some important parameters of parental constitution, pregnancy outcome, disease incidence, or development of the fetus and newborn. Such missing parameters may include fetal body size at pre-natal check-up examinations, parental anthropometric measurements, and gestational age at birth that is specified according to the day. Ideally, surveys should, at least to some extent, occur postnatally and continue into adult life in order to properly assess the impact of parameters at birth on later development.

References

1   Guilloteau P, Zabielski R, Hammon HM, Metges CC. Adverse effects of nutritional programming during prenatal and early postnatal life, some aspects of regulation and potential prevention and treatments. *J Physiol Pharmacol*. 2009 Oct;60(suppl 3):17-35.

2   Voigt M, Rochow N, Straube S, Briese V, Olbertz D, Jorch G. Birth weight percentile charts based on daily measurements for very preterm male and female infants at the age of 154-223 days. *J Perinat Med*. 2010;38:289-295.

3   Straube S, Voigt M, Hesse V, et al. Comparison of anthropometric characteristics of German-born vs. Asian-born mothers and their neonates – an analysis of the German perinatal survey (19th communication). *Geburtsh Frauenheilk*. 2010;70:472-477.

4   Hsieh WS, Wu HC, Jeng SF, et al. Nationwide singleton birth weight percentiles by gestational age in Taiwan, 1998-2002. *Acta Paediatr Taiwan*. 2006;47:25-33.

5   Mayer M, Voigt M, Schmitt K. Analyse des Neugeborenenkollektivs der Jahre 1999–2004 der Republik Österreich. 1. Mitteilung: Neue Perzentilwerte für die Körpermaße Neugeborener (Einlinge) (German). *Monatsschr Kinderheilkd*. 2008;156:49-56.

6   Kramer MS, Platt RW, Wen SW, et al. A new and improved population-based Canadian reference for birth weight for gestational age. *Pediatrics*. 2001;108:E35.

7   Voigt M, Rochow N, Hesse V, Olbertz D, Schneider KT, Jorch G. Kurzmitteilung zu den perzentilwerten für die körpermaße der neugeborenen (German). *Z Geburtshilfe Neonatol*. 2010;214:24-29.

8   Joubert K. Magyar születeskori testtömeg- es testhossz-standardok az 1990–1996. evi orszagos elveszületesi adatok alapjan. *Magyar nöorvosok lapja*. 2000;63:155-163.

9   Davidson S, Sokolover N, Erlich A, Litwin A, Linder N, Sirota L. New and improved Israeli reference of birth weight, birth length, and head circumference by gestational age: a hospital-based study. *Isr Med Assoc J*. 2008:130-134.

10 Alshimmiri MM, Al-Saleh EA, Alsaeid K, Hammoud MS, Al-Harmi JA. Birth weight percentiles by gestational age in Kuwait. *Arch Gynecol Obstet*. 2004;269:111-116.

11 Skjaerven R, Gjessing HK, Bakketeig LS. Birthweight by gestational age in Norway. *Acta Obstet Gynecol Scand.* 2000;79:440-449.

12 Carrascosa Lezcano A, Ferrández Longás A, Yeste Fernández D, et al. [Spanish cross-sectional growth study 2008. Part I: Weight and height values in newborns of 26-42 weeks of gestational age] (Spanish). *An Pediatr (Barc).* 2008;68:544-551.

13 Olsen IE, Groveman SA, Lawson ML, Clark RH, Zemel BS. New intrauterine growth curves based on United States data. *Pediatrics.* 2010;125:e214-e224.

14 Voigt M, Schneider KT, Jährig K. [Comprehensive analysis of all the newborn during 1992 in the Federal Republic of Germany: Part 2: Multidimensional links between age, body weight, body height of the mother, and body weight at birth] (German). *Geburtsh Frauenheilk.* 1997;57:246-255.

15 Voigt M, Olbertz D, Rochow N, Hesse V, Schleussner E, Schneider KT. Geburtsgewichtsperzentilwerte für Mädchen und Knaben unter Berücksichtigung von Körperhöhe und Körpergewicht der Mütter (12 Müttergruppen) (German). In: Zabransky S, ed. *SGA-Syndrome Small for Gestational Age. IUGR Intrauterine Wachstumsrestriktion.* Interdisziplinärer SGA Workshop. July 1, 2011: Kloster Schöntal, Germany.

16 Schmelzle HR, Quang DN, Fusch G, Fusch C. Birth weight categorization according to gestational age does not reflect percentage body fat in term and preterm newborns. *Eur J Pediatr.* 2007;166:161-167.

17 Sainz RD, Urlando A. Evaluation of a new pediatric air-displacement plethysmograph for body-composition assessment by means of chemical analysis of bovine tissue phantoms. *Am J Clin Nutr.* 2003;77:364-370.

18 Fusch C, Slotboom J, Fuehrer U, et al. Neonatal body composition: dual-energy X-ray absorptiometry, magnetic resonance imaging, and three-dimensional chemical shift imaging versus chemical analysis in piglets. *Pediatr Res.* 1999;46:465-473.

19 Schmelzle HR, Fusch C. Body fat in neonates and young infants: validation of skinfold thickness versus dual-energy X-ray absorptiometry. *Am J Clin Nutr.* 2002;76:1096-1100.

Development of this book was supported by funding from Sandoz

Interference with intrauterine fetal development

Chapter 6

Fetal growth restriction: definitions, causes, and epidemiology

Siegfried Zabransky

Terminology

Gestational age and birth weight of newborns may be differentiated into three groups:

Birth weight percentile	Classification
<10th	Small for gestational age (SGA)
10th–90th	Average for gestational age (AGA)
>90th	Large for gestational age (LGA)

The limiting value of the classification of SGA may vary; the most commonly used definition of SGA is birth weight below the tenth percentile, adjusted for gestational age [1,2]. A World Health Organization (WHO) Expert Committee [3,4] recommended including the lower tenth percentile of birth weight for gestational age, sex, and multiple births; risk curves can provide valuable information [5]. Figure 6.1 demonstrates a risk curve for the classification of SGA infants [6].

To classify the symptoms related to being born SGA, birth weight related to gestational age is given priority over birth length because the measurement of birth weight is easier to determine and is generally more exact. Thus, by definition, the term SGA also includes genetically

S. Zabransky (ed.), *Caring for Children Born Small for Gestational Age*,
DOI: 10.1007/978-1-908517-90-6_6, © Springer Healthcare 2013

small newborns. On the other hand, low birth weight is defined by the WHO as birth below 2500 g (or 5 pounds, 8 ounces), irrespective of gestational age [3,4].

Distinguishing between small for gestational age and intrauterine growth restriction

The terms SGA and intrauterine growth restriction (IUGR) are often erroneously interchanged and considered synonymous. However, they are different conditions and should be strictly distinguished. Children exposed to IUGR may be encumbered with a higher morbidity and mortality rate than children born SGA and may need more diagnostic and

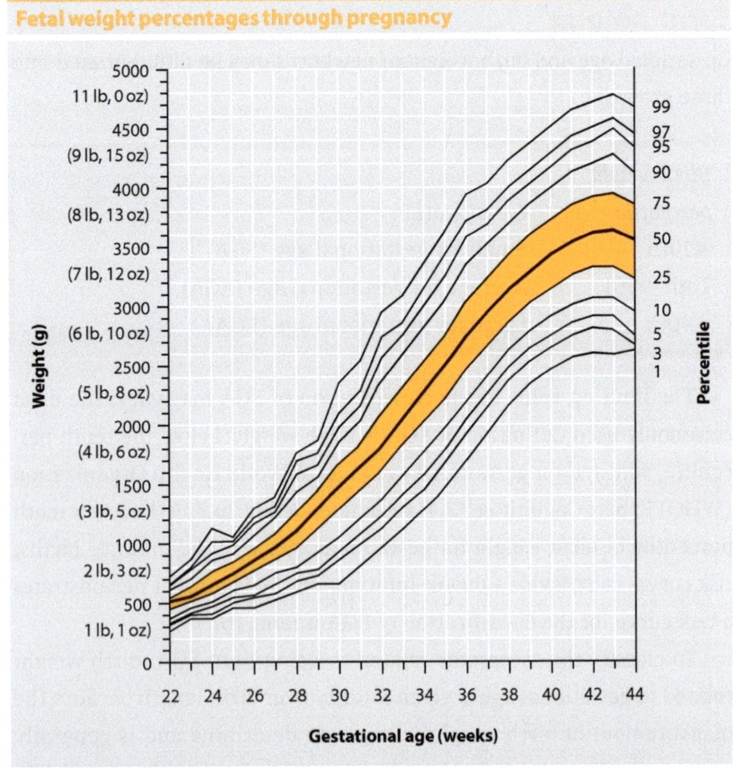

Figure 6.1 Fetal weight percentages through pregnancy. Intrauterine growth restriction identification and management. Reproduced with permission from Peleg et al [6].

therapeutic procedures [7]. The most important distinguishing feature between the two conditions is that the diagnosis of SGA is determined at birth according to adjusted birth weight, while the diagnosis of IUGR can be determined during pregnancy by fetal ultrasound. Thus, newborns born SGA may include newborn children that were also diagnosed as IUGR; however, newborns with IUGR may not always be classified as SGA. As IUGR classification is not related to birth weight, but instead to fetal intrauterine development, infants with IUGR can be SGA, AGA, or even LGA.

- The diagnosis of IUGR is made during pregnancy by repeated ultrasound evaluations of fetal growth.
- The diagnosis of SGA is made at birth and is only related to gestational, age-adjusted birth weight.

The causes of IUGR are generally related to pathological conditions (eg, infection, malnutrition, genetics, environmental factors), although a direct cause is unknown in up to 40% of cases. To describe the infant's status at birth, and also the long-term effects of being born SGA, the term 'small baby syndrome' may also be used.

Symmetrical and asymmetrical types of IUGR

In cases of insufficient nutrients and oxygen supply, the fetus is able to redistribute blood flow to sustain the function and development of vital organs. This so-called 'brain-sparing effect' favors blood flow to the brain, heart, adrenal glands, and placenta, consequently neglecting flow to other organs. These processes result in different fetal growth patterns.

In 1977, Campbell and Thoms introduced the idea of symmetric versus asymmetric growth [8]. The point in time of harm (ie, start of growth restriction) is decisive for development of these two different types of fetal growth retardation. Symmetrically small fetuses (ie, the entire body is proportionally small) are thought to have some sort of early, global insult (eg, aneuploidy, viral infection), while an asymmetrical growth in a small fetus (eg, an infant with an average head size but small waist circumference and thin limbs) is thought to be more likely due to a restriction in nutrients and gas exchange (Table 6.1) [8].

A retrospective cohort study by Dashe et al [9] of 1364 infants showed that infants born SGA with asymmetrical growth were more likely to have major anomalies than infants born SGA or AGA with symmetric growth (14%, 4%, and 3%, respectively; $P<.001$) [9]. A neonatal outcome composite that included one or more of respiratory distress, intraventricular hemorrhage, sepsis, or neonatal death was more frequent among infants born SGA with asymmetric growth when compared to infants born AGA (14% versus 5%; $P=.001$) [9].

Asymmetric growth in IUGR is associated with a higher incidence of early pregnancy-induced hypertension than symmetric IUGR, as well as more frequent cesarean-section deliveries and serious neonatal morbidities [9]. Symmetric SGA infants were not at increased risk of morbidity compared with AGA infants [9]. The infants with symmetric growth who were born SGA had outcomes very similar to the infants who were born AGA [9].

Causes of intrauterine growth restriction and small for gestational age

Fetal growth may be disturbed by fetal, maternal, or/and placental factors due to complex overlapping processes that underlie the condition [10]. Approximately 40% of infants classified as SGA are constitutionally small

Symmetrical and asymmetrical intrauterine growth restriction		
	Symmetrical IUGR	**Asymmetrical IUGR**
Proportion	Body length, weight, and head circumference are equally affected, resulting in proportionally stunted growth	Birth weight, but not length and head circumference, is considered small for gestational age
Time of growth restriction	First and second trimester; cell division and cell growth are retarded	Third trimester
Frequency	10–20% of IUGR cases	70–80% of IUGR cases
Etiology	Genetics, environmental factors (eg, toxins, nicotine, alcohol), and viral infections	Imposed restriction in nutrient and gas exchange caused by fetal malnutrition and/or placental dysfunction

Table 6.1 Symmetrical and asymmetrical intrauterine growth restriction. IUGR, intrauterine growth restriction.

babies, in that they are statistically small in size but are otherwise healthy individuals [11]. Approximately 20% of infants that are born SGA are abnormally and intrinsically small, and the remaining 40% include some larger infants that are growth-restricted but could benefit from timely and appropriate prenatal intervention [12]. In developing countries, the most important factors leading to a higher risk of IUGR and being born SGA are malnutrition, infection (eg, malaria), and insufficient prenatal care; in developed countries, cigarette smoking and alcohol abuse are the most common causes [13].

Fetal factors

Genetic factors

There is an established familial trend in birth weight. For example, a mother born SGA is 2.5–2.7 times more likely to give birth to a baby that is born SGA than a mother of average birth weight [14]. Similarly, IUGR also appears to have a genetic element and can coexist with other malformations (Table 6.2). In a population study, Khoury et al found a 22% rate of IUGR in malformed infants, with the highest frequency occurring with chromosomal anomalies [15]. For example, IUGR combined with polyhydramnion before 26 weeks gestation is caused by chromosomal abnormalities in about 20% of cases [15]. Additionally, asymmetrical IUGR at 20 weeks gestation strongly suggests fetal trisomy [16].

The first single gene defect in a child born SGA with short stature was found in the insulin-like growth factor 1 (*IGF-I*) gene [17]. In this study, a partial deletion in the *IGF-I* gene resulted in undetectable levels of serum

Intrauterine growth restriction and associated genetic conditions	
Endogen	**Genetic condition/organ system affected**
Chromosomal anomalies	Trisomy 13,18,21, Monosomy X (Ullrich-Turner syndrome)
Complex syndromes	Silver-Russell, Bloom, Cornelia de Lange IMAGE, 3-M, Lowry, Wood, GRACILE, Williams syndrome
Genetic disorders	Achondrogenesis
Malformations of several organ systems	Central nervous system, cardiovascular, renal
Metabolic inborn errors	Maternal phenylketonuria [20]

Table 6.2 Intrauterine growth restriction and associated genetic conditions.

IGF-1, extreme IUGR, severe postnatal growth failure, sensorineural deafness, and moderate learning difficulties [17].

In children with Silver-Russell syndrome (a disorder present at birth and associated with poor growth and development), no consistent cytogenetic abnormalities have been found. However, 10% of these children have inherited two copies of the maternal chromosome 7 and no paternal copy (maternal uniparental disomy for chromosome 7) [18]. Overall, it is estimated that 5–10% of fetuses are affected by chromosomal/structural anomalies or chronic intrauterine infections [19].

Maternal factors

Maternal height

In a meta-analysis by Kramer [21], the estimated weighted effect of maternal height was 7.8 g of additional birth weight for every centimeter of maternal height. A relative risk of 1.27 for IUGR was associated with a maternal height of less than 157.5–158 cm [21]. Thus, maternal height may affect infant birth weight through genetic mechanisms, as well as via physical limitations imposed on the growth of the uterus, placenta, and the fetus [21].

Maternal weight

A pre-pregnancy weight below 50 kg significantly increases the risk of giving birth to an infant that is SGA [22]. Low pre-pregnancy maternal weight and low weight gain during pregnancy may also increase the risk of IUGR [23,24]. Kramer found a sample size-weighted independent effect of 9.5 g of birth weight for every 1 kg of maternal pre-pregnancy weight [21]. Additionally, Strauss and Dietz found that low weight gain during the second and third trimester doubled the risk of IUGR [25].

Maternal malnutrition

Maternal deficiency of protein, folic acid, vitamins, zinc, calcium, magnesium, copper, or selenium may all lead to IUGR [26–29]. For example, iron-deficiency was associated with a tripling of the incidence of low birth weight [30]. Anemia is thought to cause fetal stress with increased circulation of fetal corticotropin-releasing hormone, increased cortisol production, and oxidative damage to erythrocytes, which inhibits fetal growth [30,31]. Maternal nutrition is discussed in more detail in Chapter 3.

Maternal diseases and infection

Vascular disruption associated with preeclampsia, diabetes mellitus, renal disease, or collagen vascular diseases are all common causes of IUGR [32,33]. Blood supply to the fetoplacental unit is impaired in preeclampsia. Physiological changes in the spiral arteries are restricted to the decidual segment [34].

Fetal growth can be negatively influenced by infections in either the mother or the fetus, with an estimated 5–10% of all IUGR cases thought to be caused by infection [32,35]. Depending on the type of infection, the supply of maternal nutrients may be less available to the fetus by reduction of the fetoplacental circulation and blood flow, and the structure of the placenta can be damaged to the extent that nutrient transfer is impaired. Appetite during an infection is often reduced by increased cytokines, and intestinal reabsorption may decrease, despite the resulting rise in body temperature, which can compound the problem by requiring more energy, protein, and micronutrient intake.

Maternal psychosocial and occupational effects

Maternal anxiety and depression may result in a greater risk of giving birth to an infant with low birth weight [36,37]. Heavy physical work also seems to increase the risk of IUGR [38–40]. This and other psychosocial and environmental factors are discussed in more detail in Chapter 24.

Multiple pregnancies

15–30% of twin pregnancies are associated with IUGR [32]. Monochorial twin pregnancies with intraplacental anastomoses may permit twin-to-twin transfusion [41,42]. However, the 'donor' twin often develops IUGR.

Complications after artificial reproduction techniques

Following artificial insemination, there is an increased risk of miscarriage, extrauterine gravidity (pregnancy outside of the uterus), multiple pregnancies, preeclampsia, placenta previa, prematurity, and low birth weight [43].

Low oxygenation

Maternal lung and heart diseases are also associated with an increased risk of IUGR [44]. Living in high altitude also increases IUGR risk [45] and can lead to reduced birth weight, averaging a 100 g reduction for every 1000 m altitude gain [46].

Maternal intake of harmful substances

Pharmaceutical drugs

The use of the beta-blocker atenolol at conception and during early pregnancy may increase the risk of IUGR, although this is not generally a risk during the second or third trimester [45]. High doses of gluco-corticoids may also cause IUGR [46]. In addition, warfarin treatment during pregnancy may lead to miscarriage, microencephalia, blindness, prematurity, and IUGR [47]. Immunosuppressive drugs during pregnancy may also increase risk of IUGR, prematurity, maternal hypertension, preeclampsia, and congenital anomalies [48–50].

Smoking

The toxic elements in cigarette smoke include nicotine (responsible for the addictive effect of cigarettes), carbon monoxide, cadmium and multiple carcinogens [51–54]. Smoking during pregnancy may reduce birth weight by an average of 200 g [55]. Maternal and fetal carboxy-hemoglobin levels in the blood are often lowered in a woman who has smoked and the capacity for transportation of fetal hemoglobin becomes reduced, restricting the amount of oxygen reaching fetal tissues. Fetal metabolism and growth can therefore become depressed [16]. A population-based study from Norway [56] suggested that the number of infants born SGA would be reduced by 12% if smoking was eliminated in pregnant women.

Furthermore, when a mother smokes a cigarette, the fetal pulse rate increases, causing placental circulation to decrease. After 20 minutes, fetal blood nicotine concentration is a high as maternal blood nicotine concentration. This is dangerous because the vasoconstrictive effect of nicotine may lead to contractions of the uterus, especially during the third trimester. In cord vessels, uteroplacental blood circulation can also be reduced when a mother smokes a cigarette. Endothelial damage due to the effect of nicotine can often include placental calcification and infarction (Table 6.3).

Alcohol consumption

Alcohol consumption during pregnancy has long been recognized as harmful to the fetus. In fact, even ancient texts by the Greek philosopher Aristotle mention the negative influence of alcohol consumption to the fetus [57]. In more modern times, Lemoine et al first reported the occurrence of developmental retardation in children of mothers who consumed alcohol during pregnancy in 1968 [58]. In 1973, Smith and Jones introduced the term fetal alcohol syndrome (FAS) and described the connection between alcohol-consuming mothers and physical and mental defects in their children [59,60]. Alcohol is now recognized as a teratogen that is transported rapidly from the mother's blood through the placenta to the fetus. The blood alcohol level of the fetus can be higher than the mother's level and can remain elevated for a longer period of time because it is absorbed from the fat tissue and eliminated slowly due to the immature liver of the fetus [61]. As a fetus develops, there are

Smoking-associated complications during pregnancy
Smoking leads to elevated risk of:
• spontaneous abortion; • extrauterine pregnancy; • placental ablation; • placenta previa; • preterm rupture; • premature birth; • reduced birth weight (eg, small for gestational age); • reduced head circumference and birth length; • elevated rate of malformations (eg, cleft lip-jaw-palate); • elevated perinatal mortality

Table 6.3 Smoking-associated complications during pregnancy.

critical, developmental phases for each of the organs and the extent that they can be affected by alcohol. Brain and nervous system development is particularly vulnerable to alcohol, but the development of many other organs (eg, heart, kidneys) is also negatively affected.

After the third gestational week, the embryo's beating heart and developing neural structures may be discerned. During gestational weeks 4–8, differentiation and growth of numerous organs occurs. Thus, any consumption of alcohol during these critical phases could cause specific failures in these organs [62].

During the fetal period (weeks 9–40), alcohol consumption may retard the growth of organs, affect fetal height, and induce IUGR [63]. Rapidly growing neural cells are severely affected by alcohol and alcohol consumption by the mother can lead to long-term consequences such as mental retardation, fine motor skill handicaps, and disturbed coarse motor skills in the child [62]. Thus, there is no phase during pregnancy when the fetus is protected against harmful effects of the maternal alcohol consumption. Additionally, due to genetic factors that influence maternal alcohol metabolism, there is no consensus on a permitted allowance for alcohol consumption during pregnancy.

Developmental profile of children with fetal alcohol syndrome

The range of alcohol damage during fetal development, from mild to severe, is well documented in the medical literature [64–70]. Children with FAS are generally smaller than average, underweight, have feeding problems, and are highly irritable [71]. They also tend to develop more slowly than other infants of the same age and take longer to start walking and speaking. By the age of 4–6 years, they are often still of small stature, have 'elfin' facial features, and move in a 'butterfly-like' manner (ie, flitting from one activity to another) [72]. They can have behavioral difficulties, often appearing overly talkative or aphasic [72]. Children born with FAS are at a higher risk of being hyperactive, hypersensitive to touch, misjudging dangerous/risky situations (eg, overly familiar or tactile with strangers) or having a limited attention span (attention deficit hyperactivity disorder) [72]. Coarse motor function can also be disturbed [72]. In some cases, children born with FAS require special care or must attend special schools due to severe FAS-related behavioral disturbances and learning difficulties.

Drug use

Illegal drug use (eg, methamphetamines, marijuana, opiates, cocaine) may induce IUGR by directly effecting fetal growth (although the mechanisms are still unknown). Drug use also has many indirect consequences, such as inadequate diet, lack of prenatal care, and other socioeconomic factors [32,73–76].

A summary of maternal factors that affect fetal growth can be found in Table 6.4.

Maternal factors affecting fetal growth

Maternal anamnesis
- Previously gave birth to an infant that was small for gestational age
- Previous complications during pregnancies

Maternal anthropometry
- Maternal height
- Maternal body mass index
- Pre-pregnancy weight

Obstetrics
- Parity
- Short inter-pregnancy intervals (<6 months)
- Uterine malformation
- First gravidity
- Multiple pregnancy
- Twin-to-twin-transfusions-syndrome [41]
- Assisted reproduction (eg, artificial insemination) [43]

Demographic factors
- Mother's age: (<16 years of age; >35 years of age)
- Parental ethnicity

Socioeconomic factors
- Socioeconomic determinants [77]
- Mother performing heavy physical work during pregnancy [78]
- Insufficient prenatal care

Environmental factors
- Prolonged exposure to high altitudes [45]
- Exposure to indoor air pollution

Stress
- Psychosocial stress [37]

Table 6.4 Maternal factors affecting fetal growth (continues opposite/overleaf).

Maternal factors affecting fetal growth (continued)

Maternal diseases

Diseases not associated with pregnancy:
- Renal diseases [79]
- Intestinal disease
- Autoimmune diseases [80] (eg, systemic lupus erythematosus)
- Diabetes mellitus [81]
- Hyperthyroidism [82]
- High blood pressure
- Thrombophilias
- Thalassemia [83]
- Maternal hypoxia [44] (eg, cyanotic heart disease, chronic anemia, chronic pulmonary disease, asthma)
- Bacterial infections: helicobacter pylori, malaria, toxoplasmosis, listeriosis, tuberculosis, trypanosomiasis, lues
- Viral infections: cytomegalovirus, herpes simplex virus, HIV, varicella, adenovirus, rubella, parvo virus; peridontal infections [84]

Pregnancy-associated diseases:
- Pregnancy-associated hypertension
- Preeclampsia
- Gestational diabetes mellitus
- Premature membrane rupture

Maternal nutritional status

- Inadequate protein intake
- Inadequate caloric intake
- Deficiency of vitamins
- Iron deficiency (anemia)
- Low weight before pregnancy
- Low weight gain during pregnancy
- Maternal malnutrition

Harmful substances

- Alcohol
- Nicotine [85]
- Drugs (eg, opiates, amphetamines, cocaine)
- Pharmaceutical drugs:
    - phenytoine, cyclosporine, anti-epileptic drugs [86,87]
    - warfarin [49]
    - glucocorticoids [88]
    - immunosuppressive drugs [50]

Table 6.4 Maternal factors affecting fetal growth (continued).

Placental and cord-related factors

In most cases, the placenta is genetically identical to the fetus. However, in 1–2% of pregnancies, confined placental mosaicism, in which a cytogenetic abnormality is detected in the placenta but not in the fetus, occurs [89,90]. Despite being rare, up to 20% of 'idiopathic' SGA full-term deliveries have confined placenta mosaicism (the cause of which remain unknown) [90,91].

Pregnancies with one umbilical artery may be associated with chromosome defects, IUGR, and increased fetal mortality [92,93]. Velamentous umbilical cord insertion occurs in 0.24–1.5% of all singleton pregnancies and is associated with circulating disturbances and IUGR [94]. Placenta and cord-related factors that may affect fetal growth are listed in Table 6.5.

Placentitis

Treponema pallidum (syphilis), *Toxoplasma gondii,* listeriosis, rubella, *staphylococcus, streptococcus, enterococcus, Escherichia coli, Chlamydia trachomatis,* and cytomegalovirus may infect the placenta through maternal or fetal blood or an ascending infection, which is the most common route for intrauterine infections. Less commonly, infectious agents enter the uterus as a result of invasive procedures (eg, amniocentesis, fetoscopy, cordocentesis, chorionic villus sampling) or via the fallopian tubes from an infectious process in the peritoneal cavity.

Epidemiology

Low birth weight (including infants affected by SGA and IUGR) rates vary by country. For example, in the US, low birth weight occurs in approximately 10% of all births and, of these, one-third constitute IUGR [35]. In Europe,

Placental and cord-related factors affecting fetal growth
Cord anomalies
• Single cord artery, abnormal cord insertion
Structural and functional anomalies of the placenta
• Disturbed placenta (with or without uterine pathology) • Low placental weight and surface • Placenta previa, placenta velamentosa, placenta bilobata • Low located placenta • Placental hemangioma • Placental infarction • Focal placental lesions • Premature placental separation
Confined placental mosaicism
Infections

Table 6.5 Placental and cord-related factors affecting fetal growth.

IUGR incidence in newborns occurs in 3–7% of total pregnancies [95]. For example, in Spain, IUGR occurs in approximately 5% of births, representing a progressively higher incidence during the last decade [95].

The rate of children born with a low birth weight is approximately six times higher in developing countries than in developed countries [96]. Low birth weight (as defined as <2500 g) affects 16.4% of all newborns born in developing countries (or about 20.5 million infants) each year [96,97]. According to de Onis et al, IUGR was reported to occur in about 24% of newborns in developing countries; thus, it is estimated that approximately 30 million infants suffer from IUGR every year [96,98]. The burden of IUGR is concentrated mainly in Asia (especially in the southern regions), which accounts for nearly 75% of all affected infants in developing countries; Africa and Latin America account for 20% and 5% of IUGR cases, respectively [96]. For example, in India, low birth weight has been reported in 26% of births [98], while the proportion of IUGR has been found to be 54% of those born with a low birth weight [6,99]. The incidence of low birth weight in neighboring Pakistan has been estimated to be around 25% [96]. However, the true incidence of IUGR in South Asia is not currently known, as a majority of deliveries occur at home and approximately two-thirds of children are not weighed at birth [100–102]. Thus, these high rates may still potentially underestimate the true extent and magnitude of the problem.

The observed IUGR and low birth weight rates in 17 datasets from developing countries, compared to the incidence of IUGR and low birth weight estimated using the regression model, shows that the incidence rate of IUGR without low birth weight is consistently higher than that of IUGR with low birth weight by a mean difference of approximately 15% (95% CI). The mean IUGR rate in developing countries is 23.8%, ranging from 9.4% in China to 54% in India [99].

Intrauterine growth restriction sequelae

IUGR is associated with significant morbidity in the form of meconium aspiration syndrome, hypoglycemia, hyaline membrane disease, early onset sepsis, intrapartum asphyxia, stillbirth, and mortality during the first postnatal year [103,104]. Long-term effects include growth restriction in children (if catch-up growth does not occur), detrimental neurodevelopmental progress, and pubertal disturbances. Long-term consequences of IUGR may last into adulthood and predispose individuals to developing metabolic syndrome, which can manifest as obesity, hypertension, hypercholesterolemia, cardiovascular disease, and type 2 diabetes, as well as emotional, behavioral, and social problems [105,106].

References

1. Resnik R. Intrauterine growth restriction. *Obstet Gynecol*. 2002;99:490-496.

2. Lee PA, Chernausek SD, Hokken-Kalega ACS, Czernichow P, et al. International Small for Gestational Age Advisory Board Consensus Development Conference Statement: Management of short children born small for gestational age. *Pediatrics*. 2003;111:1253-1261.

3. World Health Organization (WHO). *Physical status: the use and interpretation of anthropometry*. WHO Expert Committee. Geneva: WHO;1995:121-160.

4. de Onis M, Habicht JP. Anthropometric reference data for international use: recommendations from a World Health Organization Expert Committee. *Am J Clin Nutr*.1996;64:650-658.

5. Williams RL, Creasy RK, Cunningham GC, Hawes WE, Norris FD, Tashiro M. Fetal growth and perinatal viability in California. *Obstet Gynecol*. 1982;59:624-632.

6. Peleg FD, Kennedy CM, Hunter SK. Intrauterine growth restriction: identification and management. *Am Fam Physician*. 1998;58:453-460.

7. Low JA, Galbraith RA, Muir D, et al. Intrauterine growth retardation: a study of long-term morbidity. *Am J Obstet Gynecol*. 1982;142:670-677.

8. Campbell S, Thoms A. Ultrasound measurement of the fetal head to abdomen circumference ratio in the assessment of growth retardation. *Br J Obstet Gynaecol*. 1977;84:165-174.

9. Dashe JS, McIntire DD, Lucas MJ, Leveno KJ. Effects of symmetric and asymmetric fetal growth on pregnancy outcomes. *Obstet Gynecol*. 2000;96:321-327.

10. Severi FM, Rizzo G, Bocchi C, et al. Intrauterine growth retardation and fetal cardiac function. *Fetal Diagn Ther*. 2000;15:8-19.

11. Wollmann HA. Intrauterine growth restriction: definition and etiology. *Horm Res*. 1998;49(suppl 2):1-6.

12. Ross MG, Mansano RZ. Fetal growth restriction. Medscape Reference: Drugs, Diseases and Procedures. Emedicine.medscape.com/article/261226_overview. Accessed February 20, 2013.

13. Kramer MS, Seguin L, Lydon J, Goulet L. Socio-economic disparities in pregnancy outcome: why do the poor fare so poorly? *Paediatr Perinat Epidemiol*. 2000;14:194-210.

14. Wang X, Zuckerman B, Coffman GA, et al. Familial aggregation of low birth weight among whites and blacks in the United States. *N Engl J Med*. 1995;333:1744-1749.

15. Khoury MJ, Erickson JD, Cordero JF, McCarthy BJ. Congenital malformations and intrauterine growth retardation: a population study. *Pediatrics*. 1988;82:83-90.

16. Snijders RJ, Sherrod C, Gosden CM, Nicolaides KH. Fetal growth retardation: associated malformations and chromosomal abnormalities. *Am J Obstet Gynecol*. 1993;168:547-555.

17. Woods KA, Camacho-Hubner C, Savage MO, et al. Intrauterine growth retardation and postnatal growth failure associated with deletion of the insulin-like growth factor I gene. *N Engl J Med*. 1996;335:1363-1367.

18. Eggermann T, Wollmann HA, Kuner R, et al. Molecular studies in 37 Silver-Russell syndrome patients: frequency and etiology of uniparental disomy. *Hum Genet*. 1997;100:415-419.

19. Manning FA. General principles and applications of ultrasonography. In, Creasy RK, Resnik R, eds. *Maternal-fetal medicine: principles and practice*. Philadelphia: Saunders; 2004.

20   Ilsinger S, Das AM. Impact of selected inborn errors of metabolism on prenatal and neonatal development. *IUMB Life.* 2010;62:403-413.

21   Kramer MS. Determinants of low birth: methodological assessment and meta-analysis. *Bull World Health Org.* 1987;65:663-737.

22   Bakketeig LS, Jacobsen G, Hoffman HJ, et al. Pre-pregnancy risk factors of small-for-gestational age births among parous women in Scandinavia. *Acta Obstet Gynecol Scand.* 1993;72:273-279.

23   Dawes MG, Grudzinskas JG. Repeated measurement of maternal weight during pregnancy. Is this a useful practice? *Br J Obstet Gynaecol.* 1991;98:189-194.

24   Lawton FG, Mason GC, Kelly KA, Ramsay IN, Morewood GA. Poor maternal weight gain between 28 and 32 weeks gestation may predict small-for- gestational-age infants. *Br J Obstet Gynaecol.* 1988;95:884-887.

25   Strauss RS, Dietz WH. Low maternal weight gain in the second or third trimester increases the risk for intra-uterine growth retardation. *J Nutr.* 1999;129:988-993.

26   Neggers YH, Goldenberg RL, Tamura T, Cliver SP, Hoffman HJ. The relationship between maternal dietary intake and infant birthweight. *Acta Obstet Gynecol Scand Suppl.* 1997;165:71-75.

27   Lechtig A, Yarbrough C, Delgado H, Martorell R, Klein RE, Behar M. Effect of moderate maternal malnutrition on the placenta. *Am J Obstet Gynecol.* 1975;123:191-201.

28   Ramakrishnan U, Manjrekar R, Rivera J, Gonzales-Cossio T, Martorell R. Micronutritients and pregnancy outcome: a review of the literature. *Nutr Res.* 1999;19:103-159.

29   Bendich A. Micronutrients in women's health and immune function. *Nutrition.* 2001;17:858-867.

30   Scholl TO, Hediger ML, Fischer RL, Shearer JW. Anemia vs iron deficiency: increased risk of preterm delivery in a prospective study. *Am J Clin Nutr.* 1992;55:985-988.

31   Allen LH. Biological mechanisms that might underlie iron's effects on fetal growth and preterm birth. *J Nutr.* 2001;131:581-589.

32   Lin CC, Santolaya-Forgas J. Current concepts of fetal growth restriction: part I. Causes, classification, and pathophysiology. *Obstet Gynecol.* 1998;92:1044-1055.

33   Brodszki J, Hernandez-Andrade E, Gudmundsson S, et al. Can the degree of retrograde diastolic flow in abnormal umbilical artery flow velocity waveforms predict pregnancy outcome? *Ultrasound Obstet Gynecol.* 2002;19:229-234.

34   Khong TY, De Wolf F, Robertson WB, Brosens I. Inadequate maternal vascular response to placentation in pregnancies complicated by pre-eclampsia and by small-for-gestational age infants. *Br J Obstet Gynaecol.* 1986;93:1049-1059.

35   Vandenbosche RC, Kirchner JT. Intrauterine growth retardation. *Am Fam Physician.* 1998;58:1384-1390.

36   Hoffman S, Hatch MC. Depressive symptomatology during pregnancy: evidence for an association with decreased fetal growth in pregnancies of lower social class women. *Health Psychol.* 2000;19:535-543.

37   Rauchfuss M. *Bio-psycho-soziale Prädiktoren der Frühgeburtlichkeit und Differentialdiagnose zur intrauterinen fetalen Retardierung – Ergebnisse einer prospektiven Studie.* Habilitationsschrif. Charité - Universitätsmedizin Berlin; 2003.

38   McDonald AD, McDonald JC, Armstrong B, Cherry NM, Nolin AD, Robert D. Prematurity and work in pregnancy. *Br J Ind Med.* 1988;45:56-62.

39   Spinillo A, Capuzzo E, Baltaro F, Piazza G, Nicola S, Iasci A. The effect of work activity in pregnancy on the risk of fetal growth retardation. *Acta Obstet Gynecol Scand.* 1996;75:531-536.

40   Mozurkewich EL, Luke B, Avni M, Wolf FM. Working conditions and adverse pregnancy outcome: a meta-analysis. *Obstet Gynecol.* 2000;95:623-635.

41   Burkhardt T. Vergleich des Nabelschnur-Resistence-Index von monochorialen and dichorialen Geminischwangerschaften. Dissertation. Berlin, Med. Fakultät Charite, 2003.

42   Taylor MJ, Govender L, Jolly M, Wee L, Fisk NM. Validation of the Quintero staging system for twin-twin transfusion syndrome. *Obstet Gynecol.* 2002;100:1257-1265.

43   Diedrich K, Banz-Jansen C, Ludwig AK. Schwangerschaft und Outcome der Kinder nach ART. *Speculum Zeitschrift für Gynäkologie und Geburtshilfe.* 2011;29:17-22.

44   Pollack RN, Divon MY. Intrauterine growth retardation: definition, classification, and etiology. *Clin Obstet Gynecol.* 1992;35:99-107.

45   Goldenberg RL, Cutter GR, Hoffman HJ, Foster JM, Nelson KG, Hauth JC. Intrauterine growth retardation: standards for diagnosis. *Am J Obstet Gynecol.* 1989;161:271-277.

46   Jensen GM, Moore LG. The effect of high altitude and other risk factors on birthweight: independent or interactive effects? *Am J Public Health.* 1997;87:1003-1007.

47   Lip GY, Beevers M, Churchill D, Shaffer LM, Beevers DG. Effect of atenolol on birth weight. *Am J Cardiol.* 1997;79:1436-1438.

48   Little BB. Immunosuppressant therapy during gestation. *Semin Perinatol.* 1997;21:143-148.

49   Ramin SM, Ramin KD, Gilstrap LC. Anticoagulants and thrombolytics during pregnancy. *Semin Perinatol.* 1997;21:149-153.

50   Prevot A, Martini S, Guignard JP. In utero exposure to immunosuppressive drugs. *Biol Neonate.* 2002;81:73-81.

51   US Department of Health and Human Services (US DHHS). *Fetal Alcohol Spectrum Disorders Center for Excellence: FASD – the course.* www. fasdcenter.samhsa.gov/educationTraining/courses/FASDTheCourse/index.cfm. Accessed February 20, 2013.

52   Miller NS, Cocores JA. Nicotine dependence: Diagnosis, chemistry, and pharmacologic treatments. *Pediatr Rev.* 1993;14:275-279.

53   Daunderer M. *Klinische toxikologie.* Landsberg: Ecomed. 1998;124.

54   World Health Organization (WHO). *Tobacco smoking and tobacco smoke.* Geneva, Switzerland: WHO Press, IARC Monographs; 2002.

55   Bull J, Mulvihill, Quigel R. Prevention of low birth weight: assessing the effectiveness of smoking cessation and nutritional interventions. NHS evidence briefing. London: Department of Health; 2003. www.nice.org/uk/niceMedia/documents/low_birth_weight_evidence_briefing.pdf. Accessed February 20, 2013.

56   Rasmussen S, Irgens LM. The effects of smoking and hypertensive disorders on fetal growth. *BMC Pregnancy Childbirth.* 2006;6:16-23.

57   Abel EL. Was the fetal alcohol syndrome recognized by the Greeks and Romans? *Alcohol.* 1999;34:868-872.

58   Lemoine P, Harousseau H, Borteyru JP, Menuet JC. Les enfants des parents alcoholiques: anomolies observees a propos de 127 cas [the children of alcoholic parents: anomalies observed in 127 cases] (French). *Ouest Med.*1968;8:476-482.

59   Jones KL, Smith DW, Ulleland C, Streissguth AP. Pattern of malformation in offspring of chronic alcoholic mothers. *Lancet.* 1973:1267-1271.

60   Jones KL, Smith DW. Recognition of the fetal alcohol syndrome in early infancy. *Lancet.* 1973;2:999-1001.

61   Hoyme E, May PA, Kalberg WO, et al. A practical clinical approach to diagnosis of fetal alcohol spectrum disorders: clarification of the 1996 institute of medicine criteria. *Pediatrics.* 2005;115:39-47.

62   Spohr H-L, Steinhausen H-C, eds. *Alcohol, Pregnancy, and the Developing Child.* Cambridge, UK: Cambridge University Press; 1996.

63   Lundsburg LA, Bracken MB, Saftlas AF. Low-to-moderate gestational alcohol use and intrauterine growth restriction, low birthweight, and preterm delivery. *Ann Epidemiol.* 1997;498-508.

64   Aase JM. Clinical recognition of FAS: difficulties of detection and diagnosis. *Alcohol Health Res World.* 1994;18:5-9.

65   Schöneck U, Spohr HL, Willms J, Steinhausen HC. Alkoholkonsum und intauterine dystrophie. *Monatsschr kinderheilkd.* 1992;140:34-41.

66 Sokol RJ, Clarren SK. Guidelines for use of terminology describing the impact of prenatal alcohol on the offspring. *Alcohol Clin Exp Res*.1989;13:597-598.

67 Spohr HL, Willms J, Steinhausen HC. Prenatal alcohol exposure and longterm developmental consequences. *Lancet*. 1993;341:907-910.

68 Stratton KR, Howe CJ, Battaglia FC. *Fetal alcohol syndrome:diagnosis, epidemiology, prevention, and treatment*. Washington, DC: National Academy Press; 1996.

69 Streissguth AP, Aase JM, Clarren SK et al. The fetal alcohol syndrome in adolescence and adults. *JAMA*. 1991;265:1961-1967.

70 Streissguth A, Barr H, Sampson PD, Bookstein FL. Prenatal alcohol and offspring development: the first 14 years. *Drug Alcohol Depend*. 1994;36:89-99.

71 American Academy of Pediatrics. Committee on substance abuse and committee on children with disabilities. Fetal alcohol syndrome, and alcohol related neurodevelopmental disorders. *Pediatrics*. 2000;106:358-361.

72 Astley SJ, Clarren SK. Diagnosing the full spectrum of fetal alcohol-exposed individuals: introducing the 4-digit diagnostic code. *Alcohol*. 2000;35:400-410.

73 Fajemirokun-Odudeyi O, Sinha C, Tutty S, et al. Pregnancy outcome in women who use opiates. *Eur J Obstet Gynecol Reprod Biol*. 2006;126:170-175.

74 Fulroth R, Phillips B, Durand DJ. Perinatal outcome of infants exposed to cocaine and/or heroin in utero. *Am J Dis Child*. 1989;143:905-910.

75 Kuhn L, Kline J, Ng S, Levin B, Susser M. Cocaine use during pregnancy and intrauterine growth retardation: new insights based on maternal hair tests. *Am J Epidemiol*. 2000;152:112-119.

76 Little BB, Snell LM, Klein VR, Gilstrap LC, III. Cocaine abuse during pregnancy: maternal and fetal implications. *Obstet Gynecol*. 1989;73:157-160.

77 Kramer MS. Socioeconomic determinants of intrauterine growth retardation. *Eur J Clin Nutr*. 1998:S29-S32.

78 Bell JF, Zimmemann FJ, Diehr PK. Maternal work and birth outcome disparities. *J Matern Child Health*. 2008;12:415-426.

79 Mazor-Dray E, Levy A, Schlaeffer F et al. Maternal urinary tract infection: is it independently associated with adverse pregnancy outcome? *Matern Fetal Neonatal Med*. 2009;22:124-128.

80 Bear JR, Lincoln D, Donoghue, et al. Socioeconomic and maternal determinants of small for gestational age births: patterns of increasing disparity. *Acta Obstet Gynecol Scand*. 2009;88:575-583.

81 Howarth C, Gazis A, James D. Association of type 1 diabetes mellitus, maternal vascular disease and complications of pregnancy. *Diabet Med*. 2007;224:1229-1234.

82 Luewan S, Chakkabut P, Tongsong T. Outcomes of pregnancy complicated with hyperthyroidism: a cohort study. *Arch Gynecol Obstet*. 2011;283:243-247.

83 Traisrisilp K, Luwan S, Tongsong T. Pregnancy outcomes in women complicated by thalassemia syndrome at Maharaj Nakorn Chiang Mai Hospital. *Arch Gynecol Obstet*. 2009;279:6685-6689.

84 Pizzo G, La CM, Conti NM, Guiglia R. Periodontitis and preterm delivery. A review of the literature. *Minerva Stomatol*. 2005;54:1-14.

85 Aliyu MH, Wilson RE, Zoorob R, et al. Prenatal alcohol consumption and fetal growth restriction: potentiation effect by concomitant smoking. *Nicotine Tob Res*. 2009;11:36-43.

86 Hösli I, Tercanli S, Holzgreve W. Epilepsy and pregnancy. *Z Geburtshilfe Neonatol*. 1999;203:90-95.

87 Battino D, Granata T, Binelli S, et al. Intrauterine growth in the offspring of epileptic mothers. *Acta Neurol Scand*. 1992, 86:555-557.

88 Ain A, Canham LN, Soares MJ. Dexamethasone-induced intrauterine growth restriction impacts the placental prolactin family, insulin-like growth factor-II and the Akt signaling pathway. *J Endocrinol*. 2005;185:253-263.

89 Lestou VS, Kalousek DK Confined placental mosaicism and intrauterine fetal growth. *Arch Dis Child Fetal Neonatal*. 1998;79:F223-F226.

90 Kalousek DK, Dill FJ. Chromosomal mosaicism confined to the placenta in human conceptions. *Science*. 1983;221:665-667.

91 Wilkins-Haug L, Roberts DJ, Morton CC. Confined placental mosaicism and intrauterine growth retardation: a case-control analysis of placentas at delivery. *Am J Obstet Gynecol*. 1995;172:440-450.

92 Bryan EM, Kohler HG. The missing umbilical artery. II. Paediatric follow-up. *Arch Dis Child*. 1975;50:714-718.

93 Rinehart BK, Terrone DA, Taylor CW, Isler CM, Larmon JE, Roberts WE. Single umbilical artery is associated with an increased incidence of structural and chromosomal anomalies and growth restriction. *Am J Perinatol*. 2000;17:229-232.

94 Sepulveda W, Rojas I, Robert JA, Schnapp C, Alcalde JL. Prenatal detection of velamentous insertion of the umbilical cord: a prospective color Doppler ultrasound study. *Ultrasound Obstet Gynecol*. 2003;21:564-569.

95 Romo A, Carceller R, Tobajas J. Intrauterine growth retardation (IUGR): epidemiology and etiology. *Pediatr Endocrinol Rev*. 2009;(suppl 3):332-336.

96 de Onis M, Blossner M, Villar J. Levels and patterns of intrauterine growth retardation in developing countries. *Eur J Clin Nutr*. 1998;52:S83-S93.

97 Imdad A, Yakoob MY, Siddiqui S, Bhutta ZA. Screening and triage of intrauterine growth restriction (IUGR) in general population and high risk pregnancies: a systematic review with a focus on reduction of IUGR related stillbirths. *BMC Public Health*. 2011;11:S1.

98 Saleem T, Sajjad N, Fatima S, Habib N, Ali SR, Qadir M. Intrauterine growth retardation - small events, big consequences. *Ital J Pediatr*. 2011;37:41.

99 World Health Organization (WHO). *The World Health Report 1995: Bridging the gaps*. www.who.int/whr/1995/en/index.html. Accessed February 20, 2013.

100 Antonisamy B, Sivaram M, Richard J, Rao PSS. Trends in intrauterine growth of aingle live births in southern india. *J Trop Pediatr*. 1996;42:339-341.

101 The United Nations Children's Fund (UNICEF) and World Health Organization (WHO). *Low birthweight: country, regional and global estimates 2004*. www.unicef.org/publications/index_24840.html. Accessed February 20, 2013.

102 World Health Organization (WHO). Maternal anthropometry and pregnancy outcomes. A WHO Collaborative Study: introduction. *Bull World Health Organ*. 1995;73:S1-S98.

103 Malhotra N, Chanana C, Kumar S, Roy K, Sharma JB. Comparison of perinatal outcome of growth-restricted fetuses with normal and abnormal umbilical artery Doppler waveforms. *Indian J Med Sci*. 2006;60:311-317.

104 Sheridan C. Intrauterine growth restriction–diagnosis and management. *Aust Fam Physician*. 2005;34:717-723.

105 Durousseau S, Chavez GF. Associations of intrauterine growth restriction among term infants and maternal pregnancy intendedness, initial happiness about being pregnant, and sense of control. *Pediatrics*. 2003;111:1171-1175.

106 Dahl LB, Kaaresen PI, Tunby J, Handegard BH, Kvernmo S, Ronning JA. Emotional, behavioral, social, and academic outcomes in adolescents born with very low birth weight. *Pediatrics*. 2006;118:e449-e459.

Development of this book was supported by funding from Sandoz

Chapter 7

Obstetrical aspects

Ralf L Schild

Classification

Being born small for gestational age (SGA) is classified as being born with a fetal weight or an abdominal circumference below the 10th percentile for gestational age [1]. In the past, a variety of cutoffs have been used, adding some uncertainty to the value of individual definitions of SGA. Of note, the diagnosis of SGA does not allow a distinction between infants who are constitutionally small, growth-restricted and small, or growth-restricted but not small [2]. In general, up to 70% of infants are considered constitutionally small due to maternal ethnicity, parity, body mass index, and female gender, and thus are not at risk of increased morbidity and mortality [3]; it is important to realize that fetal size is not equivalent to fetal growth. Therefore, a single fetal biometry will not be able to reliably distinguish between SGA and intrauterine growth restriction (IUGR).

Diagnosing fetal growth restriction

Work-up of a fetus suspected of being SGA should include a complete medical history and physical examination of the pregnant patient. Factors contributing to fetal growth disturbance include drug abuse, medication, tobacco use, and pre-existing maternal disease such as thrombophilia, all of which should be addressed. Importantly, accurate assessment of gestational age is critical to the diagnosis. The optimal method to

S. Zabransky (ed.), *Caring for Children Born Small for Gestational Age*, 77
DOI: 10.1007/978-1-908517-90-6_7, © Springer Healthcare 2013

reliably determine gestational age is by first trimester fetal biometry via a transvaginal or transabdominal route. Several large studies have demonstrated that sonographic estimation of gestational age is superior to dating based on the last menstrual period [4–6].

A detailed fetal anatomic survey, including echocardiography, is recommended in all cases in order to rule out congenital anomalies (present in approximately 10% of pregnancies). Among the anomalies associated with fetal growth disturbance are severe heart defects, skeletal dysplasia, disruption of the abdominal wall, and diaphragmatic hernia. Polyhydramnios associated with IUGR is an ominous sign, as it strongly suggests fetal syndromes (ie, trisomy 18) [7]. Should the anatomic survey reveal suspicious findings, invasive fetal testing is often indicated to rule out underlying aneuploidy.

Two forms of fetal growth restriction have been described. First, the symmetric form, which is caused by early growth impairment and comprises 20–30% of all IUGR cases; second, the asymmetric form, which is characterized by a relatively greater decrease in abdominal size, develops late, and is responsible for 70–80% of cases [8]. To determine the degree of fetal growth disturbance, accurate estimation of fetal weight is the primary goal. However, fetal biometry is neither accurate nor reliable. A multitude of different formulas have been described and, in most equations, fetal measurements such as biparietal diameter, head circumference, abdominal circumference, and femur length are incorporated, thus including two or more morphometric body measurements.

In general, weight estimations are within 10% of the actual birth weight in 75% of patients in whom IUGR is suspected [9]. However, in a population of very low-birth weight (VLBW) infants, error rates of fetal weight determination were high, even in formulas specifically designed for this weight category [10]. Mongelli et al found a false-positive rate for IUGR in excess of 10% with biometry at 2-week intervals, increasing to higher rates late in the third trimester [11]. If regular fetal biometry is indicated for clinical reasons, the most recent measurement should be compared with the measurement taken 3 weeks previously, rather than the measurement taken the previous week [11]. Newer approaches have considered variables known to affect fetal weight, such as fetal gender, maternal parity, ethnicity, height, weight, and age of the patient. When tested, these customized growth curves proved to be superior to population-based weight centiles in identifying fetuses at risk of perinatal death and neonatal morbidity [12]. However, national guidelines on SGA are still characterized by noticeable variances in diagnosis and management, with only a few similar articles being cited by different committees [13].

Monitoring

Doppler sonography is the most important non-invasive investigative tool used to diagnose IUGR and evaluate maternal and fetal hemodynamics. A meta-analysis of randomized studies demonstrated a significant reduction in the number of antenatal admissions, inductions of labor, and caesarean sections for fetal distress in the Doppler group [14]. Also, the clinical action guided by Doppler ultrasonography of umbilical artery waveforms significantly reduced the odds of perinatal death [14].

Deterioration in venous Doppler parameters commonly occurs after changes on the arterial side. Measurement of flow parameters in the ductus venous was shown to be the best predictor of perinatal outcome. This measurement may be particularly useful in the prenatal management of severe IUGR, improving perinatal outcome, even at an earlier gestational age at delivery [15]. Doppler velocimetry of the ductus venosus was able to identify preterm IUGR fetuses at high risk for adverse outcome (particularly stillbirth) at least 1 week before delivery, independent of the uterine artery waveform [16]. Conversely, normal venous Doppler parameters allow expectant management at an early gestational age, even if arterial Doppler values are already abnormal. Importantly, gestational age greater than 27 weeks and 6 days provided the best prediction of survival, and gestational age of 29 weeks and 2 days proved to be the best predictor of intact survival without major morbidity [17].

Conventional antepartum fetal heart rate monitoring has a high sensitivity (but low specificity) in detecting fetal hypoxemia. The computerized cardiotocogram (cCTG) is able to determine fetal heart rate parameters, such as the short-term variation, that cannot be visually assessed but provide a more reliable prediction of fetal acidemia. The cCTG performed best when combined with venous Doppler [18].

Timing of delivery

There is little consensus about the optimal timing of delivery of the growth restricted fetus [19]. The results of the TRial of Umbilical and Fetal FLow in Europe (TRUFFLE) study are eagerly awaited, as they may shed more light on this question [20]. The decision to choose expectant management or to deliver depends on several key aspects such as gestational age, estimated fetal weight, Doppler flow parameters, antepartum fetal heart rate testing, associated maternal disease, and maternal medical history. The growth-restricted fetus should be delivered if the risk of fetal death exceeds the risk of neonatal death. Indications of impending fetal acidemia can be found in a negative A-wave of the ductus venosus and/or a significantly reduced short-term variation in the cCTG. Importantly, if delivery has to be effected before 34 weeks of gestation, antenatal steroids should be given to reduce fetal morbidity and mortality.

If IUGR is of mild severity and routine antenatal tests demonstrate no evidence of fetal compromise, delivery may be postponed until closer to term. However, preliminary work on mild IUGR suggests that the blood flow pattern in both the middle cerebral artery and the aortic arch isthmus may, if abnormal, indicate pregnancies at risk of adverse outcome (and thus requiring earlier delivery) [21]. The hypothesis behind this new evidence is that abnormal aortic isthmus impedance indices are an intermediate step between placental insufficiency-hypoxemia and cardiac decompensation [21].

Delivery method

IUGR may be associated with chronic oxygen and substrate deprivation, which are held responsible for abnormal antepartum test results. Fetal heart abnormalities as related to hypoxia are higher than in the normal population. Nevertheless, spontaneous or induced labor may be safely allowed provided antenatal testing is reassuring and intrapartum monitoring is continuous. Immediate skilled neonatal care is required, as growth-restricted fetuses are at higher risk of neonatal morbidity and mortality.

References

1   Chang TC, Robson SC, Boys RJ, Spencer JA. Prediction of the small for gestational age infant: which ultrasonic measurement is best? *Obstet Gynecol*. 1992;80:1030-1038.

2   Chard T, Costeloe K, Leaf A. Evidence of growth retardation in neonates of apparently normal weight. *Eur J Obstet Gynecol Reprod Biol*. 1992;45:59-62.

3   Ott WJ. The diagnosis of altered fetal growth. *Obstet Gynecol Clin North Am*. 1988;15:237-263.

4   Mongelli M, Wilcox M, Gardosi J. Estimating the date of confinement: ultrasonographic biometry versus certain menstrual dates. *Am J Obstet Gynecol*. 1996;174:278-281.

5   Neilson JP. Ultrasound for fetal assessment in early pregnancy. *Cochrane Database Syst Rev*. 2000;(02)CD000182.

6   Yang H, Kramer MS, Platt RW, et al. How does early ultrasound scan estimation of gestational age lead to higher rates of preterm birth? *Am J Obstet Gynecol*. 2002;186:433-437.

7   Mendez H. Introduction to the study of pre- and postnatal growth in humans: a review. *Am J Med Genet*. 1985;20:63-85.

8   Resnik R. Intrauterine growth restriction. *Obstet Gynecol*. 2002;99:490-496.

9   Guidetti DA, Divon MY, Braverman JJ, Langer O, Merkatz IR. Sonographic estimates of fetal weight in the intrauterine growth retardation population. *Am J Perinatol*. 1990;7:5-7.

10 Jouannic JM, Grange G, Goffinet F, Benachi A, Carbrol D. Validity of sonographic formulas for estimating fetal weight below 1,250 g: a series of 119 cases. *Fetal Diagn Ther*. 2001;16:254-258.

11 Mongelli M, Ek S, Tambyrajia R. Screening for fetal growth restriction: a mathematical model of the effect of time interval and ultrasound error. *Obstet Gynecol*. 1998;92:908-912.

12 Gardosi J, Francis A. A customized standard to assess fetal growth in a US population. *Am J Obstet Gynecol*. 2009;201:25.e1-7.

13 Chauhan SP, Gupta LM, Hendrix NW, Berghella V. Intrauterine growth restriction: comparison of American College of Obstetricians and Gynecologists practice bulletin with other national guidelines. *Am J Obstet Gynecol*. 2009;200:409.e1-e6.

14 Alfirevic Z, Neilson JP. Doppler ultrasonography in high-risk pregnancies: systematic review with meta-analysis. *Am J Obstet Gynecol*. 1995;172:1379-1387.

15 Bilardo CM, Wolf H, Stigter RH, et al. Relationship between monitoring parameters and perinatal outcome in severe, early intrauterine growth restriction. *Ultrasound Obstet Gynecol*. 2004;23:119-125.

16 Baschat AA. Doppler application in the delivery timing of the preterm growth-restricted fetus: another step in the right direction. *Ultrasound Obstet Gynecol*. 2004;23:111-118.

17 Baschat AA, Cosmi E, Bilardo CM, et al. Predictors of neonatal outcome in early-onset placental dysfunction. *Obstet Gynecol*. 2007;109:253-261.

18 Turan S, Turan OM, Berg C, et al. Computerized fetal heart rate analysis, Doppler ultrasound and biophysical profile score in the prediction of acid-base status of growth-restricted fetuses. *Ultrasound Obstet Gynecol*. 2007;30:750-756.

19 GRIT Study Group. A randomised trial of timed delivery for the compromised preterm fetus: short term outcomes and Bayesian interpretation. *BJOG*. 2003;110:27-32.

20 TRUFFLE multicentre group. TRial of Umbilical and Fetal FLow in Europe (TRUFFLE) Study. www.trufflestudy.org/truffle/index.htm. Accessed February 20, 2013.

21 Kennelly MM, Farah N, Turner MJ, Stuart B. Aortic isthmus Doppler velocimetry: role in assessment of preterm fetal growth restriction. *Prenat Diagn*. 2010;30:395-401.

Development of this book was supported by funding from Sandoz

Chapter 8

Placental function in intrauterine growth restriction

Berthold Huppertz

Introduction

Appropriate fetal growth in utero depends on a variety of factors including:

- paternally- and maternally-derived fetal genetic factors;
- maternal nutritional and hormonal factors;
- uterine environment, including the placenta.

An imbalance between paternal and maternal genetic factors, suboptimal nutritional supply from the mother to the fetus, and a dysregulation of placental development may all cause intrauterine growth restriction (IUGR). During pregnancy, the placenta is the decisive organ between mother and fetus and brings the blood systems of both individuals in close vicinity to one another to insure appropriate nutrient and oxygen supply to the fetus.

Features of growth restriction

IUGR affects approximately 5% of all pregnancies and is the second leading cause of perinatal mortality and morbidity [1,2]. As mentioned in previous chapters, there is often confusion in defining appropriate fetal growth, leading to the terms small for gestational age (SGA) and IUGR being used synonymously. However, SGA is a 'soft term' that includes all newborns with a birth weight below the tenth percentile. A number of these babies have used their appropriate growth potential

S. Zabransky (ed.), *Caring for Children Born Small for Gestational Age*, 83
DOI: 10.1007/978-1-908517-90-6_8, © Springer Healthcare 2013

and are genetically small, but otherwise normal [3]. By contrast, IUGR is a pathological subgroup within SGA: for all infants born SGA with a birth weight below the tenth percentile for gestational age, only 30% can also be classified as IUGR [4]. A clear delineation between SGA and IUGR was achieved by extending the definition of IUGR to include infants with a birth weight below the tenth percentile, as well as an abdominal circumference below the tenth percentile, or a longitudinal decrease in the growth of the abdominal circumference of more than 40 percentiles independently from the age-specific size curve [5].

Additionally, typical features of IUGR, such as alterations of blood flow in the uterine and umbilical arteries are now also used to classify IUGR [5,6]. Blood flow alterations within the maternal uterine arteries have been attributed to an inadequate invasion and transformation of the downstream spiral arteries [5]. Hence, partial vasomotor control of these vessels by the mother remains and results in pulsatile flow of maternal blood towards the placenta [7]. Even more disadvantageous for fetal growth and overall well-being are alterations of blood flow within the umbilical arteries. Such changes may result in an increased systole/diastole ratio in cases with still preserved end diastolic flow. Further alterations may lead to the absence of end diastolic flow velocity in these arteries or end diastolic flow may even be reversed [6]. The causes of such alterations of umbilical arterial blood flow include problems such as malformations of the villous tree, resulting in increased peripheral resistance of placental vessels.

Early trophoblast development

During human embryonic development the trophoblast lineage develops as the first cell lineage. First, trophoblast cells appear at the blastocyst stage with the trophectoderm covering the inner cell mass and the blastocyst cavity. During implantation, further differentiation of the trophoblast into the mononucleated cytotrophoblast and the multinucleated syncytiotrophoblast is crucial for the invasion of the early embryo into uterine tissues. Both trophoblast subpopulations further develop into various subtypes (Figure 8.1), establishing all trophoblast populations necessary for proper placental and fetal development. The two major

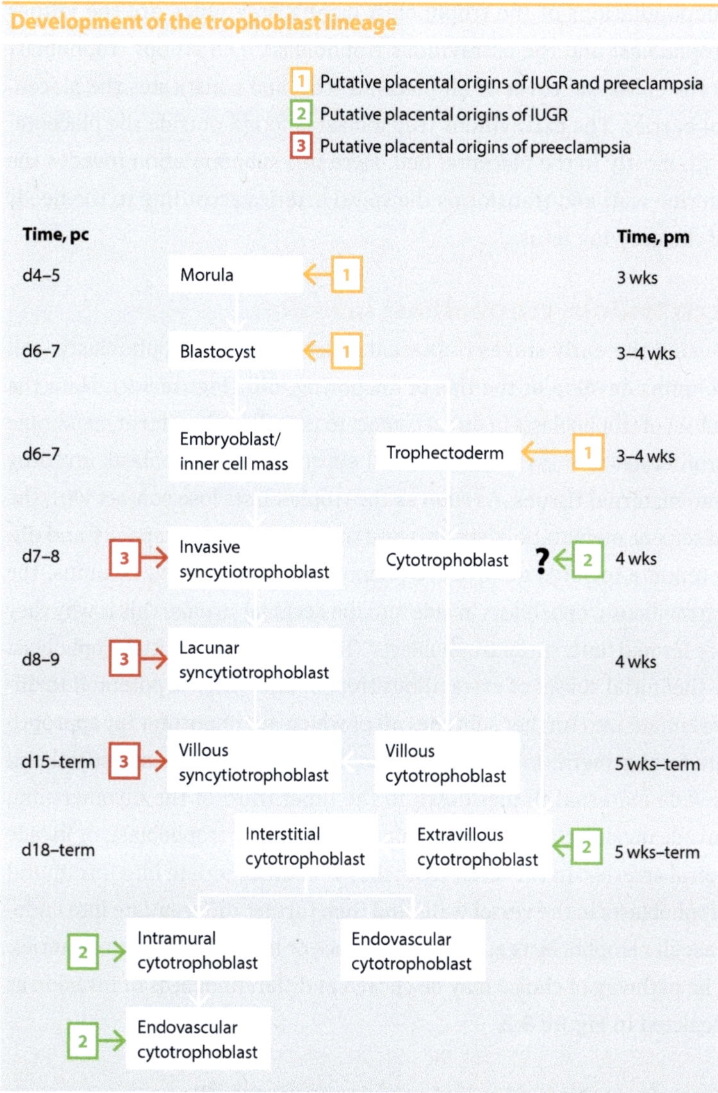

Figure 8.1 Development of the trophoblast lineage. The time of appearance can be found with day post-conception on the left and week post-menstruation (pm) on the right. The numbers in colored boxes indicate the putative insults or dysregulation of trophoblast development causing IUGR and/or preeclampsia: 1, Very early defects will affect all trophoblast subtypes and cause IUGR and preeclampsia; 2, Defects of the extravillous trophoblast in certain subtypes of this population will cause idiopathic IUGR. Defects in the cytotrophoblast, rather than only the extravillous trophoblast, may cause idiopathic IUGR; 3, Defects in the development of the syncytiotrophoblast at various stages will cause preeclampsia. IUGR, intrauterine growth restriction.

subpopulations of the trophoblast during pregnancy are the villous trophoblast and the extravillous trophoblast. The villous trophoblast is the epithelial cover of all placental villi and constitutes the placental barrier. The extravillous trophoblast is found outside the placental villi, mostly in the placental bed. Here this subpopulation invades the uterine wall and transforms the spiral arteries according to the needs of the growing fetus.

Extravillous trophoblast invasion

During the early stages of placental development, trophoblastic cell columns develop at the tips of anchoring villi (Figure 8.2). Here the subset of trophoblasts in direct contact to the villous basement membrane proliferates and is the source of all extravillous trophoblasts invading into maternal tissues. As soon as the trophoblasts lose contact with the basement membrane, they also lose their proliferative capacity and differentiate towards an invasive phenotype. From the cell columns, the extravillous trophoblasts invade into the decidual stroma; this is why they are termed 'interstitial trophoblasts' (Figure 8.2). Interstitial trophoblast is the initial subset of extravillous trophoblast with the potential to differentiate into further subtypes all of which are important for appropriate fetal growth. Interstitial trophoblasts may remain interstitial and invade maternal tissues down to the inner third of the myometrium, invade uterine glands and become endoglandular trophoblast, or invade spiral arteries. In the latter case, they first differentiate into intramural trophoblasts in the vessel walls and then further differentiate into endovascular trophoblasts at the inner surface or in the lumen of the arteries. The pathway of choice may be chosen at different depths of invasion as depicted in Figure 8.2.

Transformation of spiral arteries by extravillous trophoblast invasion

Three stages of spiral artery transformation have been identified that subsequently enable adequate supply of the placenta and fetus:

Stage 1: Vascular changes within the uterine wall independent of trophoblast invasion. Maternal vessels within the uterine walls are initially modified by the mother as soon as she becomes pregnant. Such modifications comprise widespread perturbations of the spiral arteries, vacuolation, and basophilia of the endothelium, disorganization of the vascular smooth muscle cells, and dilation of the vessel lumen [8]. These vessel modifications occur throughout the whole uterus and are not directly linked to trophoblast invasion [8].

Stage 2: Remodeling of spiral arteries by interstitial trophoblasts in close vicinity to the vessel wall. This step has been described in the guinea pig and is anticipated to occur in the human as well [9–11]. Those interstitial trophoblasts that come into close vicinity to spiral arteries secrete factors such as nitric oxide to further remodel the vessel wall and to widen the lumen. Additionally, these secreted factors further reduce the number of smooth muscle cells in the vessel wall, leading to the deposition of fibrinoid in the media prior to infiltration by endomural trophoblasts. Hence, this step comprises changes of cell numbers and extracellular matrix composition in the vessel walls [12].

Stage 3: Infiltration of the vessel wall and establishment of the endovascular trophoblast. After priming the walls of the spiral arteries, intramural trophoblasts infiltrate the vessel wall and further reduce the number of smooth muscle cells and elastic fibers [13,14]. The lumen of the spiral arteries now becomes dilated, reaching several times the original diameter of the untransformed spiral artery [15–17]. The intramural trophoblasts finally reach the endothelial basement membrane, pass this layer, and replace the endothelial cover of the vessels. These vessels are now lined by endovascular trophoblasts that start to crawl along the endothelial lining to further replace this layer. By means of deep interstitial trophoblast invasion and subsequent infiltration of vessels, trophoblasts transform spiral arteries down to the inner third of the myometrium.

Invasion of intramural and endovascular trophoblasts is a crucial step to convert maternal spiral arteries into large-bore conduits that mediate the adequate supply of oxygen and nutrients to the placenta and thus the fetus [17,18]. This supply of oxygen and nutrients is only established at the end of the first trimester [19]. During the first 10–12 weeks of gestation, endovascular trophoblasts not only replace the endothelial

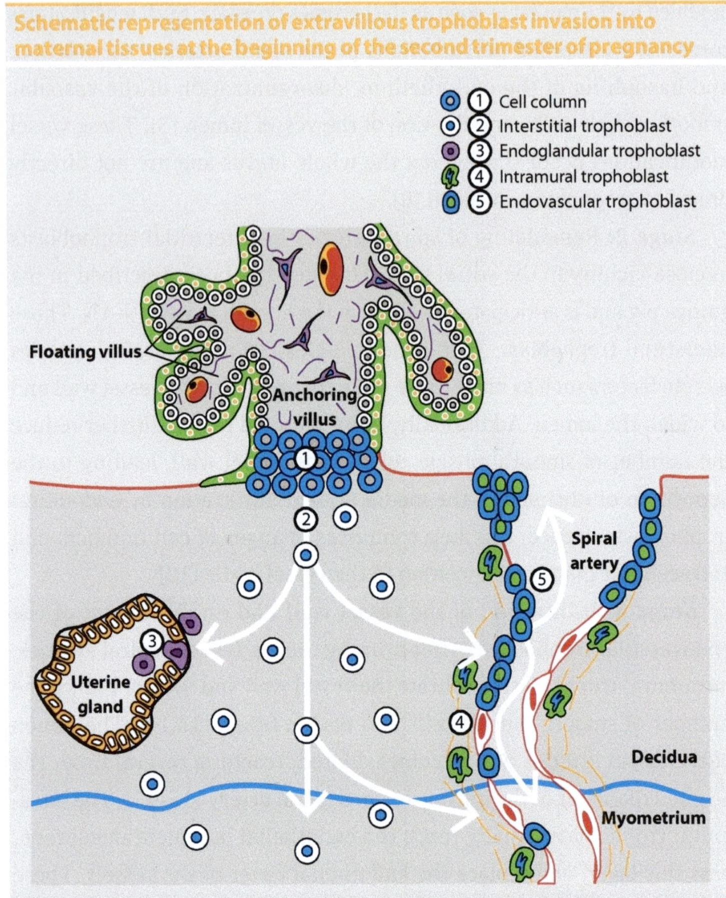

Figure 8.2 Schematic representation of extravillous trophoblast invasion into maternal tissues at the beginning of the second trimester of pregnancy. 1, Anchoring villi are attached to the decidua by trophoblast cell columns, which are the source of all extravillous trophoblasts; 2, As soon as invasive interstitial trophoblasts detach from the cell columns, they start invade into the decidual stroma, finally reaching the inner third of the myometrium. Alternative routes of invasion originating from the interstitial trophoblast go towards uterine glands; 3, endoglandular trophoblast, or towards spiral arteries; 4, intramural trophoblast; 5, endovascular trophoblast.

lining of spiral arteries but generate large aggregates of cells that plug up the vessel lumen. By this means, no maternal blood cells can enter the intervillous space and the placental villi are submerged by a lake of plasma, ultrafiltrated by the trophoblast aggregates in the lumen of the spiral arteries. Adequate nutrition of the embryo during the first trimester of pregnancy is supplied by plasma and secretion products of the uterine glands (histiotrophic nutrition), which are eroded by endoglandular trophoblasts [20] and opened towards the intervillous space [19,21]. After 10–12 weeks of gestation, the plugs of endovascular trophoblasts become permeable and only now can maternal blood cells enter the intervillous space and establish the maternal blood flow to the placenta (hemotrophic nutrition).

Thus, during the first half of pregnancy, uterine spiral arteries within the placental bed go through a series of pregnancy-specific modifications comprising:

- replacement of smooth muscle cells in the vessel media by endomural trophoblast and loss of vasomotor control;
- degradation of elastic fibers and loss of elasticity;
- widening into dilated, incontractile tubes; and
- replacement of endothelial cells by the endovascular trophoblast [22].

Transformation of spiral arteries results in a dramatic decrease in the velocity of blood flow towards the intervillous space from 1–2 m/s to approximately 10 cm/s and only has a modest impact on total blood volume flowing into the placenta [7]. At the same time, loss of maternal vasomotor control, as well as loss of contractility, assures sufficient blood supply from the mother to the placenta at any time [10,17]. Transformation of maternal uterine spiral arteries into uteroplacental vessels is vital for normal fetal growth and development.

Intrauterine growth restriction and alterations of trophoblast and placenta

Due to the close correlation between abnormal uterine artery Doppler waveforms and development of IUGR, there is general agreement that IUGR is directly linked to impaired trophoblast invasion and subsequent failure of transformation of spiral arteries.

Alterations of the extravillous trophoblast

The link between inadequate trophoblast invasion and IUGR with preeclampsia was first reported in 1972 [23]. Since then, trophoblast invasion has remained one of the major foci in placental research. Today, it is generally accepted that in cases with IUGR, it is mostly the invasion of the spiral arteries rather than the general interstitial invasion that is affected. In cases with IUGR, the interstitial trophoblast is reduced in number, but apoptosis is not increased. By contrast, the intramural and endovascular trophoblast are not only reduced in number but also show significantly increased rates of apoptosis [24]. Reduction of both trophoblast subtypes can explain why the respective vessels show a constricted lumen compared to normally invaded vessels. Moreover, maternal macrophages in close vicinity to intramural trophoblasts may further decrease the number of trophoblasts by secretion of tumor necrosis factor-alpha and indolamine-2,3-dioxygenase, a tryptophan degrading enzyme [25].

Besides this impaired invasion into the decidua, deep invasion into the inner third of the myometrium is reduced in cases with IUGR, especially into the walls of spiral arteries in this area. Here, a highly contractile segment of the spiral arteries can be found, which is inactivated during normal invasion. In IUGR, this segment is still active, causing spontaneous vasoconstrictions and intermittent, rather than uninterrupted, perfusion of the placenta [7]. It has to be stressed that the aforementioned observations have been seen in the placental bed after delivery [7]. We can only speculate on the causes and pathways that lead to these changes, but clear observations on how these alterations developed are not yet available.

Effects of alterations of trophoblast invasion

In a normal pregnancy, only the final endings of the spiral arteries are widened, while the deeper parts of the uterine arterial system remain unchanged. The major effect of this widening is to reduce the velocity of blood flow into the placenta by a factor of 100–200, to velocities of about 10 cm/s. Under such conditions, maternal blood enters the intervillous space uninterrupted and with a laminar flow [7].

Interestingly, impaired invasion of spiral arteries by extravillous trophoblasts in IUGR only has a modest impact on the blood volume flowing into the placenta [7]. Accordingly, the availability of nutrients and oxygen in the intervillous space should not be different compared to normal blood flow. Hence, placental hypoxia cannot be deduced from such a flow pattern [26]. At the same time, problems in fetoplacental circulation can still cause fetal hypoxia without any signs of placental hypoxia.

Impaired invasion of the uteroplacental arteries causes a dramatic increase in the velocity of maternal blood flowing into the intervillous space, reaching a speed of 1–2 m/s [7]. In this scenario, maternal blood enters the intervillous space with high speed and a turbulent flow pattern. This change in flow velocity has dramatic consequences for the villous trees.

Damage of the villous architecture

The epithelial cover of the floating villi (villous syncytiotrophoblast) is a very fragile layer and may be damaged by the high velocity of blood in direct contact with this layer. This damage can be visualized after delivery by a thickening of the villous basement membrane, increased deposition of fibrin-type fibrinoid, and villous infarction [27].

Rupture of anchoring villi

In the presence of an increased velocity of maternal blood flowing into the placenta, it is thought that anchoring villi break off from the decidua and the respective trophoblast cell columns disintegrate [9]. Destruction of the cell columns subsequently results in a reduction in the pool of extravillous trophoblasts and may explain the reduced number of interstitial trophoblasts at delivery.

Increased peripheral resistance in placental vessels

The increased velocity of maternal blood flow into the placenta also leads to a partial increase in pressure in the intervillous space, which will have an impact on the fragile placental villi; their capillary system cannot withstand the increased pressure and thus will reduce in width. This causes increased peripheral resistance in the placental vasculature, which may have an adverse impact on the fetal vascular system [5,6]. This may result in reduced flow in the umbilical arteries, which is a common feature associated with IUGR.

Alterations of the villous trophoblast in intrauterine growth restriction

On the level of the villous cytotrophoblast, IUGR cases show significant differences compared to age-matched controls in terms of total cytotrophoblast volume, total number of cytotrophoblasts, and total number of Ki-67 positive cytotrophoblasts as a measure of cytotrophoblast proliferation [28]. Hence, the villous cytotrophoblast shows obvious alterations in cases of IUGR.

In cases of IUGR, the lower number of villous cytotrophoblasts directly affects the syncytiotrophoblast by reducing its volume and total number of nuclei. Interestingly, the aforementioned alterations are not present in cases of pure preeclampsia [28]. Such defects in villous trophoblast growth may have an impact on the transport of nutrients from maternal to fetal blood. Also, the increased velocity of maternal blood passing the placental villi may reduce the ability of the trophoblast to take up a sufficient amount of nutrients to guarantee an appropriate feeding of the fetus.

It still needs to be clarified if the alterations found in the villous trophoblast are direct effects of idiopathic IUGR and represent a defect in the development of the trophoblast lineage. The alternative explanation would favor a secondary impact due to the alterations of blood flow in the intervillous space as described above. The second scenario would place an impact on the development of only the extravillous trophoblast and a subsequent impact on the villous trophoblast due to changes in blood flow.

Alterations of the placenta in intrauterine growth restriction

Placentae from healthy controls and placentae from patients with pure preeclampsia do not differ in regards to total placental volume and total volume of all placental villi [29,30]. Also, the volumes of specific types of villi (eg, stem, intermediate, and terminal) do not show any significant differences. By contrast, in idiopathic IUGR cases, all of the above values are significantly reduced. The placentae are smaller, there are less and smaller villi, and there is a trend towards more fibrinoid deposition in the placenta, indicating more damage to the tissues [28–30].

Placental origins of intrauterine growth restriction and preeclampsia

Dysregulation at various stages of development of the trophoblast and its subtypes, may result in an inadequate differentiation of the respective subtype (Figure 8.1). Dysregulation during the early establishment of the trophoblast lineage will have an impact on all subpopulations of the trophoblast, especially villous and extravillous trophoblasts (Figure 8.1). Alterations may already occur prior to blastocyst formation (ie, on the level of sperm and/or egg, zygote, or the first blastomeres prior to development of the morula), or at the time of blastocyst formation. Dysregulation of trophoblast differentiation may also occur slightly later when the first cytotrophoblasts are formed, which subsequently develop into villous and extravillous cytotrophoblasts. In all of these scenarios, any major dysregulation of trophoblast development will have an impact on placental development as a whole. Accordingly, the result may be a combination of preeclampsia and IUGR and could explain the severe early onset cases of patients suffering from both preeclampsia and IUGR.

Dysregulation of the extravillous pathway of trophoblast development may lead to idiopathic IUGR (Figure 8.1). In this scenario, trophoblast invasion is inadequate and transformation of spiral arteries may not be sufficient. This alteration may only occur on the level of the subtype of endomural/endovascular trophoblast, while the other subtypes of extravillous trophoblast may not show major alterations. Hence, the typical features of IUGR – failure of trophoblast invasion and missing transformation of the uterine arteries – could be explained with this scenario. In Figure 8.1, one defect causing IUGR is labeled with a question mark. This is to illustrate that it is not clear yet whether there is general defect of the cytotrophoblast subpopulation in IUGR or whether only the extravillous type of trophoblast is affected.

Dysregulation of the villous pathway of trophoblast development may lead to preeclampsia (Figure 8.1). Dysregulation of villous syncytiotrophoblast during early stages of gestation may result in malfunction and abnormal turnover, resulting in the discharge of nonapoptotic (ie, necrotic or aponecrotic) trophoblastic particles that are already affecting the mother at this stage of pregnancy [31,32]. Quantification of the preeclampsia-specific biomarker placental protein 13 (PP13) has revealed that alterations in serum PP13 can be detected at 7 weeks gestation [33]. In this scenario, only the villous trophoblast is affected, resulting in the initiation of an inflammatory response in the mother and thus, the clinical symptoms of preeclampsia. The extravillous pathway of trophoblast development is not affected in preeclampsia, since only a small subset of preeclampsia cases (ie, less than 20%) are further affected by IUGR and inadequate trophoblast invasion [33].

Conclusion

IUGR remains a major cause of fetal mortality and morbidity during pregnancy. It appears that dysregulation in the development of the extravillous trophoblast can explain most of the placental alterations that are typical for idiopathic IUGR. At the same time, it has become clear that IUGR and preeclampsia are indeed different entities that may occur at the same time, placing an even stronger burden on mother and baby. A thorough analysis and comparison of both syndromes is mandatory to decipher the different etiologies of preeclampsia and IUGR.

References

1   Neerhof MG. Causes of intrauterine growth restriction. *Clin Perinatol*. 1995;22:375-385.
2   Neerhof MG, Thaete LG. The fetal response to chronic placental insufficiency. *Semin Perinatol*. 2008;32:201-205.
3   Bernstein I, Gabbe SG. Intrauterine growth restriction. In: Gabbe SG, Niebyl JR, Simpson JL, Annas GJ, eds. *Obstetrics: normal and problem pregnancies*. 3rd ed. New York: Churchill Livingstone;1996:863-886.
4   Ott WJ. The diagnosis of altered fetal growth. *Obstet Gynecol Clin North Am*. 1988;15:237-263.
5   Cetin I, Alvino G. Intrauterine growth restriction: implications for placental metabolism and transport. A review. *Placenta*. 2009;30 (suppl A):S77-S82.
6   Sibley CP, Pardi G, Cetin I, et al. Pathogenesis of intrauterine growth restriction (IUGR) - conclusions derived from a European Union Biomed 2 Concerted Action project 'Importance of oxygen supply in intrauterine growth restricted pregnancies,' a workshop report. *Placenta*. 2002;23 (suppl A):S75-S79.
7   Burton GJ, Woods AW, Jauniaux E, Kingdom JC. Rheological and physiological consequences of conversion of the maternal spiral arteries for uteroplacental blood flow during human pregnancy. *Placenta*. 2009;30:473-482.
8   Craven CM, Morgan T, Ward K. Decidual spiral artery remodelling begins before cellular interaction with cytotrophoblasts. *Placenta*. 1998;19:241-252.
9   Hees H, Moll W, Wrobel KH, Hees I. Pregnancy-induced structural changes and trophoblastic invasion in the segmental mesometrial arteries of the guinea pig (Cavia porcellus L). *Placenta*. 1987;8:609-626.

10 Moll W, Nienartowicz A, Hees H, Wrobel K-H, Lenz A. Blood flow regulation in the uteroplacental arteries. *Trophoblast Res*. 1988;3:83-96.

11 Nanaev AK, Chwalisz K, Frank HG, Kohnen G, Hegele-Hartung C, Kaufmann P. Physiological dilation of uteroplacental arteries in the guinea pig depends on nitric oxide synthase activity of extravillous trophoblast. *Cell Tissue Res*. 1995;282:407-421.

12 Harris LK. IFPA Gabor Than Award lecture: Transformation of the spiral arteries in human pregnancy: key events in the remodelling timeline. *Placenta*. 2011;32 (suppl 2):S154-S158.

13 Robertson WB, Manning PJ. Elastic tissue in uterine blood vessels. *J Pathol*. 1974;112:237-243.

14 Robertson WB. Uteroplacental vasculature. *J Clin Pathol*. 1976;29 (suppl):9-17.

15 Brosens IA, Robertson WB, Dixon HG. The physiological response of the vessels of the placental bed to normal pregnancy. *J Pathol Bacteriol*. 1967;93:569-579.

16 Hirano H, Imai Y, Ito H. Spiral artery of placenta: development and pathology – immunohistochemical, microscopical, and electron-microscopic study. *Kobe J Med Sci*. 2002;48:13-23.

17 Benirschke K, Kaufmann P, Baergen R. *Pathology of the human placenta*. New York: Springer; 2006.

18 Pijnenborg R, Bland JM, Robertson WB, Brosens I. Uteroplacental arterial changes related to interstitial trophoblast migration in early human pregnancy. *Placenta*. 1983;4:397-413.

19 Jauniaux E, Watson AL, Hempstock J, Bao YP, Skepper JN, Burton GJ. Onset of maternal arterial bloodflow and placental oxidative stress; a possible factor in human early pregnancy failure. *Am J Pathol*. 2000;157:2111-2122.

20 Moser G, Gauster M, Orendi K, Glasner A, Theuerkauf R, Huppertz B. Endoglandular trophoblast, an alternative route of trophoblast invasion? Analysis with novel confrontation co-culture models. *Hum Reprod*. 2010;25:1127-1136.

21 Burton GJ, Jauniaux E, Charnock-Jones DS. Human early placental development: potential roles of the endometrial glands. *Placenta*. 2007;28 (suppl A):S64-69.

22 Kaufmann P, Black S, Huppertz B. Endovascular trophoblast invasion: implications for the pathogenesis of intrauterine growth retardation and preeclampsia. *Biol Reprod*. 2003;69:1-7.

23 Brosens IA, Robertson WB, Dixon HG. The role of the spiral arteries in the pathogenesis of preeclampsia. *Obstet Gynecol Annu*. 1972;1:177-191.

24 Kadyrov M, Kingdom JC, Huppertz B. Divergent trophoblast invasion and apoptosis in placental bed spiral arteries from pregnancies complicated by maternal anemia and early-onset preeclampsia/intrauterine growth restriction. *Am J Obstet Gynecol*. 2006;194:557-563.

25 Reister F, Frank HG, Kingdom JC, et al. Macrophage-induced apoptosis limits endovascular trophoblast invasion in the uterine wall of preeclamptic women. *Lab Invest*. 2001;81:1143-1152.

26 Huppertz B. Placental pathology in pregnancy complications. *Thromb Res*. 2011;127 (suppl 3):S96-99.

27 Vedmedovska N, Rezeberga D, Teibe U, Melderis I, Donders GG. Placental pathology in fetal growth restriction. *Eur J Obstet Gynecol Reprod Biol*. 2011;155:36-40.

28 Widdows K. *Gestational related morphological abnormalities in placental villous trophoblast turnover in compromised pregnancies*. PhD thesis. Brunel University, Uxbridge, UK; 2010.

29 Mayhew TM, Ohadike C, Baker PN, Crocker IP, Mitchell C, Ong SS. Stereological investigation of placental morphology in pregnancies complicated by pre-eclampsia with and without intrauterine growth restriction. *Placenta*. 2003;24:219-226.

30 Mayhew TM, Wijesekara J, Baker PN, Ong SS. Morphometric evidence that villous development and fetoplacental angiogenesis are compromised by intrauterine growth restriction but not by pre-eclampsia. *Placenta*. 2004;25:829-833.

31 Huppertz B, Sammar M, Chefetz I, Neumaier-Wagner P, Bartz C, Meiri H. Longitudinal determination of serum PP13 during development of preeclampsia. *Fetal Diagn Therapy*. 2008;24:230-236.

32 Huppertz B. Biology of the placental syncytiotrophoblast - Myths and facts. *Placenta*. 2010;31 (suppl):S75-81.

33 Huppertz B. Placental origins of preeclampsia: challenging the current hypothesis. *Hypertension*. 2008;51:970-975.

Development of this book was supported by funding from Sandoz

Chapter 9

Placental function: predicting impairment

Anja Tzschoppe, Regina Trollmann, Fabian Fahlbusch,
Kai-Dietrich Nüsken, Eva Nüsken, Jörg Dötsch, Ellen Struwe,
Ralf Schild

Introduction

Our understanding of the function (and dysfunction) of the human placenta, a complex organ that is needed for only a relatively short period of time, is still incomplete. Historically, in some cultures, it was thought that parts of the human soul survived in placental tissue, giving rise to traditions such as ceremonial placental burials in various cultures around the world throughout history, including China, ancient Palestine, the aborigines in Australia, and across Europe [2]. It was not until the 18th century that the unit connecting the mother and fetus started to be scientifically evaluated [3] and the exact role of the placenta in the transport of oxygen, nutrients, and waste products was not fully understood until the 20th century.

During the last few decades, scientists have further evaluated placental function and have been able to demonstrate a close interaction between the placenta and the fetus [4–6]. It was discovered that the placenta supplies the fetus with nutrients and oxygen from the mother, whereas fetal and maternal genomes control placental transport capacity and supply of nutrients. There may also be a permanent exchange of signals between fetus and placenta to ensure synergy between both systems.

S. Zabransky (ed.), *Caring for Children Born Small for Gestational Age*,
DOI: 10.1007/978-1-908517-90-6_9, © Springer Healthcare 2013

Intrauterine growth restriction and perinatal programming

Traditionally, the term small for gestational age (SGA) has been used to describe a fetus or a neonate whose birth weight and/or birth length is below the third percentile or greater than two standard deviations below the mean for the infant's gestational age and sex. By contrast, intrauterine growth restriction (IUGR) implies an underlying pathological process that prevents the fetus from achieving its growth potential. Among the various causes of growth restriction, placental dysfunction associated with poor placental perfusion and hypoxia is one factor for idiopathic IUGR [7].

Low birth weight has been associated with an increased risk for short stature, insulin resistance, childhood obesity, premature adrenarche, hypertension, and renal disease [8–10]. The process leading to these diseases in later childhood and/or adulthood is known as fetal programming [11]. The concept of fetal programming implies that metabolic alterations in the fetal milieu might influence the regulation of endocrine function later in life [11]. In IUGR, an adverse intrauterine environment seems to trigger adaptations that improve fetal survival [12]. If prenatal and postnatal environments are discrepant, these adaptations become a disadvantage and may lead to diseases related to the metabolic syndrome in adult life [13]. In this context, environmental changes leading to persistent alterations in the fetus should also be reflected in the placenta. Therefore, the analysis of placental tissue, which is completely accessible after birth, could help to predict disorders later in life.

Generally, there are the principle way of getting assessing placental endocrine function with possible relevance for the fetus is an examination of maternal serological markers during pregnancy, which can be used to reflect placental pathology (eg, the evaluation of angiogenic factors may help to predict the risk of evolving preeclampsia) and possible secondary fetal involvement.

Disease prediction

Oxygen deprivation and disease

One of the most serious birth complications is prenatal oxygen deprivation to the fetus (prenatal asphyxia), which may lead to hypoxic ischemic encephalopathy (HIE). The least severe grade of HIE (HIE I) only lasts for several hours to a few days, whereas the most severe grade (HIE III) can lead to serious sequelae such as cerebral palsy [14]. At present there are no parameters at birth that allow for a reliable prediction of health outcome after asphyxia. In view of the ever-increasing therapeutic options for HIE, a prediction of the outcome is of paramount importance [15]. Because the placenta is responsible for transporting oxygen from mother to fetus, it is possible that the placenta will reflect, at least partly, oxygen deprivation experienced by the fetus.

In this context, two factors counteracting the harmful consequences of oxygen deprivation in the placenta – adrenomedullin and vascular endothelial growth factor – have been shown to be predictive for the development of cerebral palsy [16–18]. Moreover, hypoxia inducible transcription factor (HIF)-dependent genes, immediate early genes, apoptosis-promoting factors, genes involved in angiogenesis/cell differentiation, mRNA processing, and embryonic development have been identified as early indicators of fetoplacental tissue hypoxia [19].

In this respect, early hypoxia-induced genomic response by the placenta mirrors that of a developing brain in a (temporarily) parallel manner [19]. Therefore, early determination of these and other factors in the placenta may allow for an early identification of neonates at risk and early commencement of adequate treatment and intervention.

Intrauterine growth restriction and disease

Another frequent fetal complication is IUGR. For a number of years, predictors for evolving IUGR have been successfully described [20–22]. Preeclampsia, a serious complication during pregnancy, can now be partially predicted by laboratory tests that measure angiogenic factors in maternal serum or urine [23,24]. With regard to the fetus, associated IUGR can also be predicted in some cases [25].

This is significant because IUGR is not only associated with an increased risk for perinatal morbidity and mortality, but can also lead to short stature, metabolic and cardiovascular disorders, increased hypothalamic-pituitary-adrenal axis reactivity, and increased anxiety-related behavior in adult life [8,9,26,27]. In this respect, it is now well-recognized that the central role of the placenta in the early programming process is to moderate fetal exposure to maternal factors [11]. Thus far, various placental endocrine regulators have been linked to IUGR including leptin, 11ß-hydroxysteroid dehydrogenase type 2 (11b-HSD2), and insulin-like growth factor-binding protein-1 (IGFBP-1) [28–31]. However, differences in gene expression were dependent on the placental sampling site [32].

Although current research is focusing on potential mechanisms and development of metabolic disorders after IUGR, major questions remain:

- Are patients at risk of developing a disease that is directly associated with an adverse intrauterine environment?
- Could infants profit from close monitoring of their prenatal and postnatal health status?
- Are there options to prevent potential disease? (Figure 9.1).

The concept of predicting diseases later in life on the basis of the feto-placental unit involves assuming that adverse environmental conditions for the fetus are prevalent in the placenta and the fetus at the same time.

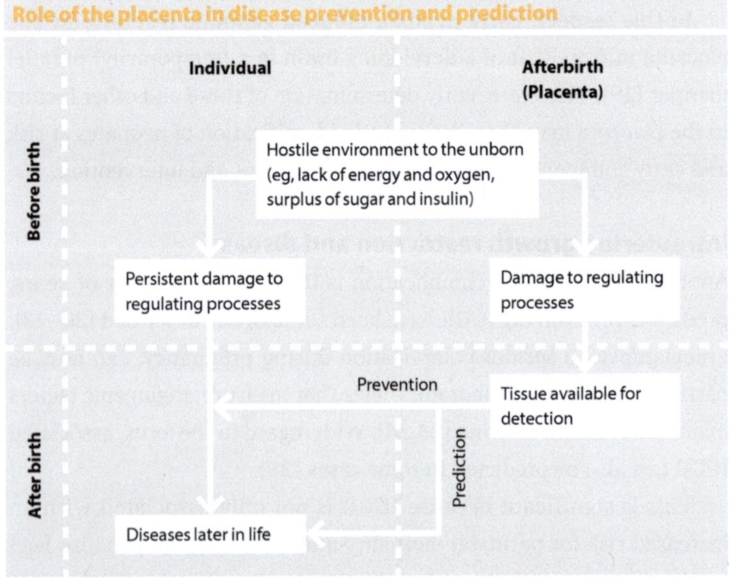

Figure 9.1 Role of the placenta in disease prevention and prediction. Reproduced with permission from Dötsch J et al [1].

Disease-predisposing alterations in the fetus are therefore reflected by the placenta. Placental tissue is available for the detection of these changes (while fetal tissue is not).

Alterations of essential regulatory processes that may lead to metabolic disease in adult life have been found to be present as early as childhood. For example, children born SGA with spontaneous catch-up growth showed a hyperinsulinemic and hypoadiponectinemic variant of visceral adiposity (without being overweight) by the age of 6 years, which predisposes a patient to develop diabetes mellitus [33]. Additionally, children born SGA have been found to have aggravated visceral adiposity and hypoadiponectinemia between 6–8 years of age [34]. However, it is still unknown whether an individual growth-restricted newborn baby will have a higher probability of developing metabolic disease later in life.

Prediction of later disease via placenta analysis

Based on the hypothesis of alterations in fetal programming, a prospective multicenter study (Fetal programming-Intrauterine growth restriction-Placenta Study [FIPS]) has been established to identify placental genes that are predictive for the development of obesity and metabolic disorders after IUGR [32]. As IUGR is diagnosed by anomalous placental Doppler velocimetry (in addition to low birth weight), all IUGR pregnancies in the FIPS study have experienced placental insufficiency [32]. In annual follow-up examinations, clinical and biochemical characteristics of the enrolled infants (especially with regard to childhood obesity, growth failure, hypertension, kidney function, and glucose tolerance) were monitored until the age of 6 years (Figure 9.2). The data were then related to placental regulating systems that may have been altered during intrauterine nutrient deprivation. It remains to be seen whether certain markers turn out to be predictive of later health. One first hint at the potential usefulness of this concept is the observation that the enzyme 11b-HSD2 (which converts active cortisol into inactive cortisone) is inversely correlated with growth velocity in the first year of life after IUGR [35].

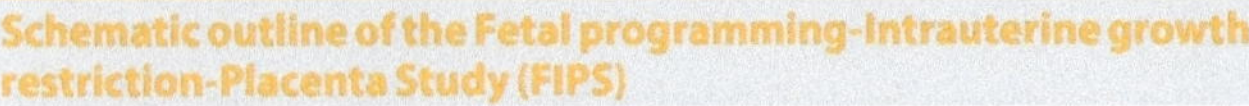

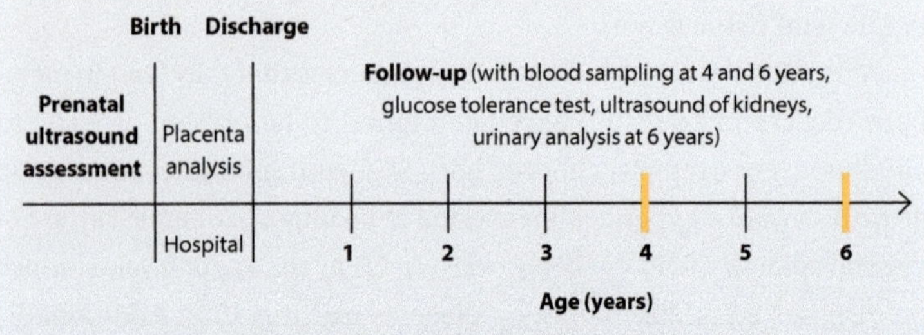

Figure 9.2 Schematic outline of the Fetal programming-Intrauterine growth restriction-Placenta Study (FIPS). It is the aim of the study to predict the probability of long-term disease after intrauterine nutrient deprivation by analyzing placental regulatory systems and relating them to clinical follow-up examinations.

Conclusion

The information provided by the placenta may act as a mirror for intrauterine life and may have the potential to reflect future disease-predisposing conditions. An early revelation of the placental biochemical properties might even help to prevent certain diseases in later life.

References

1 Dötsch J SR, Struwe E. Can the afterbirth play a role after birth? *Hum Ontogenet*. 2008;2:25-28.
2 Murray M. The bundle of life. *Ancient Egypt III*. 1930:65-73.
3 Hunter W. *The anatomy of the human gravid uterus exhibited in figures*. Birmingham, UK: John Baskerville; 1774.
4 Osada H, Watanabe Y, Nishimura Y, Yukawa M, Seki K, Sekiya S. Profile of trace element concentrations in the feto-placental unit in relation to fetal growth. *Acta Obstet Gynecol Scand*. 2002;81:931-937.
5 Constancia M, Hemberger M, Hughes J, et al. Placental-specific IGF-II is a major modulator of placental and fetal growth. *Nature*. 2002;417:945-948.
6 Angiolini E, Fowden A, Coan P, et al. Regulation of placental efficiency for nutrient transport by imprinted genes. *Placenta*. 2006;27(suppl A):S98-S102.
7 Mayhew TM, Wijesekara J, Baker PN, Ong SS. Morphometric evidence that villous development and fetoplacental angiogenesis are compromised by intrauterine growth restriction but not by pre-eclampsia. *Placenta*. 2004;25:829-833.
8 Ibanez L, Potau N, Francois I, de Zegher F. Precocious pubarche, hyperinsulinism, and ovarian hyperandrogenism in girls: relation to reduced fetal growth. *J Clin Endocrinol Metab*. 1998;83:3558-3562.
9 Levy-Marchal C, Czernichow P. Small for gestational age and the metabolic syndrome: which mechanism is suggested by epidemiological and clinical studies? *Horm Res*. 2006;65(suppl 3):123-130.
10 Plank C, Östreicher I, Dittrich K, et al. Low birth weight, but not postnatal weight gain, aggravates the course of nephrotic syndrome. *Pediatr Nephrol*. 2007;22:1881-1889.

11 Plagemann A. Perinatal nutrition and hormone-dependent programming of food intake. *Horm Res.* 2006;65(suppl 3):83-89.

12 Hales CN, Barker DJ. The thrifty phenotype hypothesis. *Br Med Bull.* 2001;60:5-20.

13 Gluckman PD, Hanson MA. Living with the past: evolution, development, and patterns of disease. *Science.* 2004;305:1733-1736.

14 Khot S, Tirschwell DL. Long-term neurological complications after hypoxic-ischemic encephalopathy. *Semin Neurol.* 2006;26:422-431.

15 Jacobs S, Hunt R, Tarnow-Mordi W, Inder T, Davis P. Cooling for newborns with hypoxic ischaemic encephalopathy. *Cochrane Database Syst Rev.* 2007;(4):CD003311.

16 Trollmann R, Schoof E, Beinder E, Wenzel D, Rascher W, Dotsch J. Adrenomedullin gene expression in human placental tissue and leukocytes: a potential marker of severe tissue hypoxia in neonates with birth asphyxia. *Eur J Endocrinol.* 2002;147:711-716.

17 Trollmann R, Amann K, Schoof E, et al. Hypoxia activates the human placental vascular endothelial growth factor system in vitro and in vivo: up-regulation of vascular endothelial growth factor in clinically relevant hypoxic ischemia in birth asphyxia. *Am J Obstet Gynecol.* 2003;188:517-523.

18 Trollmann R, Klingmuller K, Schild RL, Rascher W, Dötsch J. Differential gene expression of somatotrophic and growth factors in response to in vivo hypoxia in human placenta. *Am J Obstet Gynecol.* 2007;197:e1-e6.

19 Trollmann R, Rehrauer H, Schneider C, et al. Late-gestational systemic hypoxia leads to a similar early gene response in mouse placenta and developing brain. *Am J Physiol Regul Integr Comp Physiol.* 2010;299:R1489-R1499.

20 Ness RB, Bass D, Hill L, Klebanoff MA, Zhang J. Diagnostic test characteristics of placental weight in the prediction of small-for-gestational-age neonates. *J Reprod Med.* 2007;52:793-800.

21 Thame M, Osmond C, Wilks R, Bennett FI, Forrester TE. Second-trimester placental volume and infant size at birth. *Obstet Gynecol.* 2001;98:279-283.

22 Poon LC, Zaragoza E, Akolekar R, Anagnostopoulos E, Nicolaides KH. Maternal serum placental growth factor (PlGF) in small for gestational age pregnancy at 11(+0) to 13(+6) weeks of gestation. *Prenat Diagn.* 2008;28:1110-1115.

23 Moore Simas TA, Crawford SL, Solitro MJ, Frost SC, Meyer BA, Maynard SE. Angiogenic factors for the prediction of preeclampsia in high-risk women. *Am J Obstet Gynecol.* 2007;197:244 e1-e8.

24 Aggarwal PK, Jain V, Sakhuja V, Karumanchi SA, Jha V. Low urinary placental growth factor is a marker of pre-eclampsia. *Kidney Int.* 2006;69:621-624.

25 Chafetz I, Kuhnreich I, Sammar M, et al. First-trimester placental protein 13 screening for preeclampsia and intrauterine growth restriction. *Am J Obstet Gynecol.* 2007;197:e1-e7.

26 Welberg LA, Seckl JR. Prenatal stress, glucocorticoids and the programming of the brain. *J Neuroendocrinol.* 2001;13:113-128.

27 Weinstock M. The long-term behavioural consequences of prenatal stress. *Neurosci Biobehav Rev.* 2008;32:1073-1086.

28 Abuzzahab MJ, Schneider A, Goddard A, Grigorescu F, Lautier C, Keller E, et al. IGF-I receptor mutations resulting in intrauterine and postnatal growth retardation. *N Engl J Med.* 2003;349:2211-2222.

29 Dotsch J, Nusken KD, Knerr I, Kirschbaum M, Repp R, Rascher W. Leptin and neuropeptide Y gene expression in human placenta: ontogeny and evidence for similarities to hypothalamic regulation. *J Clin Endocrinol Metab.* 1999;84:2755-2758.

30 Struwe E, Berzl GM, Schild RL, et al. Simultaneously reduced gene expression of cortisol-activating and cortisol-inactivating enzymes in placentas of small-for-gestational-age neonates. *Am J Obstet Gynecol.* 2007;197:43

31 Struwe E, Berzl G, Schild R, et al. Microarray analysis of placental tissue in intrauterine growth restriction. *Clin Endocrinol (Oxf).* 2009;72:241-247.

32 Tzschoppe AA, Struwe E, Dorr HG, et al. Differences in gene expression dependent on sampling site in placental tissue of fetuses with intrauterine growth restriction. *Placenta.* 2010;31:178-185.

33 Ibanez L, Suarez L, Lopez-Bermejo A, Diaz M, Valls C, de Zegher F. Early development of visceral fat excess after spontaneous catch-up growth in children with low birth weight. *J Clin Endocrinol Metab.* 2008;93:925-928.

34 Ibanez L, Lopez-Bermejo A, Diaz M, Suarez L, de Zegher F. Low-birth weight children develop lower sex hormone binding globulin and higher dehydroepiandrosterone sulfate levels and aggravate their visceral adiposity and hypoadiponectinemia between six and eight years of age. *J Clin Endocrinol Metab.* 2009;94:3696-3699.

35 Tzschoppe A, Struwe E, Blessing H, Fahlbusch F, Liebhaber G, Dorr HG, et al. Placental 11beta-HSD2 gene expression at birth is inversely correlated with growth velocity in the first year of life after intrauterine growth restriction. *Pediatr Res.* 2009;65:647-653.

Development of this book was supported by funding from Sandoz

Chapter 10

The role of genetics and epigenetics in growth restriction

Thomas Eggermann

Introduction

Human growth is a complex process, with both genetic and environmental factors thought to contribute in equal parts. Intrauterine growth is characterized by a high rate of cell division and differentiation, while postnatal growth mainly consists of cell expansion. Differentially expressed hormones and a complex interaction of growth factors are responsible for regular intrauterine cellular proliferation and differentiation, whereas systemic acting hormones such as growth hormone (GH) regulate postnatal growth. In both prenatal and postnatal growth, genetic factors and predispositions play a pivotal role.

The following chapter is a review of fetal genetic factors that influence intrauterine growth and its disturbances. This chapter will provide the reader with an introduction to this complex and dynamic field, with a recommendation for consulting the Online Mendelian Inheritance in Man database (www.ncbi.nlm.nih.gov/omim) and other public databases for further comprehensive information [1].

Genetic determinants of fetal growth

The determinants influencing fetal growth can be separated into two groups: maternal and fetal. Approximately 50% of fetal growth factors are regarded as 'maternal determinants', which can be traced to

S. Zabransky (ed.), *Caring for Children Born Small for Gestational Age*,
DOI: 10.1007/978-1-908517-90-6_10, © Springer Healthcare 2013

exogenous, genetic predisposition, or maternal diseases that affect the fetal growth [2]. Genetic maternal-effect factors include diabetes and preeclampsia, both of which have been associated with intrauterine growth restriction (IUGR) [3,4]. For instance, several studies indicate a profound contribution of genetic predispositions to the etiology of preeclampsia [5–7].

Among fetal determinants, genetic disturbances are the main causes of IUGR. The general influence of genetic predisposition to intrauterine growth and end-height of an individual can be seen in twin studies, which indicate that 70–90% of end-height measurements can be attributed to familial height measurements [8–10]. Familial height should also be considered when comparing biometry results at birth. Three types of genetic disturbances in IUGR (and postnatal growth) have been identified:

- submicroscopic chromosomal disturbances;
- monogenic causes for IUGR;
- epigenetic alterations.

Chromosomal disturbances

In general, growth disturbances are an unspecific feature of chromosomal aberrations. Up to 40% of children with numerical and structural aberrations show an IUGR; conversely, in 10% of fetuses with IUGR, chromosomal disturbances can be detected [2]. The majority of human chromosomal aberrations are associated with IUGR (Table 10.1). Therefore, IUGR that is associated with further fetal malformations provides evidence for a fetal chromosomal imbalance.

Until recently, standard cytogenetic karyotyping was indicated in children exhibiting intrauterine and/or postnatal growth restriction, congenital malformations, craniofacial dysmorphisms, and mental retardation. However, with conventional karyotyping, only aberrations of less than five megabases (Mb) become visible due to limited microscopic resolution. Therefore, many smaller chromosomal rearrangements can remain undetected. With the development of molecular high-resolution techniques (eg, array comparative genomic hybridization, single nucleotide polymorphism arrays), a fine resolution down to several kilobases is possible (Figure 10.1).

Examples of chromosomal aneuploidies and structural aberrations associated with intrauterine growth restriction

Syndrome	Localization	Conventional cytogenetic findings*	Only detectable by microarray*
Cornelia de Lange-Syndrome	3q26.3	Selection, translocation, duplication	In some cases
Wolf-Hirschhorn syndrome	4p16.3	Deletion	In some cases
Cri-du-Chat syndrome	5p	Deletion	In some cases
Silver-Russell syndrome	7p12-p14 11p15	Duplications	In the majority of cases
Williams-Beuren syndrome	7q11.2	–	Microdeletion
12q14 microdeletion syndrome	12q14	–	Yes
Pätau syndrome	13	Trisomy 13	No
Prader-Willi syndrome	15q11-q12	Deletion	In some cases
IGF-1R deletion	15q26.3	Ring chromosomes	Microdeletion
18p- syndrome	18p	Deletion	In some cases
18q- syndrome	18q	Deletion	In some cases
Edwards syndrome	18	Trisomy 18	No
Down syndrome	21	Trisomy 21	No
Turner syndrome	X	Monosomy X; 45,X	No

Table 10.1 Examples of chromosomal aneuploidies and structural aberrations associated with intrauterine growth restriction. *Depending on the size (<5 megabases) of the aberrant fragment the aberration might not be detectable by conventional cytogenetics.

Several new microdeletion syndromes have been identified using genomic array technology [11], but the search for genomic imbalances has nearly always been focused on patients with mental retardation and facultative clinical features. In a recent patient cohort, up to 19% of patients showed a pathogenic copy number variation [12]. The need to screen patients (prenatally) with growth restriction, but without mental retardation, for submicroscopic chromosomal imbalances was recently illustrated by the identification of patients with Silver-Russell syndrome features carrying deletions or duplications of 1.1Mb–2.7Mb [13,14].

Molecular karyotyping should be considered in cases with preexisting and persisting postnatal growth restriction and only minor dysmorphisms (ie, without mental retardation). In addition to the confirmation of a clinical diagnosis, the identification of chromosomal imbalances is

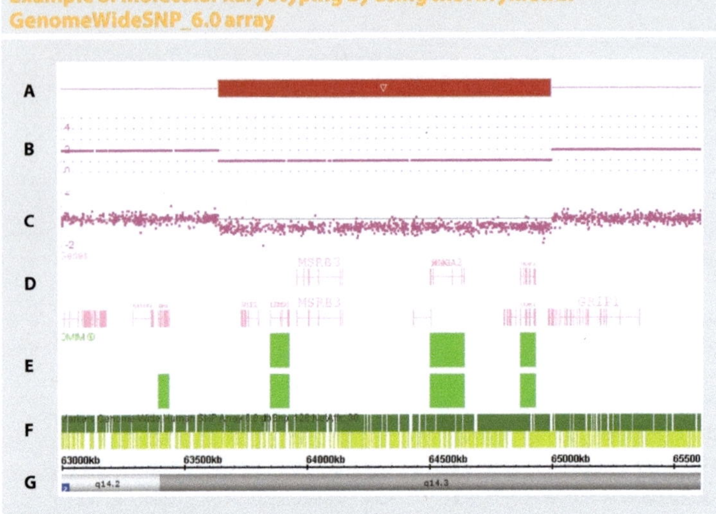

Figure 10.1 Example of molecular karyotyping by using the Affymetrix GenomeWideSNP_6.0 array. A, Schematic presentation of the copy number segments; B, Illustration of the copy number state; C, Intensity of signal markers in the affected area; D, Overview on the genes in the affected 12q14 region; E, List of Online Mendelian Inheritance in Man disorders localized within the region 12q14; F, Marker coverage of the used array system; G, Physical position and chromosomal band at 12q14.

important for genetic counseling. Many chromosomal imbalances are associated with structural imbalances and might have been inherited from a chromosomally-balanced parent. In these families, a predisposition for a structural chromosomal aberration can be delineated and appropriate risk figures can be calculated [15].

Monogenic causes of intrauterine growth restriction

Whereas the influence of chromosomal disturbances on fetal growth is well known, only a limited number of reports exist that describe mutations in single genes associated with IUGR and postnatal growth restriction (Table 10.2).

Less than 1% of children under the third percentile for height carry mutations in the members of the GH–insulin-like growth factor 1 (IGF-1) axis (or have a GH deficiency) [2]. Mutations have been described in the genes that encode growth factors and their receptors,

Examples of single gene defects/monogenic disorders associated with intrauterine growth restriction

Gene	Chromosomal localization	Patient group
Pituitary-specific transcription factor 1	3p11	Combined pituitary hormone deficiency
Homeobox gene expression in embryonic stem cells	3p21	Combined pituitary hormone deficiency
Prophet of PIT-1	5q31.2	Combined pituitary hormone deficiency
Growth hormone receptor	5p13	Laron syndrome
Growth-hormone- releasing hormone receptor	7p14	Single families
LIM homeobox 3	9q34	Combined pituitary hormone deficiency
High-mobility group AT-hook 2 (HMGA2)*	12q14	Intrauterine growth restriction
		Postnatal growth restriction
		Further features
Insulin-like growth factor 1 (IGF-1)	12q22	Intrauterine growth restriction
		Postnatal growth restriction
		Sensorineuronal deafness
		Mental retardation
Insulin-like growth factor 1 receptor	15q25	Intrauterine growth restriction
		Postnatal growth restriction
Growth hormone 1	17q23	Isolated growth hormone deficiency, Typ IA, IB, II
Short stature homeobox gene (SHOX)	Xp22.3	Isolated intrauterine growth restriction
		Small for gestational age
		Postnatal growth restriction
		Turner syndrome
		Léri-Weill dyschondrosteosis
		Langer mesomelic dysplasia

Table 10.2 Examples of single gene defects/monogenic disorders associated with intrauterine growth restriction. The order of genes corresponds to their chromosomal localization. Generally, these monogenic disorders are rare (except SHOX mutations). *The phenotype of HMGA2 deletion carriers depends on extent of the 12q14 microdeletion.

as well as in proteins which regulate the expression of growth factors (eg, pituitary-specific positive transcription factor 1, prophet of PIT1) [16,17]. However, mutations in these genes are rare and have only been reported in single patients. Therefore, it was surprising that mutations in the short stature homeobox gene (SHOX) gene, which were initially identified in syndromic growth retardation, were observed to contribute to a significant proportion of idiopathic short stature [18]. These disturbances (eg, deletions and point mutations resulting in SHOX haploinsufficiency) account for 2% of children with short stature and are found in 1 in 2000 children. For the sake of comparison, it should be noted that classic GH deficiency is present in 1 in 3500 children, and Turner syndrome in 1 in 2500 girls [18]. SHOX testing should be considered in children with low biometric parameters at birth but within the lower normal range (eg, not with severe IUGR), those with short stature that persists in later life, and a positive family history [19].

Evidence for a further genetic contribution to IUGR and postnatal growth restriction (PNGR) have been obtained in a study that conducted a detailed molecular analysis of patients with different microdeletions in chromosome 12q14 [20]. While the extent of the deletion and the clinical course was different, all patients sharing deletions of the *HMGA2* gene were prenatally and postnatally growth-restricted, thus confirming the role of this gene in human growth [20]. However, point mutations in *HMGA2* have not yet been reported [14].

Consistent with the situation in chromosomal aberrations, the identification of a genomic mutation causing a clinical phenotype and its significance for the carrier and their family makes genetic counseling of the patient and close relatives necessary, as many of the known mutations are inherited and therefore specific risk figures can be delineated.

Epigenetic influences on human growth

Central members in the growth factor axis are regulated epigenetically (eg, by insulin-like growth factor 2, growth factor receptor-bound protein 10) and thereby reflect the importance of imprinting for correct mammalian ontogenesis. These so-called 'imprinted' genes are expressed on only one chromosome from one parent. Generally, paternally-expressed genes enhance fetal growth, whereas maternally-expressed genes suppress it. Based on this observation, a genetic conflict theory has been hypothesized [20] to explain the evolution of imprinted paternally-derived genes that aim to extract more resources from the mother, whereas maternally-derived genes balance the nutrient provision to the current fetus with that of potential future fetuses from the same mother.

With the identification of human diseases caused by epigenetic mutations, the significance of a balanced expression of imprinted genes becomes obvious. In these imprinting disorders, different classes of mutations can be observed. In addition to classical genetic mutations such as deletions/duplications and point mutations, aberrant methylation patterns at the regions regulating the expression of genes or uniparental disomies contribute to the mutation spectrum.

Silver-Russell syndrome

The majority of congenital imprinting disorders are characterized by disturbed growth; among them, Silver-Russell syndrome (SRS) is the most prominent growth restriction syndrome with epigenetic mutations [21]. SRS is a clinically and genetically heterogeneous disorder that is mainly characterized by severe IUGR, PNGR, and a small triangular face [21]. The disease is also associated with a failure to thrive and additional dysmorphic features, including fifth-finger clinodactyly and hemihypoplasia [21]. Although a clinical scoring system to assist the diagnosis has recently been suggested [22], the accuracy of diagnosis is influenced by the experience of the clinical investigator. Furthermore, the clinical picture of SRS in adulthood is less clear than in early childhood and, therefore, pictures from early childhood should be included in a careful anamnestic workup.

The clinical heterogeneity is reflected by the heterogeneous genetic and epigenetic findings in SRS patients; in about 10% of cases, a maternal uniparental disomy of chromosome 7 (UPD(7)mat) can be detected, whereas approximately 38% carry a methylation defect in the telomeric imprinted region on chromosome 11p15 [21]. Indeed, the 11p15 epimutation carriers often show the more typical SRS phenotype, while UPD(7)mat carriers are generally mildly affected [23]. Nevertheless, many exceptions have been reported, thereby making a strict genotype-phenotype correlation impossible [22,23]. In addition to these two major disturbances, several SRS patients carry submicroscopic structural aberrations affecting numerous chromosomes [13]. Furthermore, as many SRS features are unspecific, the clinical transition to other inborn disorders (eg, 12q14 microdeletion syndrome) is fluid.

The regulation of gene expression by epigenetic mechanism is not yet completely understood; currently, we are only beginning to decipher the epigenome and its regulators. An impressive example of the complexity of genomic imprinting is the 11p15 region (Figure 10.2). In 11p15, two imprinting control regions (ICR) are localized, each of which regulate the expression of different genes. Whereas ICR1 controls the expression of *H19* and *IGF2*, ICR2 regulates the expression of *CDKN1C*. Of these, *IGF2* and *CDKN1C* have been shown to influence human growth [15]. Therefore, aberrant methylation, or other mutations of the ICR1 or the ICR2 in 11p15, influence the expression of *IGF2* and *CDKN1C,* and thereby cause growth restriction or overgrowth in SRS or Beckwith Wiedemann syndrome (Table 10.2). While the unambiguous association between

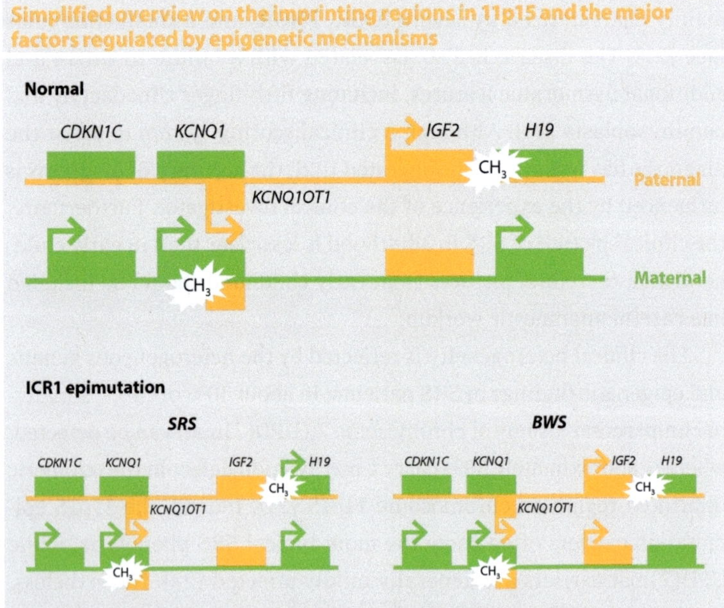

Figure 10.2 Simplified overview on the imprinting regions in 11p15 and the major factors regulated by epigenetic mechanisms. Whereas *CDKN1C, H19,* and *KCNQ1* are expressed from the maternal allele, *IGF2* and the non-coding ribonucleic acid *KCNQ1OT1* are expressed from the paternal copy. The regulated expression is mediated by CpG methylation and chromatide organization (not shown). Aberrant methylation might affect both regions. Here the hypo- or hypermethylation at the ICR1 is illustrated resulting in SRS or BWS. However, further types of mutations and epimutations also exist. BWS, Beckwith-Wiedemann syndrome; CpG, cytosine-phosphate-guanine; ICR1, imprinting control region 1; SRS, Silver-Russell syndrome.

aberrant methylation at specific imprinted loci and distinct imprinting disorders has been widely accepted, it has recently been brought into question by the identification of methylation defects at multiple imprinted loci (MLMD) [24]. Strikingly, in different imprinting disorders, the same MLMD patterns can be observed, making an epigenotype-phenotype correlation more difficult.

Application of high-throughput technologies

Previously, the identification of the genetic basis of congenital disorders was mainly hampered by technical limitations, making the discovery of disease-causing mutations possible mainly through functional approaches (eg, delineation of a candidate gene by its functional properties), identifying chromosomal aberrations with breakpoints in disease genes, or by linkage analysis. All of these strategies require extensive and detailed clinical and molecular analysis.

This situation has changed with the development of high-throughput techniques for the identification of genomic alterations. For example, initial array studies for the detection of submicroscopic chromosomal imbalances (eg, 'DNA chips,' molecular karyotyping) were focused on patients with mental retardation as the main clinical feature, resulting in increased detection rates [11]. However, pilot studies reporting on single patients with growth-restriction and cryptic imbalances, but without mental retardation, show that loss or gain of genomic fragments with a size of several Mbs does not automatically cause intellectual incapacities [13,14]. Indeed, genomic copy number alterations should generally be considered in patients with IUGR, PNGR, and other minor further anomalies that have normal intelligence.

With the development of next-generation, high-throughput sequencing, highly effective and exhaustive whole genome analyses has become possible. As outlined for the application of array-typing in molecular karyotyping, these techniques allow the analysis of complete genomes within a short time and at a relatively low cost. In the previous few years, the power of next-generation sequencing to decipher the genetic basis of specific congenital disorders has been impressively documented [25,26]. In the future, these strategies will help us to discover the general contribution of genomic variants to the pathophysiology of numerous disorders and conditions, including IUGR. Furthermore, they will provide us with a huge amount of information that requires extensive bioinformatics expertise and data memory capacity. Additionally, the interpretation of these data is a significant challenge, as pathogenic mutations have to be differentiated from apathogenic variants or predisposing factors. In a routine array application, this interpretation is already difficult, leaving the physiological significance of several microdeletions and duplications unclear [12]. Indeed, recent studies indicate that humans have an exceptionally high per-generation mutation rate, which complicates the interpretation of de novo variants [27]. However, with the growing knowledge on mutation rates, their significance for human pathology, and the increasing number of variants in public databases, this problem will likely be resolved.

As a result of these revolutionizing techniques, whole genome analysis of an individual, independent from initial clinical diagnosis, is possible. With these strategies, it is possible that genetic alterations which would have been previously neglected in a classical candidate gene approach due to their unexpected functional properties can now be discovered. However, after identification of these 'unexpected' genetic disturbances, a careful genotype–phenotype correlation will be necessary to understand the pathophysiological mechanism as the basis for therapeutic approaches. Furthermore, these tests should be embedded in genetic counseling to provide the patient with the maximum amount of information.

Technically, the new strategies are applicable in prenatal diagnostics. Their implementation in postnatal genetic testing is ongoing, but in prenatal diagnosis their use must be considered with caution. To circumvent the identification of numerous genetic variants of unknown significance, prenatal testing should be restricted to those genomic regions with a well-known clinical significance (eg, tiling path resolution mapping, as described for the 1p36 deletion syndrome) [28]. However, even in well-known aberrations, an unambiguous prognosis might not be possible, as illustrated in DiGeorge (or 15q13 microdeletion) syndrome [29]. For both genomic imbalances, severely affected (as well as healthy) carriers of the same aberration have been reported. In cases such as these, genetic counseling is a relevant prerequisite prior to laboratory testing.

References

1 Online Mendelian Inheritance in Man (OMIM) database. www.ncbi.nlm.nih.gov/omim. Accessed February 20, 2013.

2 Wollmann HA. Intrauterine wachstumsretardierung. *Monatsschr Kinderhlkd*. 1998;146:714-726.

3 Cross JC. The genetics of pre-eclampsia: a feto-placental or maternal problem? *Clin Genet*. 2003;64:96-103.

4 Park JH, Stoffers DA, Nicholls RD, Simmons RA. Development of type 2 diabetes following intrauterine growth retardation in rats is associated with progressive epigenetic silencing of Pdx1. *J Clin Invest*. 2008;118:2316-2324.

5 Chappell S, Morgan L. Searching for genetic clues to the causes of pre-eclampsia. *Clin Sci*. 2006;110:443-458.

6 Williams PJ, Pipkin FB. The genetics of pre-eclampsia and other hypertensive disorders of pregnancy. *Best Pract Res Clin Obstet Gynaecol*. 2011;25:405-417.

7 Vitoratos N, Vrachnis N, Iavazzo C, Kyrgiou M. Preeclampsia: molecular mechanisms, predisposition, and treatment. *J Pregnancy*. 2012;2012:145487.

8 Phillips K, Matheny AP. Quantitative genetic analysis of longitudinal trends in height: preliminary results from the Louisville twin study. *Acta Genet Med Gemellol*. 1990;39:143-163.

9 Preece MA. The genetic contribution to stature. *Horm Res*. 1996;45:56-58.

10 Silventoinen K, Kaprio J, Lahelma E, Koskenvuo M. Relative effect of genetic and environmental factors on body height: differences across birth cohorts among Finnish men and women. *Am J Public Health*. 2000;90:627-630.

11 Shaffer LG, Bejjani BA, Torchia B, Kirkpatrick S, Coppinger J, Ballif BC. The identification of microdeletion syndromes and other chromosome abnormalities: cytogenetic methods of the past, new technologies for the future. *Am J Med Genet*. 2007;145C:335-345.

12 Miller DT, Adam MP, Aradhya S, et al. Consensus statement: chromosomal microarray is a first-tier clinical diagnostic test for individuals with developmental disabilities or congenital anomalies. *Am J Hum Genet*. 2010;86:749-764.

13 Bruce S, Hannula-Jouppi K, Puoskari M, et al. Submicroscopic genomic alterations in Silver-Russell syndrome and Silver-Russell-like patients. *J Med Genet*. 2010;47:816-822.

14 Spengler S, Schönherr N, Binder G, et al. Submicroscopic chromosomal imbalances in idiopathic Silver-Russell syndrome (SRS): the SRS phenotype overlaps with the 12q14 microdeletion syndrome. *J Med Genet*. 2010;47:356-360.

15 Eggermann T, Eggermann K, Schönherr N. Growth retardation versus overgrowth: Silver-Russell syndrome is genetically opposite to Beckwith-Wiedemann syndrome. *Trends Genet*. 2008;24:195-204.

16 Kant SG, Wit JM, Breuning MH. Genetic analysis of short stature. *Horm Res*. 2003;60:157-165.

17 Walenkamp MJE, Wit JM. Genetic disorder in the growth hormone – insulin-like growth factor I axis. *Horm Res*. 2006;66:221-230.

18 Leka SK, Kitsiou-Tzeli S, Kalpini-Mavron A, et al. Familial growth and skeletal features associated with SHOX haploinsufficiency. *J Pediatr Endocrinol Metab*. 2003;16:987-996.

19 Lynch SA, Foulds N, Thuresson AC, et al. The 12q14 microdeletion syndrome: six new cases confirming the role of HMGA2 in growth. *Eur J Hum Genet*. 2011;19:534-539.

20 Moore T, Haig D. Genomic imprinting in mammalian development: a parental tug-of-war. *Trends Genet*. 1991;17:45-49.

21 Eggermann T, Spengler S, Bachmann N, et al. Chromosome 11p15 duplication in Silver-Russell syndrome due to a maternally inherited translocation t(11;15). *Am J Med Genet A*. 2010;152:1484-1487.

22 Bartholdi D, Krajewska-Wolazek M, Dunap K, et al. Epigenetic mutations of the imprinted IGF2-H19 domain in Silver-Russell syndrome (SRS): results from a large cohort of patients with SRS and SRS-like phenotypes. *J Med Genet*. 2009;46:192-197.

23 Kotzot D. Maternal uniparental disomy 7 and Silver-Russell syndrome – clinical update and comparison with other subgroups. *Eur J Med Genet*. 2008;51:444-451.

24 Eggermann T, Leisten I, Binder G, Begemann M, Spengler S. Disturbed methylation at multiple imprinted loci: an increasing observation in imprinting disorders. *Epigenomics*. 2011;3:625-637.

25 Hoischen A, van Bon BW, Gilissen C, et al. De novo mutations of SETBP1 cause Schinzel-Giedion syndrome. *Nat Genet*. 2010;42:483-485.

26 Becker J, Semler O, Gilissen C, et al. Exome sequencing identifies truncating mutations in human SERPINF1 in autosomal-recessive osteogenesis imperfecta. *Am J Hum Genet*. 2011:88:62-371.

27 Roach JC, Glusman G, Smit AF, et al. Analysis of genetic inheritance in a family quartet by whole-genome sequencing. *Science*. 2010:328:636-639.

28 Redon R, Rio M, Gregory SG, et al. Tiling path resolution mapping of constitutional 1p36 deletions by array-CGH: contiguous gene deletion or "deletion with positional effect" syndrome? *J Med Genet*. 2005;42:166-171.

29 van Bon BW, Mefford HC, Menten B, et al. Further delineation of the 15q13 microdeletion and duplication syndromes: a clinical spectrum varying from non-pathogenic to a severe outcome. *J Med Genet*. 2009;46:511-523.

Development of this book was supported by funding from Sandoz

Chapter 11

Fetal programming

Thomas Harder and Andreas Plagemann

Introduction

In recent years, an overwhelming number of epidemiological, clinical, and experimental data have shown that exposures during prenatal and early postnatal life influence the risk of developing chronic diseases during childhood and adulthood (eg, obesity, type 2 diabetes, cardiovascular disease). For these phenomena, the term 'perinatal programming' has been proposed [1]. Although the general concept was introduced in the 1970s by Dörner [2], it did not receive much attention until the formulation of the 'thrifty phenotype' hypothesis in 'small baby syndrome' some 20 years later [3].

Small baby syndrome hypothesis and match-mismatch paradigm

The 'small baby syndrome' hypothesis, as introduced by Hales and Barker, was proposed as a result of studies showing that individuals with low birth weight (LBW) have an increased risk of developing symptoms of metabolic syndrome, type 2 diabetes, and cardiovascular diseases [3]. This 'thrifty phenotype' hypothesis has two premises: 1) LBW is an indicator of maternal and, consequently, fetal undernutrition; and 2) phenotypic characteristics that lead to increased energy storage must be beneficial for the individual. Essentially, Hales and Barker proposed that prenatal undernutrition leads to decreased insulin secretion and,

S. Zabransky (ed.), *Caring for Children Born Small for Gestational Age*, 117
DOI: 10.1007/978-1-908517-90-6_11, © Springer Healthcare 2013

simultaneously, insulin resistance in the fetus which, in turn, slows down weight gain [3]. Moreover, they proposed that this phenotype resulted from active fetal adaptations and is preserved for the lifespan of affected individuals [3]. Later in life, such a phenotype must be 'thrifty' and help affected individuals to cope better with conditions of food shortage. However, under affluent conditions in modern western societies where there are rarely periods of food shortage, this 'advantage' soon becomes a disadvantage and leads to metabolic syndrome, type 2 diabetes, and cardiovascular diseases [3].

Hanson and Gluckman have considerably expanded upon the evolutionary context of this hypothesis and proposed the existence of respective predictive adaptive responses [4], a term that is more often seen in developmental psychology. The authors suggested that the fetus makes reactive adaptations to features of the intrauterine environment (eg, prenatal malnutrition). However, their adaptive value is not realized immediately and only becomes apparent later in life, as the signals that lead to the adaptation are predictions of the conditions of the postnatal lifespan environment. Therefore, if the predictions turn out to be correct, the adaptations will confer a survival advantage; if not, they can lead to a higher risk of metabolic disease. Ultimately, Gluckman and Hanson formulated a generalization of this theoretical framework and suggested the 'mismatch' paradigm theory [5,6]. This concept claims that a mismatch between prenatal conditions and the later-life environment increases the risk of developing diseases, while a 'match' (eg, deprivation in utero followed by nutrient deprivation later in life) prevents disease due to a beneficial adaptation to prospective life conditions [5,6].

A critical appraisal

In the 1990s, a number of concerns were raised about the thrifty phenotype hypothesis [7,8], which was the initial foundation of this theoretical framework. Firstly, a potential role of important confounders and/ or mediators in the observed associations between LBW and risk of later diseases has not been considered adequately in the majority of studies that address 'small baby syndrome'. In particular, most studies performed did not adequately adjust for the potential influence of gestational age (ie, they did not convincingly characterize subjects who were small for gestational age [SGA]).

Similarly, parental body weight and maternal disease during pregnancy were not considered. Furthermore, they did not consider the potential role of neonatal nutrition and general rearing conditions for babies with LBW and the development of disease later in life [9,10] (Figure 11.1).

Neonatal nutrition

In recent years, neonatal overnutrition has increasingly been considered a causal mechanism underlying an increased risk of metabolic and cardiovascular alterations in LBW children [7]. A number of epidemiological and clinical studies speak in favor of the critical role of neonatal overnutrition for the long-term outcome of small babies. For example, Hofman et al showed that children born with LBW (no matter if they were term newborns who were SGA or if they were preterm newborns who were average for gestational age [AGA]) had reduced insulin sensitivity, indicating an increased risk of developing type 2 diabetes [11]. The finding that the risk among AGA children who were born prematurely is similar to the risk among full-term children born SGA argues strongly against diminished prenatal food supply as a causal factor for later outcome [9].

Rather, it has been suggested that increased weight gain in early infancy as a result of neonatal overnutrition might lead to an increased risk of developing metabolic and cardiovascular disturbances later on

Major problems and inconsistencies with the 'small baby syndrome'/ 'thrifty phenotype' hypothesis and respective studies and interpretations

Major problems with the 'small baby syndrome' hypothesis

- Failure to adjust for potential prenatal confounders (eg, gestational age, maternal diseases, parental body mass index)
- Inappropriate adjustment for potential mediators (eg, childhood)
- Body mass index as an adult
- Failure to adjust for potential neonatal confounders (eg, overnutrition/ formula feeding) and increased neonatal weight gain
- Biological plausibility: does undernutrition lead to insulin resistance?

Figure 11.1 Major problems and inconsistencies with the 'small baby syndrome'/'thrifty phenotype' hypothesis and respective studies and interpretations.

[12,13]. Remarkably, this hypothesis has been supported by results from animal models. For example, in a recent study, rats born SGA were found to have a greater risk of developing diabetogenic disturbances (eg, hyperinsulinemia) when exposed to neonatal overnutrition [14]. However, one of the most obvious problems with these hypotheses arises from the fact that obesity is the most important risk factor for developing metabolic syndrome and type 2 diabetes, and maternal obesity has been linked to LBW. Consequently, one would expect that LBW would be an independent risk factor for obesity in later life.

However, this is not the case; a systematic literature review showed that, to date, no study exists in which an inverse association between birth weight and risk of becoming overweight later in life has been found. By contrast, 89% of all published studies found a linear positive relation; that is, the higher the birth weight, the higher the risk of becoming overweight in later life [15] (Figure 11.2).

Moreover, an inverse linear relation between birth weight and risk of type 2 diabetes in later life, which is one of the most important predictions of the 'thrifty phenotype' hypothesis [3], is not observable. By meta-analysis, our group showed that the relation between birth weight and risk of type 2 diabetes is rather 'U-shaped,' with both LBW and high birth weight (HBW) leading to an increased risk of developing type 2 diabetes [9,16,17]. Similar findings apply to type 1 diabetes risk, which is increased after HBW (but not LBW) [18]. An independent relation between LBW and later hypertension is still debatable [19].

A further important concern with regard to the 'small baby syndrome' hypothesis relates to the fact that there is no animal model that convincingly shows that LBW caused by prenatal undernutrition leads to the full spectrum of disorders of metabolic syndrome. To the contrary, Hales and colleagues were unable to find adipogenic or diabetogenic alterations in terms of metabolic syndrome in later life of rats perinatally exposed to maternal undernutrition [20,21]. Even after dietary provocation by a 'cafeteria diet' in adult life, offered to simulate the modern western lifestyle, no increased adipogenic or diabetogenic risk occurred, and even the contrary [20]. Accordingly, in perinatally underfed animals, life expectancy actually increased [22].

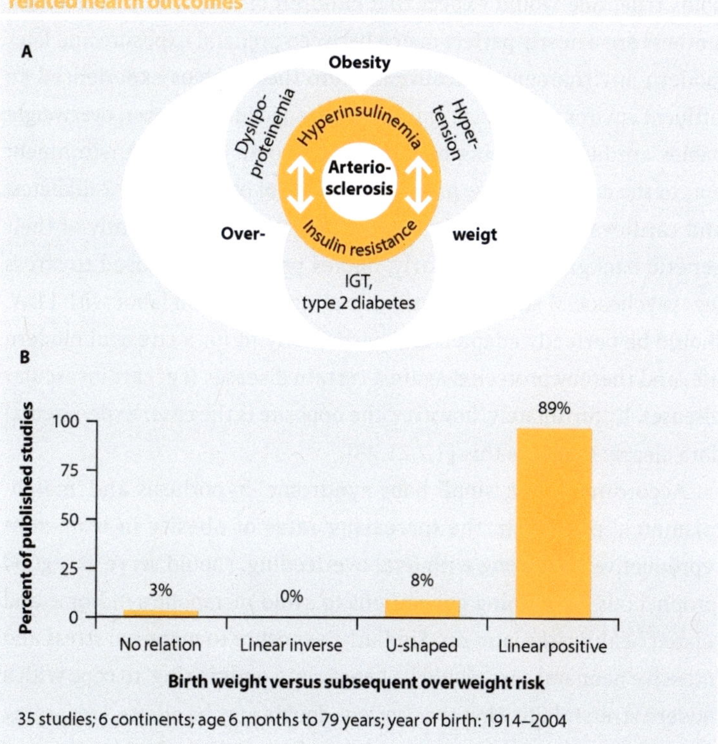

Figure 11.2 A and B Relationship between birth weight and risk of becoming overweight and related health outcomes. A, The main outcome proposed by the 'small baby syndrome'/'thrifty phenotype' hypothesis is the metabolic syndrome, critically characterized by the pathophysiological link between overweight and insulin resistance, leading to metabolic and cardiovascular endpoints. B, A systematic review of respective studies globally shows that high but not low birth weight is strongly related to later overweight. IGT, impaired glucose tolerance.

The 'match-mismatch' paradigm: a general hypothesis?

In a similar manner, the generalization of the aforementioned hypotheses in the form of the mismatch paradigm ultimately leads to inconsistencies within epidemiological, clinical, and experimental data. For example, exposure to maternal diabetes mellitus in utero, which leads to prenatal (glucose) overfeeding and, pathognomonically, accelerated growth and fat deposition, is followed by an increased risk of obesity and diabetes later in life [23–27]. Given that the mismatch paradigm holds true, one would expect that children of diabetic or overweight mothers are a nearly perfect match between prenatal exposure and later modern environments, because in utero these babies experienced an 'affluent environment' that continues later on in life. However, overweight babies are far from being better adapted to an affluent environment but, to the contrary, have an increased risk of obesity, type 2 diabetes, and cardiovascular diseases later in life (even independently of their genetic background). Similarly, babies prenatally exposed to stress (eg, psychosocial stress, infection) leading to preterm labor with LBW, should be perfectly adapted and particularly fit for a stressful modern life, and thereby protected against certain diseases (eg, cardiovascular disease). Unfortunately, however, the opposite is the case. Experimental data clearly supports this [1,7,21,28].

According to the 'small baby syndrome' hypothesis and 'match-mismatch' paradigm, the increasing rates of obesity in women at reproductive age, along with fetal overfeeding, should serve as a good 'prophylaxis' for coming generations to avoid metabolic syndrome and related health risks later on. Similarly, exposure to maternal stress and intensive neonatal care would be beneficial 'conditioning' to cope with a modern stressful life. However, serious doubts may be allowed regarding these scenarios, more so against the background of a large amount of contradictory data [28].

Conclusion

Taken together, there is overwhelming evidence from epidemiological and clinical studies clearly indicating that a phenomenological association exists between LBW and an increased risk of developing chronic diseases, especially in terms of metabolic syndrome. On the other hand, despite its undisputable intellectual attractiveness, neither the 'small baby syndrome' hypotheses, nor the 'mismatch' paradigm appear to be suitable theories to explain these phenomena. In particular, prenatal undernutrition is highly unlikely to be the decisive, causative risk factor responsible for disorders in later life in terms of metabolic syndrome. Therefore, and most importantly, a generalization of these concepts might even have unfavorable consequences for developing respective public health policies.

While the existence and impact of the biomedical phenomenon of perinatal programming is now generally accepted [28], exploration of practical preventive strategies to cope with increased long-term risks in babies born with LBW needs further causally-orientated research. There should be a focus on preventive measures against intrauterine growth restriction (IUGR) and improvement of neonatal rearing conditions in LBW babies to avoid deleterious neonatal programming of affected children [28].

References

1   Plagemann A. 'Fetal programming' and 'functional teratogenesis': on epigenetic mechanisms and prevention of perinatally acquired lasting health risks. *J Perinat Med*. 2004;32:297-305.
2   Dörner G. Perinatal hormone levels and brain organization. In: Stumpf W, Grant LD, eds. *Anatomical neuroendocrinology*. Basel, Switzerland: Karger; 1975:245-252.
3   Hales CN, Barker DJP. Type 2 (non-insulin-dependent) diabetes mellitus: the thrifty phenotype hypothesis. *Diabetologia*. 1992;35:595-601.
4   Gluckman PD, Hanson MA. The conceptual basis for the developmental origins of health and disease. In: Gluckman P, Hanson M, eds. *Developmental origins of health and disease*. Cambridge: Cambridge University Press; 2006:33-50.
5   Gluckman PD, Hanson MA, Cooper C, et al. Effect of in utero and early-life conditions on adult health and disease. *N Engl J Med*. 2008;359:61-73.
6   Gluckman PD, Hanson MA. *Mismatch: the lifestyle diseases timebomb*. Oxford, UK: Oxford University Press; 2008.
7   Dörner G, Plagemann A. Perinatal hyperinsulinism as possible predisposing factor for diabetes mellitus, obesity and enhanced cardiovascular risk in later life. *Horm Metab Res*. 1994;26:213-221.
8   Lucas A, Fewtrell MS, Cole TJ. Fetal origins of adult disease - the hypothesis revisited. *BMJ*. 1999;319:245-249.
9   Plagemann A, Harder T. Premature birth and insulin resistance (letter). *N Engl J Med*. 2005;352:939-940.
10 Plagemann A, Rodekamp E, Harder T. To: Hales CN, Ozanne SE. For debate: fetal and early postnatal growth restriction lead to diabetes, the metabolic syndrome and renal failure (letter). *Diabetologia*. 2004;47:1334-1335.
11 Hofman PL, Regan F, Jackson WE, et al. Premature birth and later insulin resistance. *N Engl J Med*. 2004;351:2179-2186.
12 Crowther NJ, Trusler J, Cameron N, et al. Relation between weight gain and beta-cell secretory activity and non-esterified fatty acid production in 7-year-old African children: results from the Birth to Ten study. *Diabetologia*. 2000;43:978-985.
13 Fewtrell MS, Doherty C, Cole TJ, et al. Effects of size at birth, gestational age and early growth in preterm infants on glucose and insulin concentrations at 9-12 years. *Diabetologia*. 2000;43:714-717.
14 Neitzke U, Harder T, Plagemann A. Intrauterine growth restriction and developmental programming of the metabolic syndrome: a critical appraisal. *Microcirculation*. 2011;18:304-311.
15 Harder T, Schellong K, Stupin J, et al. Where is the evidence that low birth weight leads to obesity? *Lancet*. 2007;369:1859.

16 Harder T, Rodekamp E, Schellong K, et al. Birth weight and subsequent risk of type 2 diabetes: a meta-analysis. *Am J Epidemiol*. 2007;165:849-857.

17 Plagemann A, Harder T. Birth weight and risk of type 2 diabetes. *JAMA*. 2009;301:1540.

18 Harder T, Roepke K, Diller N, et al. Birth weight, early weight gain and subsequent risk of type 1 diabetes: systematic review and meta-analysis. *Am J Epidemiol*. 2009;169:1428-1436.

19 Huxley RR, Neil A, Collins R. Unravelling the fetal origins hypothesis: is there really an inverse association between birth weight and subsequent blood pressure? *Lancet*. 2002;360:659-665.

20 Petry CJ, Ozanne SE, Wang CL, et al. Early protein restriction and obesity independently induce hypertension in 1-year-old rats. *Clin Sci*. 1997;93:147-152.

21 Plagemann A. Fetale programmierung und funktionelle teratologie: ausgewählte mechanismen und konsequenzen. In: Gortner L, Dudenhausen JW, eds. *Vorgeburtliches Wachstum und gesundheitliches*. Frankfurt: Med Verl-Ges Umwelt und Medizin; 2001:65-78.

22 Ozanne SE, Hales CN. Lifespan: catch-up growth and obesity in male mice. *Nature*. 2004;427:411-412.

23 Pettitt DJ, Baird HR, Aleck KA, et al. Excessive obesity in offspring of Pima Indian women with diabetes during pregnancy. *N Engl J Med*. 1983;308:242-245.

24 Silverman BL, Rizzo T, Green OC, et al. Long-term prospective evaluation of offspring of diabetic mothers. *Diabetes*. 1991;40(suppl 2):121-125.

25 Plagemann A, Harder T, Kohlhoff R, et al. Overweight and obesity in infants of mothers with long-term insulin-dependent diabetes or gestational diabetes. *Int J Obes*. 1997;21:451-456.

26 Weiss PAM, Scholz HS, Haas J, et al. Long-term follow-up of infants of mothers with type 1 diabetes: Evidence for hereditary and nonhereditary transmission of diabetes and precursors. *Diabetes Care*. 2000;23:905-911.

27 Dabelea D, Hanson RL, Lindsay RS, et al. Intrauterine exposure to diabetes conveys risks for type 2 diabetes and obesity: a study of discordant sibships. *Diabetes*. 2000;49:2208-2211.

28 Plagemann A. Toward a unifying concept on perinatal programming: vegetative imprinting by environment-dependent biocybernetogenesis. In: Plagemann A, ed. *Perinatal programming - the state of the art*. Berlin: Walter De Gruyter; 2011:243-282.

Development of this book was supported by funding from Sandoz

Long-term consequences

Chapter 12

Premature infants

Martijn JJ Finken

Introduction

Among preterm infants, three maturity levels are distinguished by the World Health Organization (WHO) [1] according to gestational age:

- preterm (<37 weeks);
- very preterm (<32 weeks);
- extremely preterm (<28 weeks).

However, a classification according to birth weight is often adopted in countries where a reliable estimate of gestational age is not always available [1]. Low birth weight (LBW) infants are those with a birth weight under 2500 g, which may be due to prematurity, being born small for gestational age (SGA), or both [1]. Those with a birth weight under 1500 g are labeled very low-birth-weight (VLBW) infants, while those with a birth weight under 1000 g are considered extremely low-birth-weight (ELBW) infants [1]. In general, there is an over-representation of infants born SGA in VLBW and ELBW study populations [2]. Therefore, caution must be exercised in extrapolating findings from study populations to general groups of preterm infants.

In most industrialized countries, there is a rising incidence in the number of preterm births, which is attributed to an older maternal age at first birth and the increased application of assisted reproductive technologies (leading to more twin gestations) [3,4]. Owing to improvements in perinatal management (eg, widespread use of antenatal

S. Zabransky (ed.), *Caring for Children Born Small for Gestational Age*, 127
DOI: 10.1007/978-1-908517-90-6_12, © Springer Healthcare 2013

glucocorticoids and synthetic surfactant), neonatal mortality of very preterm infants has declined from approximately 30% in the early 1980s to an estimated 10% by the mid-1990s [3,4]. The past decade has been characterized by advances in neonatal resuscitation techniques [5], ventilatory strategies [6], and nutrition [7], resulting in a greater number of infants born at the border of viability (23–24 weeks) that go on to survive, although often with chronic conditions and handicaps [8,9]. Therefore, results from studies in older populations of preterm infants cannot be automatically generalized and applied to the current generation of preterm survivors.

Recent evidence suggests that, from mid-childhood onwards, the endocrine-metabolic state of preterm individuals resembles that of subjects born SGA [10,11]. The first evidence for an elevated type 2 diabetes risk in survivors of preterm birth came from a small study which showed that prepubertal children born very preterm had reduced insulin sensitivity during an intravenous glucose tolerance test [10]. Similar findings were subsequently reported in adult populations [11].

Evidence for an association between preterm birth and type 2 diabetes was provided by several population-based studies in middle-aged subjects whose birth data (eg, weight, length, gestational age) were known [12–14]. The risk of diabetes doubled in subjects who were born preterm [12], whereas another study found that the relative risk (RR) for developing type 2 diabetes was 1.67 (95% CI, 1.33–2.11) after very preterm birth [13]. Another study found that preterm birth was associated with type 2 diabetes and with higher glucose and insulin levels during an oral glucose tolerance test [14]. The associations found in these studies were irrespective of the size at birth [10,11,13,14]. In addition, individuals born preterm were found to have higher blood pressure in adolescence/young adulthood [15–20].

Growth

Early growth

After an initial weight loss, birth weight is usually regained somewhere between the end of the first and third week of life, depending on the infant's gestational age, birth weight, morbidity, and nutrition [7,21].

Once birth weight is regained, the growth velocity increases to a level which approaches the intrauterine growth rate. However, the rate of weight gain during hospital stay was shown to be slower in infants with acute illnesses and chronic lung disease [21–23]. Postnatal growth failure has also been associated with shorter gestational age, lower birth weight standard deviation score (SDS), longer duration of respiratory support, and postnatal dexamethasone therapy [23].

A likely explanation for these associations relates to increased energy expenditure. However, the importance of practice decisions in nutritional support should not be overlooked, since it has been suggested that the perceived health status plays a crucial role in these decisions, with healthier infants receiving more nutritional support during the first weeks of life than those who are ill [24]. In comparisons between neonatal intensive care units, differences in the postnatal weight gain were often explained by variations in neonatal nutrition practices [25,26].

Evidence from randomized trials and observational studies has shown that strategies providing early nutritional support increased energy levels, reduced nutritional deficits, and improved neonatal growth and neurodevelopmental outcomes, without increasing the risk of adverse clinical outcomes [7].

Childhood growth

A considerable proportion of very preterm infants have a weight and/or length under –2 standard deviations (SD) from the mean at 40 weeks postmenstrual age [27–29]. As soon as their clinical condition improves, catch-up growth in weight, length, and head circumference is initiated and is often achieved within the first 2 years of life. Continuing catch-up growth throughout childhood and adolescence is not unusual [30–33].

On average, very preterm subjects attain an adult stature that lies 0.5 SD below the population-specific reference mean [31,33–36] (Table 12.1). There is controversy as to whether this reduction could be explained by earlier pubertal development. Earlier menarche, bone-age advancement, and younger age at initiation of the pubertal growth spurt have been reported [33,37,38], while in other studies markers of pubertal timing did not deviate from control populations [31,32,36,39].

In a large study of 1320 VLBW children, height at 6 years of age was best predicted by their length at 1 year of age [40]; parental height, gestational age, and birth weight SDS were found to be less important predictors of childhood growth. Very preterm infants who were born appropriate for gestational age (AGA) with a length and/or weight under –2 SD at the age of 3 months post-term were found to grow in a similar way to children born SGA after a similar pregnancy duration, reaching a final height of approximately 1 SD below the population reference mean (Figure 12.1) [41]. Those with a height under –2 SD at 5 years of age were unlikely to catch up subsequently.

Body composition

Compared to term children, children born very preterm were found to have increased fat mass and abdominal fat deposition at term, in spite of a lower body weight and length [42,43]. Children who had experienced either intrauterine growth restriction (IUGR) or extrauterine growth retardation

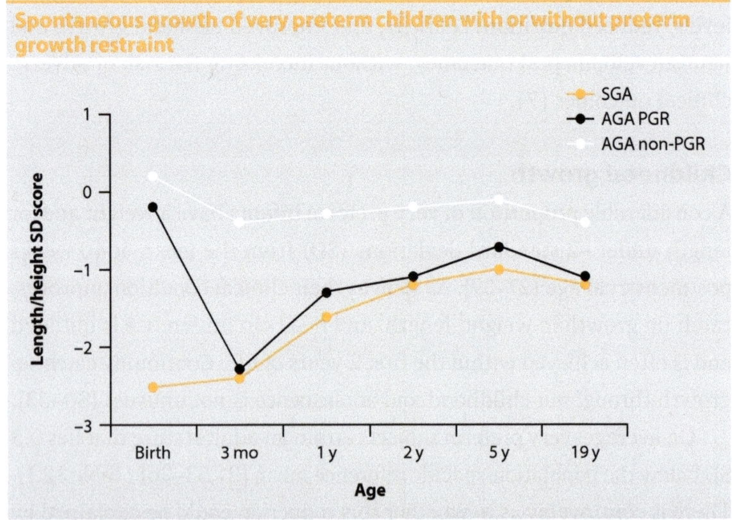

Figure 12.1 Spontaneous growth of very preterm children with or without preterm growth restraint. Growth patterns of 27 children born SGA (birth weight and/or length under –2 SD), 79 children born AGA with PGR (birth weight and length at or above -2 SD followed by a weight and/or length under –2 SD at the age of 3 months post-term), and 274 children born AGA without PGR. AGA, appropriate for gestational age; PGR, preterm growth restraint; SGA, small for gestational age; SD, standard deviation. Adapted from Finken et al [41].

(EUGR) had a lower fat-mass percentage at term than non-growth-retarded infants, but had a greater fat mass accretion in the period thereafter, so that these differences had disappeared by the age of 3 months post-term [44]. At the age of 1 year, the body composition of preterm children was still different from that of infants born at term [45].

Despite these differences in fat mass accretion after birth, preterm infants (especially those born SGA) were found to be lighter and thinner during infancy and childhood [40,46]. From mid-childhood onwards, a gradual increase in weight that exceeded increases in height was demonstrated (Table 12.1) [32,33,35,47]. There is a tendency towards a higher adult body mass index (BMI) with increasing prematurity (Table 12.1). Even with a relatively normal BMI, lower lean mass and centralization of fat distribution have been observed in young adults that were born preterm [11,34].

Growth hormone therapy

In the current SGA indication for growth hormone (GH) therapy, the nature and timing of the growth-restraining insult that has led to the SGA condition are thought to be irrelevant for determining whether or not to commence GH therapy. Regardless of whether the child's growth is retarded at birth, many very preterm infants have a weight and/or length under 2 SD at term age. It has been argued that it is illogical to exclude preterm AGA infants with EUGR from GH therapy if their small size at term evolves to a short stature in childhood [48].

Thus far, a randomized trial aimed at the long-term efficacy and safety of GH therapy in short children who had experienced EUGR after a preterm birth has not been conducted. The short-term response to GH therapy in short children born prematurely has been evaluated by a few observational studies [49–51], which have shown an average height-gain of 0.6–0.9 SD in the first year of treatment [49,50]. It is unclear whether the short-term response to GH therapy is indicative of the long-term growth response.

Assessing size at preterm birth

The use of neonatal anthropometric charts for assessing the preterm newborn's size deserves special attention. Firstly, many charts are based

Growth of very preterm or very low birth weight infants

First author	Population	Year of birth	Sex	n	Length/height (SDS)				Weight (SDS)			
					Infancy	Childhood	Adolescence	Adulthood	Infancy	Childhood	Adolescence	Adulthood
Brandt [36]	ELBW and SGA (1) with catch-up growth	1967-1978	M+F	21	–	–	–	22.8 y: +0.03 (2)	3.5 y: -0.72	5 y: -0.64	–	–
	ELBW and SGA (1) without catch-up growth	1967-1978	M+F	26	–	–	–	22.8 y: -1.89 (2)	3.5 y: -1.12	5 y: -0.98	–	–
Hack [31]	VLBW	1977-1979	M	103	8 mo.: -0.94 20 mo.: -0.55	8 y: -0.45	–	20 y: -0.44	8 mo: -1.70 20 mo.: -1.16	8 y: -0.46	–	20 y: -0.35
			F	92	8 mo.: -0.51 20 mo.: -0.16	8 y: -0.20	–	20 y: -0.26	8 mo. -1.09; 20 mo.: -0.82	8 y: -0.23	–	20 y: +0.26
Ford [32] and Doyle [35]	ELBW	1977-1982	M+F	86	2 y: -0.98	5 y: -0.67 8 y: -0.78	14 y: -0.43	20 y: -0.52 (3)	2 y: -1.27	5 y: -1.01 8 y: -0.89	14 y: -0.14	20 y: +0.14 (3)
	VLBW, not ELBW	1977-1982	M+F	120	2 y: -0.59	5 y: -0.35 8 y: -0.46	14 y: -0.11	–	2 y: -0.45	5 y: -0.43 8 y: -0.43	14 y: +0.10	–

First author	Population	Year of birth	Sex	n	Length/height (SDS)				Weight (SDS)			
					Infancy	Childhood	Adolescence	Adulthood	Infancy	Childhood	Adolescence	Adulthood
Saigal [33]	ELBW	1977–1982	M	65	1 y: -1.59 2 y: -0.92 3 y: -0.72	8 y: -0.84	11-16 y: -0.46	21.5-26.5 y: -0.86	1 y: -2.49 2 y: -1.90 3 y: -1.44	8 y: -1.05	11-16 y: -0.53	21.5-26.5 y: -0.25
			F	82	1 y: -1.04 2 y: -0.77 3 y: -0.58	8 y: -0.94	11-16 y: -0.59	21.5-26.5 y: -0.77	1 y: -1.96 2 y: -1.68 3 y: -1.16	8 y: -1.05	11-16 y: -0.24	21.5-26.5 y: -0.13
Euser [34]	Very preterm	1983	M	187	–	–	–	19 y: -0.55	3 mo.: -0.94 (M+F) 1 y: -0.98 (M+F)	–	–	19 y: -0.41
			F	216	–	–	–	19 y: -0.60	3 mo.: -0.94 (M+F) 1 y: -0.98 (M+F)	–	–	19 y: -0.48

Table 12.1 Growth of very preterm or very low birth weight infants. (1) SGA (small for gestational age) = birth weight <10th percentile; (2) Mean adult height of the entire group:= −1.02 SDS; (3) Data at 20 years of age are provided for only 43 subjects. Only studies that provided a longitudinal follow-up into adulthood are listed in the table. ELBW, extremely low birth weight; F, female; M, male; SDS, standard deviation score; VLBW, very low birth weight; y, year-of-age. Data taken from [31–36].

upon relatively small numbers of extremely preterm infants, which makes them less accurate in the lower range of gestational ages. For instance, the widely adopted Usher and McLean curve is derived from the data of 300 infants, among whom there were 33 born at a gestational age of 28 weeks or less [52].

Furthermore, neonatal anthropometric charts differ from fetal growth charts that are used in obstetrics, the latter being based upon ultrasound measurements obtained during healthy pregnancies continued until term [53]. The exclusion of preterm neonates born after pathological pregnancies does not imply that the reference data rely exclusively on completely healthy pregnancies. Even in the absence of clear pathology, a preterm birth is often preceded by a variable degree of IUGR. In other words, in the preterm range, anthropometric charts tend to underestimate the level of IUGR.

Blood pressure

Hypotension (low blood pressure) is diagnosed in up to 50% of preterm infants during the first days of life. Several definitions have been implemented in clinical practice, including a mean arterial blood pressure (MABP) of less than 30 mmHg, below the infant's gestational age in weeks and in the lower range of distribution (eg, if below the 10th percentile of MABP for birth weight and postnatal age based on normative data) [54].

In extremely preterm infants, myocardial dysfunction is thought to play a role in hypotension in the first hours after birth, during which period the immature myocardium is confronted with an abrupt increase in afterload [55]. Of greater importance is a low systemic vascular resistance, due to either a hemodynamically active shunt or abnormalities in the regulation of the vascular tone (eg, adrenocortical dysfunction).

In very preterm newborns, systemic hypotension was found to be a predictor of intraventricular hemorrhage and periventricular leukomalacia [56,57]. It has also been associated with a poorer neurological outcome [58,59]. However, many studies have failed to confirm these relations and the causality of these statistical associations has therefore been questioned [60]. An alternative explanation for these associations is confounding by factors associated with both systemic hypotension and cerebral injury (eg, asphyxia or respiratory distress syndrome).

Treatment for neonatal hypotension should be based upon the cardiovascular status and not merely on blood pressure [60]. Assessment of the heart rate, peripheral perfusion, urinary output, and other factors that limit oxygen delivery (eg, hypoxemia or anemia) should therefore not be overlooked.

Glucose availability

Because of a continuous transplacental delivery of nutrients, the endocrine milieu of the growing fetus is characterized by constantly high levels of insulin and low levels of glucagon. The situation in postnatal life is characterized by alternating periods of enteral feeding and fasting. During fasting, glucose, gluconeogenic substrates, and alternative fuels are released from energy stores, the development of which is generally confined to the third trimester of pregnancy. In the last month of gestation, there is a rapid increase in hepatic glycogen content, reaching a concentration of approximately 50 mg/g tissue at the time of birth [61].

Hypoglycemia

Hypoxia, asphyxia, hypothermia, and illness are common in preterm infants and these consequently increase the glucose demands in tissues. This, in combination with a lack of energy stores and immature responses to declining glucose concentrations, results in hypoglycemia being almost inevitable in the early postnatal course of preterm infants.

In the first week of life, circulating levels of the gluconeogenic substrates lactate and pyruvate are similar to those of full-term newborns, contrasting with the lower circulating levels of glycerol and alanine [62].

Very preterm newborns in their first week of life can only partly compensate for a sudden decline in the intravenous glucose supply with an increase in their glucose production rate [63]. In ELBW infants receiving total parenteral nutrition, the glucose production rate did not increase at all in response to a reduction in the infusion rate, and consequently the circulating level, of glucose [64]. This could be attributed to a decreased activity of glucose-6-phosphatase [65], the final step in both glycogenolysis and gluconeogenesis. Intravenous administration of glycerol was found to enhance gluconeogenesis [66], especially in conjunction with polyunsaturated free fatty acids [67]. Preterm infants are also compromised in their ability to respond adequately to declining glucose levels with an increase in counter-regulatory hormones such as catecholamines and cortisol [63,68].

Lipolysis and ketogenesis are severely impaired in preterm infants in their first week of life, even at low blood glucose levels [62,63]. The lack of ketone bodies is not explained solely by small fat deposits, as it has been demonstrated in preterm infants that, for a given level of free fatty acids, the hepatic ketone production was two to three times lower than in full-term infants [69].

Hyperglycemia

Glucose disposal is dependent on the action of insulin. It has been observed that hyperglycemic preterm infants require insulin infusion at higher rates to achieve euglycemia, which is indicative of insulin resistance or lack of insulin-sensitive targets such as hepatic glucokinase, adipose tissue, and skeletal muscle [61]. In line with these observations, hepatic glucose production was not switched off during a euglycemic-hyperinsulinemic clamp [70] or glucose infusion at high rates [71,72]. There is some evidence for a partial defect in the processing of proinsulin in very preterm infants, given the high proinsulin/insulin ratio that was observed in those who became hyperglycemic [73]. Lack of insulin action leads to hyperglycemia (and if profound, to osmotic diuresis), and promotes catabolism.

Hyperglycemia is common in VLBW infants, especially in the most immature children [74]. Glucose intake should be kept between 6–12 mcg/kg/min, depending on the clinical condition, with sick infants requiring higher rates than their healthier counterparts. Insulin therapy should be considered when the blood glucose level remains greater than 10 mmol/L after the glucose intake has been optimized, and started at a relatively low rate (eg, 0.025 U/kg/hr). To avoid hypoglycemia, it is recommended to keep the glucose level at the upper range of normal [75,76].

Adrenocortical function

During the third trimester of pregnancy, the adrenal cortex changes substantially. While the fetal zone involutes, the adult zone increases in size [77]. The main product of the fetal zone is dehydroepiandrosterone sulfate (DHEAS), which serves as a precursor for the placental hormone, estriol.

Cortisol is the principal steroid from the adult zone and is necessary for the maintenance of blood pressure and glucose homeostasis. It plays a role in setting the sensitivity of the peripheral tissues to insulin, glucagon, and catecholamines. In preterm newborns, the cortisol level and the cortisol:DHEAS ratio in cord blood increase with gestational age [78,79].

The greatest impairment in adrenocortical function is observed in very preterm newborns at 1 week of age, particularly in those who require mechanical ventilation and/or inotropic support [80–82]. This is followed by a rapid adaptation of the hypothalamus-pituitary-adrenal (HPA) axis by the end of the second week, with the largest improvement in adrenocortical function being observed in ill preterm infants [80,81]. The most important rate-limiting step is probably impaired 11β-hydroxylase activity [83–85].

Antenatal glucocorticoid therapy

A single treatment course of antenatal glucocorticoids to mothers with impending preterm delivery has been shown to improve neonatal survival [86]. This is attributed to a lower incidence of the respiratory distress syndrome and complications related to hemodynamic instability, such as intraventricular hemorrhage and necrotizing enterocolitis.

Repeated treatment courses of antenatal glucocorticoids (mostly given every 7–14 days until weeks 32–34) seem to increase the risk for IUGR [87,88]. Infants exposed to at least four treatment courses were found to have a reduction of 1 SD in birth weight and length [89]. Head circumference was less affected. Rates of neurological impairment among infants aged 18–24 months who had been treated with repeated courses (74% of whom were exposed to three courses or less) did not differ from those treated only once [90]. Long-term follow-up data are not available yet.

Betamethasone and dexamethasone are used for the induction of fetal lung maturation, since these glucocorticoids are able to escape inactivation by placental 11β-hydroxysteroid dehydrogenase type 2 activity.

Betamethasone readily crosses the placenta, resulting in a high cord vein glucocorticoid bioactivity that returns to the reference level within 1 or 2 days following the last steroid dose [91,92].

In preterm newborns, the effects of antenatal glucocorticoids are likely to be more pleiotropic, at least shortly after exposure, than merely reflected in a lower incidence of the respiratory distress syndrome.

In ELBW infants, antenatal betamethasone treatment was associated with a reduced need for blood pressure support during the first 48 hours after birth [93]. Preterm newborns exposed antenatally to betamethasone had an elevation of proinsulin, insulin, and C-peptide levels in cord blood up to 48 hours after the last steroid dose, in spite of a normal glucose concentration, indicative of insulin resistance [94]. There is some preliminary evidence suggesting that betamethasone suppresses aldosterone production [95], an effect that might be mediated through inhibition of P450 side-chain cleavage.

Postnatal glucocorticoid therapy

In two placebo-controlled randomized trials in preterm infants on vasopressor support, hydrocortisone (1 mg/kg every 8 hours for 5 days) or a single dose of dexamethasone (0.25 mg/kg) successfully enabled the discontinuation of inotropics [96,97]. Comparable results were reached in case series of preterm infants with refractory hypotension and/or adrenocortical insufficiency [98–100]. Dosages of hydrocortisone of up to 6 mg/kg per day were used in these studies.

There is less experience with prophylactic glucocorticoid treatment for preterm hypotension. Both a single dose of dexamethasone (0.2 mg/kg) and hydrocortisone for 5 days (2 mg/kg/day on day 1 and day 2 and 0.6 mg/kg/day on days 3–5) seems to be effective [101,102]. A review of postnatal glucocorticoid therapy for respiratory conditions is beyond the scope of this chapter.

Thyroid function

When comparing term and preterm infants, the thyroid function of preterm newborns is characterized by a lower thyroid stimulating hormone (TSH) surge immediately after delivery and a thyroxin (T4) concentration that falls, after a smaller initial increase, over the subsequent 1 to 2 weeks (Figure 12.2). The T4 nadir on day 7 is deeper with increasing prematurity [103,104]. The triiodothyronine (T3) concentration does not decrease in parallel with T4, which is probably the result of an increase in the availability of type 1 deiodinase, as well as the loss of placental type 3 deiodinase activity.

Apparently, the causes of the decrease in T4 observed postnatally in preterm infants are multifactorial and include clearance of maternal T4 from the neonatal circulation, decreased thyroidal iodide stores, an increased vulnerability to the thyroid-suppressive effects of excess iodide, medical treatment (eg, dopamine and glucocorticoids), and differences in the availability of thyroid-binding globulin (TBG) [105]. TBG is produced in the liver and its plasma concentration increases with maturity levels and decreases during critical illnesses, thereby influencing the total T4 concentration [103]. The free T4 concentration usually remains constant in spite of fluctuations in the concentrations of TBG and total T4.

Despite a low serum T4, the TSH level usually remains within the normal range. Elevated TSH levels may be seen in the recovery phase of critically ill children, or early in the course of healthy infants in the extremely preterm range [103,106]. In the latter group, this could reflect insensitivity to TSH associated with maturity-related differences in its glycosylation [107].

Lower levels of T4 and T3 throughout the neonatal phase have been associated with increased mortality and short- and long-term morbidity, including the respiratory distress syndrome, intraventricular hemorrhage, and neuromotor and cognitive deficits [108–111]. Several trials have studied the effects of thyroid hormone supplementation in preterm infants [112]. Different treatment protocols have been used in these trials, including T4 or T3 alone, and T4 and T3 combined, as continuous or bolus injections. Overall, no effect on mortality or respiratory outcomes was observed. A trend towards a lower occurrence of patent ductus arteriosus was observed. Only one trial in infants born before 30 weeks gestation has focused on neurodevelopmental outcomes up to 10 years of age, which were improved in the most premature ones but worse in those of 29 weeks gestation [113–115].

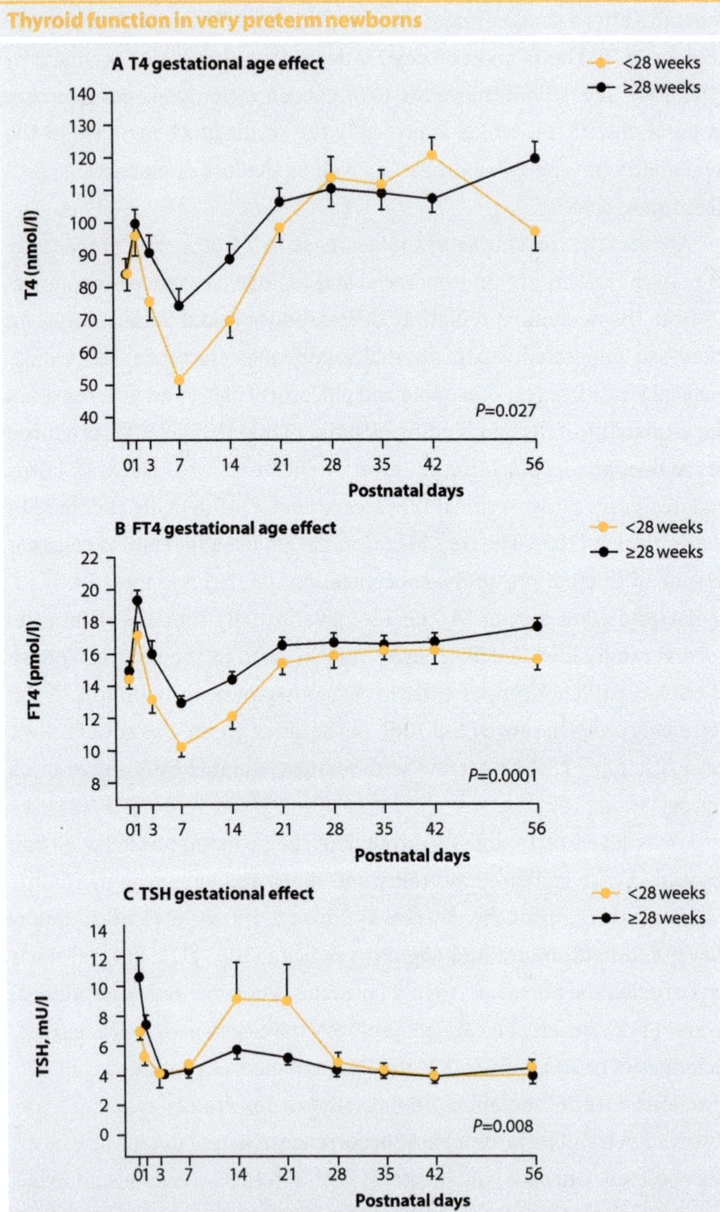

Figure 12.2 A-C Thyroid function in very preterm newborns. Thyroid function during the first 8 weeks after birth: effects of gestational age on T4 (Figure 12.2A), FT4 (Figure 12.2B), and TSH (Figure 12.2C). Adapted from Van Wassenaer et al [103].

The optimal treatment protocol remains to be defined. There are some pharmacokinetic arguments, related to TSH depression and immature tissue metabolism by deiodinases, that recommend continuous supplementation with T4 and T3, or T4 alone, rather than bolus injections or treatment with T3 alone [116–118]. Given all these uncertainties, routine treatment with thyroid hormone is not recommended in preterm infants.

Bone metabolism

Very preterm newborns carry a risk of developing metabolic bone disease with undermineralized bones, as bone mineralization, along with calcium and phosphorus accretion, mainly occurs during the third trimester of pregnancy. Although frank radiological rickets with fractures has been described, the condition is often asymptomatic and is generally detected biochemically (eg, by an elevation of serum alkaline phosphatase).

After infancy, most preterm individuals show an improvement in bone mineralization, so that their bone mass in childhood is in proportion to their body size. Some have suggested that the adverse effects of neonatal dexamethasone therapy on the bone-mass accrual in infancy [119,120] are still present in childhood [121].

Several studies have shown that once adulthood is reached, the bone mineral density (BMD) is no different to that of non-preterm individuals [122–124]. Only one study has found a decreased BMD in young adulthood [125], with the subjects in the study born at a lower gestational age (mean=29.3 weeks) than those included in the other studies. It is possible that BMD cannot be fully restored in the most immature subjects.

Long-term endocrine sequelae

It can be assumed that very preterm infants with enhanced cardiovascular responses and who mobilize their fuels more efficiently are offered short-term benefits. Traits associated with blood pressure regulation and glucose availability that predispose to later hypertension and type 2 diabetes possibly contribute to these benefits.

There is some evidence for a permanent activation of the HPA axis in survivors of very preterm births [126,127]. Whether this is a reflection of selective survival of particular sets of genotypes is hard to prove. Survivors aged 19 years old who had been treated with glucocorticoids as neonates were found to have altered allele frequencies of glucocorticoid receptor (GR) polymorphisms [128], which suggests that genotype selection by life-threatening conditions is possible.

An alternative explanation for the enhanced stress responsiveness is an environmentally-driven hypermethylation at the GR gene promoter in the brain, leading to decreased central feedback suppression. This has been demonstrated in the offspring of low-grooming rat mothers [129] and in humans who were abused as children and later committed suicide [130]. Whether this also occurs in the preterm newborn is unknown.

There is no compelling evidence for long-lasting metabolic side effects in subjects born to mothers who had been treated with a single treatment course of betamethasone [131–134]. The long-term effects of multiple courses of antenatal glucocorticoids remain to be explored.

From epidemiological data, it has been speculated that accelerated fat mass accretion in infancy and childhood, which is commonly observed after a period with suboptimal neonatal nutrition and EUGR, produces alterations in metabolic set points predisposing to insulin resistance and raised blood pressure [44,135,136]. The impact of recent improvements in early feeding upon adult metabolic health outcomes has yet to be determined.

References

1   World Health Organization. *International Statistical Classification of Diseases and Related Health Problems. 10th revision.* http://apps.who.int/classifications/icd10. Accessed February 20, 2013.

2   Euser AM, de Wit CC, Finken MJ, Rijken M, Wit JM. Growth of preterm born children. *Horm Res.* 2008;70:319-328.

3   Stoelhorst GMSJ, Rijken M, Martens SE, et al; on behalf of the Leiden Follow-up Project on Prematurity. Changes in neonatology: comparison of two cohorts of very preterm infants (gestational age <32 weeks): the Project on Preterm and Small For Gestational Age Infants 1983 and the Leiden Follow-up Project on Prematurity 1996-1997. *Pediatrics.* 2005;115:396-405.

4   Alexander GR, Kogan M, Bader D, Carlo W, Allen M, Mor J. US birth weight/gestational age-specific neonatal mortality: 1995-1997 rates for whites, Hispanics, and blacks. *Pediatrics.* 2003;111:e61-e66.

5   Schmölzer GM, Te Pas AB, Davis PG, Morley CJ. Reducing lung injury during neonatal resuscitation of preterm infants. *J Pediatr.* 2008;153:741-745.

6   Ramanathan R, Sardesai S. Lung protective ventilatory strategies in very low birth weight infants. *J Perinatol.* 2008;28(suppl 1):S41-S46.

7   Ehrenkranz RA. Early nutritional support and outcomes in ELBW infants. *Early Hum Dev.* 2010;86:S21-S25.

8   Larroque B, Bréart G, Kaminski M, et al; on behalf of the Epipage study group. Survival of very preterm infants: Epipage, a population based cohort study. *Arch Dis Child Fetal Neonatal Ed.* 2004;89:F139-F144.

9   Costeloe K, Draper E, Myles J, Hennessy E. EPICure 2: survival and early morbidity of extremely preterm babies in England: changes since 1995. *Arch Dis Child.* 2008;93:A33-A34.

10   Hofman PL, Regan F, Jackson WE, et al. Premature birth and later insulin resistance. *N Engl J Med.* 2004;351:2189-2186.

11   Hovi P, Andersson S, Eriksson JG, et al. Glucose regulation in young adults with very low birth weight. *N Engl J Med.* 2007;2053-2063.

12   Lawlor DA, Davey Smith G, Clark H, Leon DA. The associations of birthweight, gestational age and childhood BMI with type 2 diabetes: findings from the Aberdeen children of the 1950s cohort. *Diabetologia.* 2006;49:2614-2617.

13   Kaijser M, Bonamy AK, Akre O, et al. Perinatal risk factors for diabetes in later life. *Diabetes.* 2009;58:523-526.

14   Pilgaard K, Færch K, Carstensen B, et al. Low birth weight and premature birth are both associated with type 2 diabetes in a random sample of middle-aged Danes. *Diabetologia.* 2010;53:2526-2530.

15   Doyle LW, Faber B, Callanan C, Morley R. Blood pressure in late adolescence and very low birth weight. *Pediatrics.* 2003;111:252-257.

16   Kistner A, Celsi G, Vanpee M, Jacobson SH. Increased blood pressure but normal renal function in adult women born preterm. *Pediatr Nephrol.* 2000;15:215-220.

17   Leon DA, Johansson M, Rasmussen F. Gestational age and growth rate of fetal mass are inversely associated with systolic blood pressure in young adults: an epidemiologic study of 165,136 Swedish men aged 18 years. *Am J Epidemiol.* 2000;152:597-604.

18   Siewert-Delle A, Ljungman S. The impact of birth weight and gestational age on blood pressure in adult life: a population-based study of 49-year-old men. *Am J Hypertens.* 1998;11:946-953.

19   Hack M, Schluchter M, Cartar L, Rahman M. Blood pressure among very low birth weight (<1.5 kg) young adults. *Pediatr Res.* 2005;58:677-684.

20   Keijzer-Veen MG, Finken MJ, Nauta J, et al; for the Dutch POPS-19 Collaborative Study Group. Is blood pressure increased 19 years after intrauterine growth restriction and preterm birth? A prospective follow-up study in The Netherlands. *Pediatrics.* 2005;116:725-731.

21   Ehrenkranz RA, Younes N, Lemons JA, et al. Longitudinal growth of hospitalized very low birth weight infants. *Pediatrics.* 1999;104:280-289.

22   Berry MA, Abrahamowicz M, Usher RH. Factors associated with growth of extremely premature infants during initial hospitalization. *Pediatrics.* 1997;100:640-646.

23   Marks KA, Reichman B, Lusky A, Zmora E; Israel Neonatal Network. Fetal growth and postnatal growth failure in very-low-birthweight infants. *Acta Paediatr.* 2006;95:236-242.

24   Ehrenkranz RA, Das A, Wrage LA, et al; for the Eunice Kennedy Shriver National Institute of Child Health and Human Development neonatal research network. Early nutrition mediates the influence of severity of illness on extremely LBW infants. *Pediatr Res.* 2011;69:522-529.

25   Olsen IE, Richardson DK, Schmid CH, Ausman LM, Dwyer JT. Intersite differences in weight growth velocity of extremely premature infants. *Pediatrics.* 2002;110:1125-1132.

26   Blackwell MT, Eichenwald EC, McAlmon K, et al. Interneonatal intensive care unit variation in growth rates and feeding practices in healthy moderately premature infants. *J Perinatol.* 2005;25:478-485.

27   Niklasson A, Engstrom E, Hard AL, Wikland KA, Hellstrom A. Growth in very preterm children: a longitudinal study. *Pediatr Res.* 2003;54:899-905.

28   Wood NS, Costeloe K, Gibson AT, Hennessy EM, Marlow N, Wilkinson AR. The EPICure study: growth and associated problems in children born at 25 weeks of gestational age or less. *Arch Dis Child Fetal Neonatal Ed.* 2003;88:F492-F500.

29 Bertino E, Coscia A, Mombrò M, et al. Postnatal weight increase and growth velocity of very low birthweight infants. *Arch Dis Child Fetal Neonatal Ed.* 2006;91:F349-F356.

30 Knops NB, Sneeuw KC, Brand R, et al. Catch-up growth up to ten years of age in children born very preterm or with very low birth weight. *BMC Pediatr.* 2005;5:26.

31 Hack M, Schluchter M, Cartar L, Rahman M, Cuttler L, Borawski E. Growth of very low birth weight infants to age 20 years. *Pediatrics.* 2003;112:e30-e38.

32 Ford GW, Doyle LW, Davis NM, Callanan C. Very low birth weight and growth into adolescence. *Arch Pediatr Adolesc Med.* 2000;154:778-784.

33 Saigal S, Stoskopf B, Streiner D, Paneth N, Pinelli J, Boyle M. Growth trajectories of extremely low birth weight infants from birth to young adulthood: a longitudinal, population-based study. *Pediatr Res.* 2006;60:751-758.

34 Euser AM, Finken MJ, Keijzer-Veen MG, et al; for the Dutch POPS-19 Collaborative Study Group. Associations between prenatal and infancy weight gain and BMI, fat mass, and fat distribution in young adulthood: a prospective cohort study in males and females born very preterm. *Am J Clin Nutr.* 2005;81:480-487.

35 Doyle LW, Faber B, Callanan C, Ford GW, Davis NM. Extremely low birth weight and body size in early adulthood. *Arch Dis Child.* 2004;89:347-350.

36 Brandt I, Sticker EJ, Gausche R, Lentze MJ. Catch-up growth of supine length/height of very low birth weight, small for gestational age preterm infants to adulthood. *J Pediatr.* 2005;147:662-668.

37 Peralta-Carcelen M, Jackson DS, Goran MI, Royal SA, Mayo MS, Nelson KG. Growth of adolescents who were born at extremely low birth weight without major disability. *J Pediatr.* 2000;136:633-640.

38 Wehkalampi K, Hovi P, Dunkel L, et al. Advanced pubertal growth spurt in subjects born preterm: the Helsinki study of very low birth weight adults. *J Clin Endocrinol Metab.* 2011;96:525-533.

39 Powls A, Botting N, Cooke RW, Pilling D, Marlow N. Growth impairment in very low birthweight children at 12 years: correlation with perinatal and outcome variables. *Arch Dis Child Fetal Neonatal Ed.* 1996;75:F152-F157.

40 Trebar B, Traunecker R, Selbmann HK, Ranke MB. Growth during the first two years predicts pre-school height in children born with very low birth weight (VLBW): results of a study of 1,320 children in Germany. *Pediatr Res.* 2007;62:209-214.

41 Finken MJJ, Dekker FW, de Zegher F, Wit JM; for the Dutch Project on Preterm and Small-for-Gestational-Age-19 Collaborative Study Group. Long-term height gain of prematurely born children with neonatal growth restraint: parallellism with the growth pattern of short children born small for gestational age. *Pediatrics.* 2006;118:640-643.

42 Atkinson SA, Randall-Simpson J. Factors influencing body composition of premature infants at term-adjusted age. *Ann N Y Acad Sci.* 2000;904:393-399.

43 Roggero P, Giannì ML, Amato O, et al. Is term newborn body composition being achieved postnatally in preterm infants? *Early Hum Dev.* 2009;85:349-352.

44 Roggero P, Giannì ML, Liotto N, et al. Rapid recovery of fat mass in small for gestational age preterm infants after term. *PLoS One.* 2011;6:e14489.

45 Cooke RJ, Rawlings DJ, McCormick K, et al. Body composition of preterm infants during infancy. *Arch Dis Child Fetal Neonatal Ed.* 1999;80:F188-F191.

46 Bracewell MA, Hennessy EM, Wolke D, Marlow N. The EPICure study: growth and blood pressure at 6 years of age following extremely preterm birth. *Arch Dis Child Fetal Neonatal Ed.* 2007;93:F108-F114.

47 Farooqi A, Hägglöf B, Sedin G, Gothefors L, Serenius F. Growth in 10- to 12-year-old children born at 23 to 25 weeks' gestation in the 1990s: a Swedish national prospective follow-up study. *Pediatrics.* 2006;118:e1452-e1465.

48 Wit JM, Finken MJJ, Rijken M, de Zegher F. Preterm growth restraint: a paradigm that unifies intrauterine growth retardation and preterm extrauterine growth retardation and has implications for the small-for-gestational-age indication in growth hormone therapy. *Pediatrics.* 2006;117:e793-e795.

49   Boguszewski MCS, Karlsson H, Wollmann HA, Wilton P, Dahlgren J. Growth hormone treatment in short children born prematurely—data from KIGS. *J Clin Endocrinol Metab*. 2011;96:1687-1694.

50   Ranke MB, Martin DD, Ehehalt S, et al. Short children with low birth weight born either small for gestational age or average for gestational age show similar growth response and changes in insulin-like growth factor-1 to growth hormone treatment during the first prepubertal year. *Horm Res Paediatr*. 2011;76:104-112.

51   De Kort SWK, Willemsen RH, Van der Kaay DCM, Duivenvoorden HJ, Hokken-Koelega ACS. Does preterm birth influence the response to growth hormone treatment in short, small for gestational age children? *Clin Endocrinol (Oxf)*. 2009;70:582-587.

52   Usher R, McLean F. Intrauterine growth of live-born Caucasian infants at sea level: standards obtained from measurements in 7 dimensions of infants born between 25 and 44 weeks of gestation. *J Pediatr*. 1969;74:901-910.

53   Gardosi J, Chang A, Kalyan B, Sahota D, Symonds EM. Customised antenatal growth charts. *Lancet*.1992;339:283-287.

54   Cunningham S, Symon AG, Elton RA, Zhu C, McIntosh N. Intra-arterial blood pressure reference ranges, death and morbidity in very low birthweight infants during the first seven days of life. *Early Hum Dev*. 1999;56:151-165.

55   Gill AB, Weindling AM. Echocardiographic assessment of cardiac function in shocked very low birthweight infants. *Arch Dis Child*. 1993;68:17-21.

56   Miall-Allen VM, De Vries LS, Whitelaw AG. Mean arterial blood pressure and neonatal cerebral lesions. *Arch Dis Child*. 1987;62:1068-1069.

57   Børch K, Lou HC, Greisen G. Cerebral white matter blood flow and arterial blood pressure in preterm infants. *Acta Paediatr*. 2010;99:1489-1492.

58   Martens SE, Rijken M, Stoelhorst GMSJ, et al; on behalf of the Leiden Follow-up Project on Prematurity, The Netherlands. Is hypotension a major risk factor for neurological morbidity at term age in very preterm infants? *Early Hum Dev*. 2003;75:79-89.

59   Low JA, Froese AB, Galbraith RS, Smith JT, Sauerbrei EE, Derrick EJ. The association between preterm newborn hypotension and hypoxemia and outcome during the first year. *Acta Paediatr*. 1993;82:433-437.

60   Subhedar NV. Treatment of hypotension in newborns. *Semin Neonatol*. 2003;8:413-423.

61   Mitanchez D. Glucose regulation in preterm newborn infants. *Horm Res*. 2007;68:265-271.

62   Hawdon JM, Ward Platt MP, Aynsley-Green A. Patterns of metabolic adaptation for preterm and term infants in the first neonatal week. *Arch Dis Child*. 1992;67:357-365.

63   Van Kempen AAMW, Romijn JA, Ruiter AFC, et al. Adaptation of glucose production and gluconeogenesis to diminishing glucose infusion in preterm infants at varying gestational ages. *Pediatr Res*. 2003;53:628-634.

64   Chacko SK, Ordonez J, Sauer PJ, Sunehag AL. Gluconeogenesis is not regulated by either glucose or insulin in extremely low birth weight infants receiving total parenteral nutrition. *J Pediatr*. 2011;158:891-896.

65   Hume R, Burchell A. Abnormal expression of glucose-6-phosphatase in preterm infants. *Arch Dis Child*. 1993;68:202-204.

66   Sunehag AL. Parenteral glycerol enhances gluconeogenesis in very premature infants. *Pediatr Res*. 2003;53:635-641.

67   Van Kempen AAMW, van der Crabben SN, Ackermans MT, Endert E, Kok JH, Sauerwein HP. Stimulation of gluconeogenesis by intravenous lipids in preterm infants: response depends on fatty acid profile. *Am J Physiol Endocrinol Metab*. 2006;290:E723-E730.

68   Ng PC. Is there a "normal" range of serum cortisol concentration in preterm infants? *Pediatrics*. 2008;122:873-875.

69   De Boissieu D, Rocchiccioli F, Kalach N, Bougneres PF. Ketone body turnover at term and in preterm newborns in the first 2 weeks after birth. *Biol Neonate*. 1995;67:84-93.

70   Farrag HM, Nawrath LM, Healey JE, et al. Persistent glucose production and greater peripheral sensitivity to insulin in the neonate vs. the adult. *Am J Physiol*. 1997;272:E86-E93.

71   Cowett RM, Oh W, Schwartz R. Persistent glucose production during glucose infusion in the neonate. *J Clin Invest*. 1983;71:467-475.

72   Sunehag A, Gustafsson J, Ewald U. Very immature infants (≤30 wk) respond to glucose infusion with incomplete suppression of glucose production. *Pediatr Res*. 1994;36:550-555.

73   Mitanchez-Mokhtari D, Lahlou N, Kieffer F, Magny JF, Roger M, Voyer M. Both relative insulin resistance and defective islet beta-cell processing of proinsulin are responsible for transient hyperglycemia in extremely preterm infants. *Pediatrics*. 2004;113:537-541.

74   Beardsall K, Vanhaesebrouck S, Ogilvy-Stuart AL, et al. Prevalence and determinants of hyperglycemia in very low birth weight infants: cohort analyses of the NIRTURE study. *J Pediatr*. 2010;157:715-719.

75   Beardsall K, Vanhaesebrouck S, Ogilvy-Stuart AL, et al. Early insulin therapy in very-low-birth-weight infants. *N Engl J Med*. 2008;359:1873-1884.

76   Ogilvy-Stuart AL, Beardsall K. Management of hyperglycaemia in the preterm infant. *Arch Dis Child Fetal Neonatal Ed*. 2010;95:F126-F131.

77   Mesiano S, Jaffe RB. Developmental and functional biology of the primate fetal adrenal cortex. *Endocr Rev*. 1997;18:378-403.

78   Scott SM, Watterberg KL. Effect of gestational age, postnatal age, and illness on plasma cortisol concentrations in premature infants. *Pediatr Res*. 1995;37:112-116.

79   Kari MA, Raivio KO, Stenman UH, Voutilainen R. Serum cortisol, dehydroepiandrosterone sulfate, and steroid-binding globulins in preterm neonates: effect of gestational age and dexamethasone therapy. *Pediatr Res*. 1996;40:319-324.

80   Ng PC, Lam CW, Lee CH, et al. Reference ranges and factors affecting the human corticotropin-releasing hormone test in preterm, very low birth weight infants. *J Clin Endocrinol Metab*. 2002;87:4621-4628.

81   Ng PC, Lee CH, Lam CW, et al. Transient adrenocortical insufficiency of prematurity and systemic hypotension in very low birthweight infants. *Arch Dis Child Fetal Neonatal Ed*. 2004;89:F119-F126.

82   Huysman MWA, Hokken-Koelega ACS, de Ridder MAJ, Sauer PJJ. Adrenal function in sick very preterm infants. *Pediatr Res*. 2000;48:629-633.

83   Hingre RV, Gross SJ, Hingre KS, Mayes DM, Richman RA. Adrenal steroidogenesis in very low birth weight preterm infants. *J Clin Endocrinol Metab*. 1994;78:266-270.

84   Korte C, Styne D, Merritt TA, Mayes D, Wertz A, Helbock HJ. Adrenocortical function in the very low birth weight infant: improved testing sensitivity and association with neonatal outcome. *J Pediatr*. 1996;128:257-263.

85   Bolt RJ, van Weissenbruch MM, Popp-Snijders C, Sweep FGJ, Lafeber HN, Delemarre-van der Waal HA. Maturity of the adrenal cortex in very preterm infants is related to gestational age. *Pediatr Res*. 2002;52:405-410.

86   Roberts D, Dalziel S. Antenatal corticosteroids for accelerating fetal lung maturation for women at risk of preterm birth. *Cochrane Database Syst Rev*. 2006;3:CD004454.

87   Crowther CA, Haslam RR, Hiller JE, et al; for the Australasian Collaborative Trial of Repeat Doses of Steroids (ACTORDS) Study Group. Neonatal respiratory distress syndrome after repeat exposure to antenatal corticosteroids: a randomised controlled trial. *Lancet*. 2006;367:1913-1919.

88   Murphy KE, Hannah ME, Willan AR, et al; for the MACS Collaborative Group. Multiple courses of antenatal corticosteroids for preterm birth (MACS): a randomised controlled trial. *Lancet*. 2008;372:2143-2151.

89   Norberg H, Stålnacke J, Heijtz RD, et al. Antenatal corticosteroids for preterm birth: dose-dependent reduction in birthweight, length and head circumference. *Acta Paediatr*. 2011;100:364-369.

90   Asztalos EV, Murphy KE, Hannah ME, et al; for the Multiple Courses of Antenatal Corticosteroids for Preterm Birth Study Collaborative Group. Multiple courses of antenatal corticosteroids for preterm birth study: 2-year outcomes. *Pediatrics*. 2010;126:e1045-e1055.

91 Kajantie E, Raivio T, Jänne OA, Hovi P, Dunkel L, Andersson S. Circulating glucocorticoid bioactivity in the preterm newborn after antenatal betamethasone treatment. *J Clin Endocrinol Metab.* 2004;89:3999-4003.

92 Nykänen P, Raivio T, Heinonen K, Jänne OA, Voutilainen R. Circulating glucocorticoid bioactivity and serum cortisol concentrations in premature infants: the influence of exogenous glucocorticoids and clinical factors. *Eur J Endocrinol.* 2007;156:577-583.

93 Moïse AA, Wearden ME, Kozinetz CA, Gest AL, Welty SE, Hansen TN. Antenatal steroids are associated with less need for blood pressure support in extremely premature infants. *Pediatrics.* 1995;95:845-850.

94 Verhaeghe J, van Bree R, van Herck E, Coopmans W. Exogenous corticosteroids and *in utero* oxygenation modulate indices of fetal insulin secretion. *J Clin Endocrinol Metab.* 2005;90:3449-3453.

95 Kessel JM, Cale JM, Verbrick E, Parker CR Jr, Carlton DP, Bird IM. Antenatal betamethasone depresses maternal and fetal aldosterone levels. *Reprod Sci.* 2009;16:94-104.

96 Gaissmaier RE, Pohlandt F. Single-dose dexamethasone treatment of hypotension in preterm infants. *J Pediatr.* 1999;134:701-705.

97 Ng PC, Lee CH, Bnur FL, et al. A double-blind, randomized, controlled study of a "stress dose" of hydrocortisone for rescue treatment of refractory hypotension in preterm infants. *Pediatrics.* 2006;117:367-375.

98 Helbock HJ, Insoft RM, Conte FA. Glucocorticoid-responsive hypotension in extremely low birth weight newborns. *Pediatrics.* 1993;92:715-717.

99 Ng PC, Lam CW, Fok TF, et al. Refractory hypotension in preterm infants with adrenocortical insufficiency. *Arch Dis Child Fetal Neonatal Ed.* 2001;84:F122-F124.

100 Seri I, Tan R, Evans J. Cardiovascular effects of hydrocortisone in preterm infants with pressor-resistant hypotension. *Pediatrics.* 2001;107:1070-1074.

101 Kopelman AE, Moise AA, Holbert D, Hegemier SE. A single very early dexamethasone dose improves respiratory and cardiovascular adaptation in preterm infants. *J Pediatr.* 1999;135:345-350.

102 Efird MM, Heerens AT, Gordon PV, Bose CL, Young DA. A randomized-controlled trial of prophylactic hydrocortisone supplementation for the prevention of hypotension in extremely low birth weight infants. *J Perinatol.* 2005;25:119-124.

103 van Wassenaer AG, Kok JH, Dekker FW, de Vijlder JJM. Thyroid function in very preterm infants: effects of gestational age and disease. *Pediatr Res.* 1997;42:604-609.

104 Mercado M, Yu VY, Francis I, Szymonowicz W, Gold H. Thyroid function in very preterm infants. *Early Hum Dev.* 1988;16:131-141.

105 Brown RS. The thyroid. In: Brook C, Clayton P, Brown RS, eds. *Brook's Clinical Pediatric Endocrinology.* 6th ed. Chichester, UK: Wiley-Blackwell; 2009:250-282.

106 Frank JE, Faix JE, Hermos RJ, et al. Thyroid function in very low birth weight infants: effects on neonatal hypothyroidism screening. *J Pediatr.* 1996;128:548-554.

107 Gyves PW, Gesundheit N, Stannard BS, DeCherney GS, Weintraub BD. Alterations in the glycosylation of thyrotropin during ontogenesis. Analysis of sialylated and sulfated oligosaccharides. *J Biol Chem.* 1989;264:6104-6110.

108 Abassi V, Merchant K, Abramson D. Postnatal triiodothyronine concentrations in healthy preterm infants and infants with respiratory distress syndrome. *Pediatr Res.* 1977;11:802-804.

109 Paul DA, Leef KH, Stefano JL, Bartoshesky L. Low serum thyroxine on initial newborn screening is associated with intraventricular hemorrhage and death in very low birth weight infants. *Pediatrics.* 1998;101:903-907.

110 Lucas A, Morley R, Fewtrell MS. Low triiodothyronine concentration in preterm infants and subsequent intelligence quotient (IQ) at 8 year follow up. *BMJ.* 1996;312:1133-1134.

111 Den Ouden AL, Kok JH, Verkerk PH, Brand R, Verloove-Vanhorick SP. The relation between neonatal thyroxine levels and neurodevelopmental outcome at age 5 and 9 years in a national cohort of very preterm and/or very low birth weight infants. *Pediatr Res.* 1996;39:142-145.

112 van Wassenaer AG, Kok JH. Trials with thyroid hormone in preterm infants: clinical and neurodevelopmental effects. *Semin Perinatol.* 2008;32:423-430.

113 van Wassenaer AG, Kok JH, de Vijlder JJM, et al. Effects of thyroxine supplementation on neurologic development in infants born at less than 30 weeks' gestation. *N Engl J Med.* 1997;336:21-26.

114 Briët JM, van Wassenaer AG, Dekker FW, de Vijlder JJM, van Baar A, Kok JH. Neonatal thyroxine supplementation in very preterm children: developmental outcome evaluated at early school age. *Pediatrics.* 2001;107:712-718.

115 van Wassenaer AG, Westera J, Houtzager BA, Kok JH. Ten-years follow up of children born at <30 weeks' gestational age supplemented with thyroxine in the neonatal period in a randomized controlled trial. *Pediatrics.* 2005;116:e613-e618.

116 van Wassenaer AG, Kok JH, Dekker FW, Endert E, de Vijlder JJ. Thyroxine administration to infants of less than 30 weeks gestational age decreases plasma tri-iodothyronine concentrations. *Eur J Endocrinol.* 1998;139:508-515.

117 Valerio PG, van Wassenaer AG, de Vijlder JJ. A randomized, masked study of triiodothyronine plus thyroxine administration in preterm infants less than 28 weeks of gestational age: hormonal and clinical effects. *Pediatr Res.* 2004;55:248-253.

118 La Gamma EF, van Wassenaer AG, Ares S, et al. Phase 1 trial of 4 thyroid hormone regimens for transient hypothyroxinemia in neonates of <28 weeks' gestation. *Pediatrics.* 2009;124:e258-e268.

119 Shrivastava A, Lyon A, McIntosh N. The effect of dexamethasone on growth, mineral balance and bone mineralisation in preterm infants with chronic lung disease. *Eur J Pediatr.* 2000;159:380-384.

120 Ng PC, Lam CW, Wong GW, et al. Changes in markers of bone metabolism during dexamethasone treatment for chronic lung disease in preterm infants. *Arch Dis Child Fetal Neonatal Ed.* 2002;86:F49-F54.

121 Eelloo JA, Roberts SA, Emmerson AJ, Ward KA, Adams JE, Mughal MZ. Bone status of children aged 5-8 years, treated with dexamethasone for chronic lung disease of prematurity. *Arch Dis Child Fetal Neonatal Ed.* 2008;93:F222-F224.

122 Weiler HA, Yuen CK, Seshia MM. Growth and bone mineralization of young adults weighing less than 1500 g at birth. *Early Hum Dev.* 2002;67:101-112.

123 Dalziel SR, Fenwick S, Cundy T, et al. Peak bone mass after exposure to antenatal betamethasone and prematurity: follow-up of a randomized controlled trial. *J Bone Miner Res.* 2006;21:1175-1186.

124 Breukhoven PE, Leunissen RWJ, de Kort SWK, Willemsen RH, Hokken-Koelega ACS. Preterm birth does not affect bone mineral density in young adults. *Eur J Endocrinol.* 2011;164:133-138.

125 Hovi P, Andersson S, Järvenpää AL, et al. Decreased bone mineral density in adults born with very low birth weight: a cohort study. *PLoS Med.* 2009;6:e1000135.

126 Szathmári M, Vásárhelyi B, Tulassay T. Effect of low birth weight on adrenal steroids and carbohydrate metabolism in early adulthood. *Horm Res.* 2001;55:172-178.

127 Meuwese CL, Euser AM, Ballieux BE, et al. Growth-restricted preterm newborns are predisposed to functional adrenal hyperandrogenism in adult life. *Eur J Endocrinol.* 2010;163:681-689.

128 Finken MJ, Meulenbelt I, Dekker FW, et al; for the Dutch POPS-19 Collaborative Study Group. Abdominal fat accumulation in adults born preterm exposed antenatally to maternal glucocorticoid treatment is dependent on glucocorticoid receptor gene variation. *J Clin Endocrinol Metab.* 2011;96:E1650-E1655.

129 Weaver IC, Cervoni N, Champagne FA, et al. Epigenetic programming by maternal behavior. *Nat Neurosci.* 2004;7:847-854.

130 McGowan PO, Sasaki A, D'Alessio AC, et al. Epigenetic regulation of the glucocorticoid receptor in human brain associates with childhood abuse. *Nat Neurosci.* 2009;12:342-348.

131 Dessens AB, Haas HS, Koppe JG. Twenty-year follow-up of antenatal corticosteroid treatment. *Pediatrics.* 2000;105:E77.

132 Doyle LW, Ford GW, Davis NM, Callanan C. Antenatal corticosteroid therapy and blood pressure at 14 years of age in preterm children. *Clin Sci (Lond)*. 2000;98:137-142.

133 Dalziel SR, Walker NK, Parag V, et al. Cardiovascular risk factors after antenatal exposure to betamethasone: 30-year follow-up of a randomised controlled trial. *Lancet*. 2005;365:1856-1862.

134 Finken MJJ, Keijzer-Veen MG, Dekker FW, et al; for the Dutch POPS-19 Collaborative Study Group. Antenatal glucocorticoid treatment is not associated with long-term metabolic risks in individuals born before 32 weeks of gestation. *Arch Dis Child Fetal Neonatal Ed*. 2008;93:F442-F447.

135 Regan FM, Cutfield WS, Jefferies C, Robinson E, Hofman PL. The impact of early nutrition in premature infants on later childhood insulin sensitivity and growth. *Pediatrics*. 2006;118:1943-1949.

136 Rotteveel J, van Weissenbruch MM, Twisk JWR, Delemarre-Van de Waal HA. Infant and childhood growth patterns, insulin sensitivity, and blood pressure in prematurely born young adults. *Pediatrics*. 2008;122:313-321.

Development of this book was supported by funding from Sandoz

Chapter 13

Term newborns
Axel Huebler

Introduction

Being born small for gestational age (SGA) is caused by a heterogeneous array of conditions, including intrauterine growth restriction (IUGR), and has a lifelong impact on a fetus' ability to develop and survive [1]. Long-term complications that are manifested in childhood include an increased risk for short stature, neurologic disorders (including cerebral palsy), and cognitive delays and decreased academic achievement [2]. Exposure to drugs in utero is also correlated with the occurrence of IUGR [3].

Up to the middle of the last century, the World Health Organization (WHO) defined all newborns with a birth weight below 2500 g as 'preterm infants.' However, in 1961 Gruenwald reported that about one-third of all infants with a birth weight below 2500 g were not actually born preterm. He also described a relationship between IUGR and abnormalities of placental vascularity (especially avascular chorionic villi) [4].

IUGR may be classified as asymmetric, symmetric, combined, or dysmorphic [5]. The most common causes of asymmetric growth restriction are placental insufficiency, maternal hypertensive conditions, long-standing maternal diabetes, renal disease, smoking, and living at a high altitude. Symmetric growth restriction may be due to congenital infections, chromosomal abnormalities, fetal alcohol syndrome, and/or low socioeconomic status [6]. Combined IUGR has elements of both the asymmetric and symmetric varieties, while infants with dysmorphic

S. Zabransky (ed.), *Caring for Children Born Small for Gestational Age*, 151
DOI: 10.1007/978-1-908517-90-6_13, © Springer Healthcare 2013

IUGR have heads, trunks, and limbs that appear disproportionate [5]. Romo et al reviewed the different etiologic factors that contribute to IUGR and found that maternal active and passive tobacco consumption, stress level, total months worked during pregnancy, total daily working hours, time spent standing up, and height were the most significant [7].

The fetal origins hypothesis (or Barker hypothesis) proposes that IUGR and SGA originate through adaptations that the fetus makes when it is undernourished [8]. These adaptations can be cardiovascular, metabolic, or endocrine in nature and can potentially permanently change the structure and function of the body (eg, growth and height restriction) [9].

Disorders of the newborn

Neonatal management requires special attention to a number of significant morbidities that are more prone to develop in growth-restricted infants (Table 13.1) [5].

Respiratory disorders

Preterm infants with IUGR and/or born SGA are at higher risk of death due to chronic lung disease [10]. Meconium aspiration syndrome (MAS) occurs when meconium is present in the lungs during or before delivery

Common morbidities in full-term infants with intrauterine growth restriction	
Cardiopulmonary adaptations	Perinatal asphyxia
	Persistent pulmonary hypertension
	Meconium aspiration
	Pulmonary hemorrhage
Metabolism	Hypoglycemia
	Hyperglycemia
	Hypocalcemia
Temperature regulation	Temperature instability
Hematology/immunology	Polycythemia/hyperviscosity
	Thrombocytopenia
	Neutropenia
	Coagulation
	Lowered immunoglobulin G levels

Table 13.1 Common morbidities in full-term infants with intrauterine growth restriction. Data from Yu and Upadhyay [5].

and is the most common respiratory complication in newborns with IUGR [11]. Initially, chest X-ray findings of an infant with MAS will show irregular infiltrates with hyperexpansion; it may later progress to secondary surfactant deficiency, persistent pulmonary hypertension, or pulmonary hemorrhage [11]. Administration of exogenous surfactant as well as bronchoalveolar lavage may be efficacious in treating MAS [12].

Progress has been made in preventing MAS. A population cohort study conducted in Australia found that the rate of MAS in IUGR infants declined from 3.3% to 2.4% over a 10-year period between 1997 and 2007, and this reduction was associated with changes in maternal and pregnancy risk factors (eg, smoking) and an increase in protective obstetric practices (eg, induction of labor) [13].

Postnatal age-related modifications of the respiratory rhythm control are often disturbed in infants born SGA. This may be due to hypoxia associated with IUGR [14].

Asphyxia

Perinatal asphyxia is characterized by:

- a low Apgar score ($\geq$5 minutes after birth) [15];
- severe acidosis (a pH of <7 or a base deficit of $\leq$16 mmol/L) in an arterial cord blood sample during the first hour after birth [15]; and/or
- an acute perinatal event (late or variable decelerations, cord prolapse, cord rupture, uterine rupture, maternal trauma, hemorrhage, or cardiorespiratory arrest) [16].

In newborns with IUGR, the higher risk of asphyxia may be caused by lower stress tolerance during spontaneous delivery. Several randomized, controlled trials of induced hypothermia (33.5°C–34.5°C) in infants >36 weeks gestational age with moderate-to-severe hypoxic-ischemic encephalopathy found that cooling significantly reduced death and neurodevelopmental disability at 18 months of age [17]. Newborns with evolving moderate-to-severe hypoxic-ischemic encephalopathy should be given therapeutic hypothermia. Cooling should be initiated within 6 hours of birth, conducted under well-defined protocols in a neonatal intensive care facility, and continued for 72 hours, 'rewarming' over at least 4 hours [17].

Cardiovascular disorders

Severe cardiovascular dysfunction can occur in full-term infants with IUGR. For example, modified-myocardial performance index, B-type natriuretic peptide, troponin I, and early–to–late diastolic filling ratios increase with each stage of IUGR severity [18]. Koklu et al found significantly greater measurements of aortic intima-media thickness, a marker of atherosclerosis risk, and reduced serum insulin-like growth factor I in neonates with IUGR than in controls [19]. In another trial, a diminished stroke volume was seen in neonates with SGA with prenatal hemodynamic disturbances. However, left ventricular ejection times remained mostly unchanged [20].

In a study of 65 infants with IUGR compared with controls of the same age, the IUGR infants had higher heart rates (4.2 beats/min; $P=0.005$) and a 42% higher overnight cortisol/creatinine ratio ($P=0.002$). These may be precursors to hypertension and cardiovascular diseases that can manifest in adulthood, although this has not been completely proven [21]. Fetal hypoxia has also been linked to future cardiovascular problems, from the postnatal period up to adulthood. Findings from animal models of hypoxia-induced IUGR support the hypothesis that hypoxia damages the fetal cardiovascular system through myocardial hypoplasia [22]. While maternal protein restriction during gestation does not affect the number of cardiomyocytes [23], it can induce expressions of connective tissue growth factor and collagen in the aorta [24].

In infants with growth restriction, an elevated nucleated red blood cell count is a risk factor for pulmonary hemorrhage and other postnatal bleeding complications. The reason for this is unclear. Early detection and aggressive support of the coagulation system may help to prevent severe bleeding [25].

Hypoglycemia

Glucose is the most important fetal energy substrate. At birth, the transplacental transfer of energy substrates is terminated, so before the start of breastfeeding the newborn infant must be able to produce its own glucose. Fatty acids formed through lipolysis in the last trimester of pregnancy contribute to the mother's energy supply, saving glucose for the fetus to store [26]. However, in pregnancies complicated by IUGR (eg, due to maternal malnutrition), there is a loss of fetal glucose due to reduced lipolysis [27]. Thus, neonatal hypoglycemia commonly occurs in SGA neonates (and other at-risk groups such as infants of diabetic mothers) during the first days of life [28].

Clinical symptoms of hypoglycemia include irritability, seizures, apnea, cyanosis, hypothermia, and feeding difficulties [29]. Severe, prolonged neonatal hypoglycemia can cause brain injury, including cerebral lesions [30].

Because hypoglycemia can be asymptomatic, routine screening in SGA infants is recommended [31]. After birth, rapid glucose screening is necessary, followed by closely monitored clinical observation. A symptomatic neonate needs a rapid intravenous glucose infusion followed by a slow weaning of the parenteral energy supply when blood glucose is stable and enteral feeding can be tolerated. Neonates needing glucose infusions >12 mg/kg/min should be investigated for recurrent or resistant hypoglycemia [31].

Hyperglycemia

Hyperglycemia is caused by lowered insulin secretion in the first days of life (transient hyperinsulinemia). Hyperglycemia may be also observed in preterm infants because they cannot keep glucose production in check, they do not have a proper insulin secretory response, and their insulin processing is not fully developed. There is also an increased ratio of the glucose transporters GLUT1 and GLUT2 in fetal tissues, reducing the hepatocyte reaction to increments in glucose/insulin concentrations during hyperglycemia. Additionally, IUGR has been associated with increased fasting insulin levels during the postnatal period [32].

True neonatal diabetes mellitus is a rare form of insulin-dependent diabetes mellitus. Its primary clinical features are IUGR, hyperglycemia, failure to thrive, fever, dehydration, and acidosis (with or without ketonuria) [33].

Hematologic alterations

The degree of hematologic alteration in neonates with IUGR may be predicted by abnormal antenatal umbilical artery end-diastolic velocity

Doppler status. Severe placental dysfunction with absent umbilical artery end-diastolic velocity leads to higher rates of anemia and thrombocytopenia at birth, which often continue during the first week of life. Neonates with absent end-diastolic velocities required more platelet transfusions than those with positive end-diastolic velocities [34].

Polycythemia and hyperviscosity

Polycythemia is often a result of chronic intrauterine hypoxia which induces the synthesis of erythropoietin. Additionally, a transfusion from the placenta to the fetus may occur during labor, causing a shift of placental blood, and the elevated hematocrit may disturb the flow characteristics of the erythrocytes. The increased blood viscosity influences microcirculation in several organs (especially the brain and lungs) as well as cardiac function. Polycythemia is characterized by hematocrit values ≥65% and is associated with cyanosis, lethargy, muscular hypotonia, seizures, heart failure, renal vein thrombosis, hyperbilirubinemia, and feeding difficulties. Hyperviscosity also leads to a turnover of thrombocytes, with accompanying thrombocytopenia, as well as hypoglycemia and hypocalcemia. Other predispositions for hyperviscosity are smoking during pregnancy, trisomy 21, Beckwith-Wiedemann-Syndrome, and feto-fetal transfusion in twins [35].

Cytopenia

Thrombocytopenia in neonates born SGA may be due to a pronounced suppression of megakaryopoiesis coupled with increased platelet consumption [36]. Maternal pregnancy-induced hypertension is often a predisposition for increased infant thrombocytopenia and nucleated red blood cells [37]. Hohlfeld et al retrospectively studied the etiology of thrombocytopenia in blood samples from 247 fetuses and found that 28% of cases were caused by congenital infectious diseases (eg, toxoplasmosis, rubella, and cytomegalovirus), 18% by immune-related conditions (eg, alloimmunizations, immune thrombocytopenic purpura), 17% by chromosomal abnormalities (eg, trisomy 21, Turner's syndrome, triploidy), and 25% by other disorders (eg, IUGR, gestational thrombocytopenia). No specific cause could be established in the remaining 12% of cases [38].

Congenital bone marrow failure syndromes (CBMFS), which encompass several types of cytopenia, are rare in neonates. However, when neonates present with persistent cytopenia, CBMFS should be considered and tested for [39].

Immunologic deficiencies

Serum immunoglobulins in the infant are primarily derived from maternal intraplacental transfer during the third trimester. Preterm and SGA neonates have lower immunoglobulin (IgG) levels than normal [40]. One study found that umbilical levels of IgG, IgA, and IgM in infants with IUGR were significantly lower than those in infants with normal growth [41].

Neurologic function

Cerebrocortical electrophysiologic maturation is often delayed in infants born SGA. This may lead to neurocognitive deficits during childhood [42]. During the early neonatal period, nerve growth factor levels are lower in infants with IUGR than appropriate-for-gestational-age (AGA) infants, though other neurotrophin levels were similar between the two groups [43]. In a population-based case-control study of over 231,000 neonates, IUGR was associated with a five-fold increased risk for perinatal arterial stroke resulting in motor impairment [44].

Nutrition

In 1981, Brandt reported that the development of infants born SGA of very low birth weight can be supported in such a way that postnatal development is able to follow a relatively normal course. Conditions that foster healthy development include appropriate nutrition during the early growth period, a stimulating environment, and an abundance of maternal attention [45]. This is important because the nutritional energy required by infants born SGA is elevated and the appropriate feeding of infants with growth restriction is important to overcome *in utero* deficiencies [6]. However, even with adequate nutrition, approximately 10–15% of infants do not achieve catch-up growth [46].

There are neonatal and long-lasting alterations of the intestinal microbiota in infants with IUGR, complicating nutritional intake. For example, IUGR increases bacterial density at birth. Mucins and trefoil factor family 3 actively contribute to epithelium protection and healing in the colonic barrier, and since these are reduced in the IUGR neonate, this could be a factor in the higher bacterial density [47]. Rats with IUGR maintained colonic differences from controls even into adulthood (eg, harboring fewer immunomodulating *Bifidobacterium spp* and more *Roseburia intestinalis* bacteria) [48].

Intravascular supplementation can help extend the duration that IUGF fetuses spend in the womb, leading to improved survivability. Tchirikov et al reported on a case of daily intravascular supplementation with amino acids and glucose in a human fetus with IUGR at 33 weeks gestational age with oligohydramnios and placental insufficiency. Both fetal condition and fetal weight gain significantly improved. At a follow-up examination 1 year after birth, development and weight gain were comparable to those in an infant without IUGR [49].

Infant nutritional intake is influenced by sociodemographic determinants, such as obesity and unhealthy diet, as well as by breastfeeding practices in the maternity wards, as long-term breastfeeding may be supported or discouraged by active promotion (eg, giving supplemental formulas or donated milk) [50]. Longer breastfeeding durations in infants born SGA is associated with higher intelligence scores and may help to prevent some of the later neurologic and metabolic problems [51,52]. Using nutrient-enriched formulas to promote fast weight gain may enhance the risk of developing type 2 diabetes and metabolic syndrome in adulthood, so breastfeeding should be recommended whenever possible and formulas used sparingly. However, restricting nutrition in infants born SGA in order to prevent later metabolic disease is not recommended [53]. In mice, underfeeding during the early postnatal period delayed growth, whereas overfeeding hastened it. In both situations, final body size was permanently altered due to changes in pituitary growth hormone (GH), plasma insulin-like growth factor (IGF)-I, and gene expression of hypothalamic GH-releasing hormone [54].

Growth

Endocrinologic and genetic aspects of early growth regulation

Insulin-like growth factor-I and IGF-II partly determine somatic growth during fetal development, as well as in infancy and adulthood. The IGF-binding proteins (IGFBPs) are important molecules for regulating the amount of IGF-I and IGF-II that can bind to cell surface receptors [55]. It has been proposed that fetal adaptation to an adverse intrauterine environment determines altered programming of the GH–IGF axis.

In human fetuses, IGF-I and IGF-II levels have been shown to increase longitudinally during pregnancy [56], and there is a positive relationship between maternal IGF-I levels and birth weight, particularly in the last trimester [57]. The IGFs and IGFBPs are nutritionally regulated in the fetus, and fetal growth retardation causes abnormalities in the GH–IGF axis and the hypothalamic-pituitary-adrenal axis that are associated with later conditions such as hypertension and growth retardation [58,59].

Pituitary GH is present in early pregnancy in the fetal circulation and the concentrations during this time are higher than during and after birth. Because of the nearly complete GH resistance of the fetus, the metabolic effects of GH on body composition and fat and glucose metabolism may be more important than previously thought [60].

In humans, some genes are significantly differentially expressed between normal and IUGR placentas, suggesting that genomic imprinting may play a role in IUGR pathogenesis. The exact mechanisms behind this are unclear, because some imprinted genes are upregulated and other genes are downregulated [61]. While low circulating levels of IGFBPs are noted in early pregnancy, their expression in the placenta is often elevated in pre-eclampsia late in pregnancy. This upregulation may be compensation for abnormal placental development, a possible adaptive mechanism to increase local IGF levels and promote feto-placental growth [62].

Choi et al described a heterozygous mutation of the *IGFIR* gene found in 2 children with unexplained IUGR and short stature. There was haploinsufficiency of the *IGFIR* gene due to terminal 15q26.2->qte deletion. The growth deficit decreased after administration of recombinant human GH therapy, suggesting that *IGFIR* mutations restrict intrauterine and subsequent growth in humans [63]. Thus, minor genetic variations in the *IGF-I* gene could influence prenatal and postnatal growth. Another study found that children carrying allele 191 had significantly lower IGF-I levels than children who did not [64]. These genetically determined low IGF-I levels may lead to reduced birth weight, length, and head circumference and to persistent short stature and small head circumference in later life. In animal models, IUGR-affected epigenetic characteristics, particularly the histone code, along the length of the hepatic IGF-I gene in a gender-specific manner. These changes and reduced IGF-I levels persisted postnatally [65].

Umbilical levels reflect fetal, placental, and maternal influences on an infant's growth. Conversely, infant serum levels are the result of the autonomous endocrinologic regulation. In the human full-term neonate, IGFBP-1 and IGFBP-2 are the most important binding proteins for IGFs in umbilical cord plasma [66]. Umbilical IGFBP-2 has been found to have a significantly negative correlation with birth weight and birth length in full-term neonates [67], while umbilical levels of IGF-I and IGFBP-3 are positively correlated with infants' size and growth characteristics at birth (eg, being born SGA) and are influenced by additional factors such as sex and maternal smoking [57,68,69]. Studies have found no significant relationship between IGF-II levels and birth size, but there is a positive relationship between IGF-II and the IGF-II receptor and a significant correlation between their interaction and birth weight [70].

The IGF-I receptor is most likely involved in cord blood lymphocyte proliferation and the production of immunoglobulin and cytokines (eg, interferon-gamma). Therefore, it may play an important role in the modulation of immune functions [71].

Low cord blood concentrations of insulin and IGF-I and high concentrations of IGFBP-1 have been noted in twins with IUGR. A disturbance in the pathways of amino acid placental transport leads to these alterations in the fetal insulin-IGF axis causing IUGR. However, the mechanism that regulates this transport is still unclear [72].

The relative IGF-I resistance (ratio of IGF-1 to birth weight) seen in neonates with IUGR drives energy toward survival at the expense of growth [73]. Neonatal cord leptin concentrations have a direct correlation to birth weight and body mass index [74], but this is independent of the IGF system [75]. Other mechanisms may explain the associations between with fetal growth and leptin [76].

Cance-Rouzaud et al found that during the first 5 days of life, SGA infants had lower IGF-I levels and lower IGFBP-3 levels than AGA neonates [77]. Furthermore, in SGA neonates born with short stature, IGF-I levels were lower and GH levels were higher than in SGA neonates with normal stature. There appeared to be a graduation in the severity of impact of this "fetal malnutrition" on the somatotropic axis and on intrauterine growth [77]. The pattern of IGF regulation greatly changes during the first weeks of life: IGFBP-1 and IGFBP-2 are initially expressed more, but IGFBP-3 soon becomes the major serum IGFBP, a pattern which continues throughout adulthood [78] (Figure 13.1).

In childhood, functional changes of IGF-I and IGF-II may reflect early growth restriction. Studies have shown that SGA children have reduced insulin sensitivity, and one cause may be resistance to the somatotropic actions of GH and IGF-I. Elevated fasting insulin levels and reduced insulin sensitivity in SGA children with postnatal growth failure are linked with elevated levels of overnight GH secretion [79]. Data suggest that insulin sensitivity is reduced in the liver but increased peripherally [28].

Thyroid abnormalities may occur in short-stature SGA children, and it is possible that some, such as reduced thyroid-stimulating hormone levels, may be due to a different setting of the hypothalamic-hypophyseal-thyroid axis during the time in utero [80].

Growth pattern and prognosis

Results from clinical trials suggest that IUGR does not have a uniform etiology or underlying pathophysiology that can determine possible fetal risk and subsequent long-term consequences for fetal health [81]. While the exact mechanisms linking IUGR to postnatal short stature remain

Schematic presentation of the time dependency of growth factor concentrations in 229 preterm and fullterm infants during the first 8 months of life

Pole reversal hypothesis of the IGF/IGFBP-axis from fetal-to-adult regulation

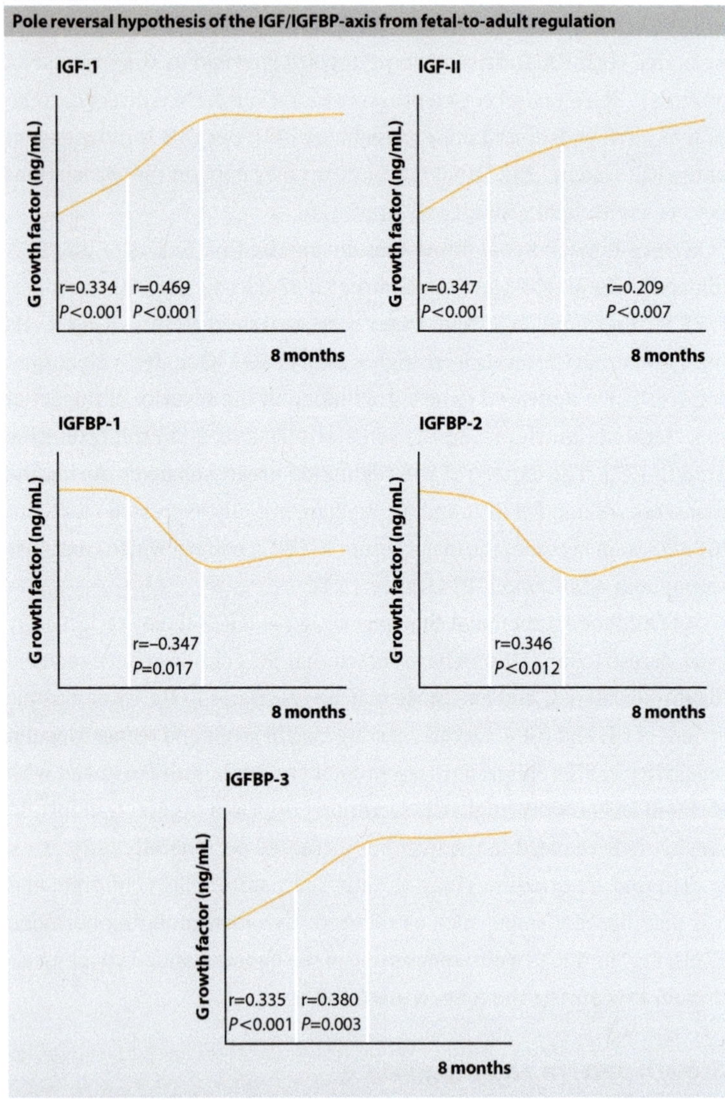

Figure 13.1 Schematic presentation of the time dependency of growth factor concentrations in 229 preterm and fullterm infants during the first 8 months of life. Bravais-Pearson correlation coefficient during 1–2 months, 3–4 months, and 5–8 months of life; upper columns: IGF-I, IGF-II; lower columns: IGFBP-1, IGFBP-2, IGFBP-3. IGF, insulin-like growth factor; IGFBP, insulin-like growth factor-binding protein.

poorly understood, gestational age, birth weight, body mass index, placental weight, and Apgar score are all significantly related to the degree of IUGR [82]. However, neonatal/gestational weight curves are often misleading in detecting low birth weight infants, as they are based only on population norms and do not take intrauterine growth or physiologic determinants of individual growth into account. It is recommended that they only be used when there are no obstetric data available [83].

In a sample representative of 12-month-old infants born AGA or SGA, maternal and postnatal factors were better predictors of developmental delays than demographic variables (eg. socioeconomic status). For example, in children born SGA, maternal smoking during pregnancy, high levels of stress associated with parenting, and low levels of satisfaction with parenting were significantly associated with developmental delays following birth [77].

Simmons et al found that in a model of asymmetric SGA, glucose transport was decreased in the lungs but not affected in the brain [84]. They further discovered that treatment with insulin and IGF-I increased glucose uptake levels of GLUT1 in the lungs and muscles of normal fetuses but not in SGA fetuses. Therefore, the maintenance of normal transporter function and expression in brain may play a role in sparing its growth in infants with IUGR [9].

Thus, the overall outcome of each child is the result of a complex interaction between intrauterine and extrauterine factors. A cohort study of 5111 children who were followed from infancy to 18 years of age found that those who were born SGA had a 7-fold higher risk for short stature compared with the non-SGA group. Birth length and mid-parental height were directly related to the magnitude of catch-up growth during infancy, childhood, and adolescence [1]. A retrospective cohort study found that despite tertiary level neonatal care and intensive fetal surveillance survival for growth-restricted fetuses before 28 weeks' gestation remained poor, with outcome primarily affected by sepsis, respiratory morbidity, and metabolic compromise [85]. Abnormal neurodevelopment in infancy is also related to low weight and acidosis at birth, indicating that the severity of fetal acidosis and malnutrition can affect long-term outcome [86].

Cardiovascular assessments in pre-adolescent patients born SGA found altered cardiac shapes, reduced stroke volume, and increased arterial stiffness (pulse wave velocity) in this group. These physiologic changes could lead to cardiovascular disease in adulthood [87,88]. Intrauterine growth restriction is also associated with poorer lung function in childhood [89].

Alterations of glucose homeostasis and increased lipid oxidation have been observed during the early pubertal stages of even nondiabetic children born SGA. These children also have altered stature and increased fat mass, which may contribute to the future development of insulin resistance [90].

Care around birth

Close collaboration between obstetricians and neonatologists is essential for the care of a fetus with growth restriction. This includes the joint determination of an optimal timing of delivery and the availability of a neonatal resuscitative team. Fetal risks should weighed against neonatal morbidity.

Intrauterine growth retardation is associated with greater stillbirth and infant mortality rates in full-term and post-term infants [5]. Krikun et al have postulated that reducing uteroplacental flow initiates a cascade of molecular effects that eventually causes hypoxia, thrombosis, and endothelial cell dysfunction, resulting in serious complications and difficult pregnancies [91]. Prescribing antenatal corticosteroids to women identified as having persistent absent end-diastolic flow in the umbilical artery may help at least partially restore that flow. Results of a retrospective cohort study of betamethasone administration in these complicated pregnancies found that fetuses who did not respond to corticosteroid therapy were at heightened perinatal risk and were more likely to require assisted ventilation and a longer duration of ventilation and supplemental oxygen [92].

It has been hypothesized that a deteriorated immune response causing leukocyte activation and tissue factor synthesis triggers a coagulation cascade, leading to a vicious cycle. This can cause worsening inflammation and placental disorders, and eventually adverse pregnant outcomes, including IUGR [93]. A high placental ratio, stemming from increased placental size and decreased birth weight, in infants born SGA is associated with a greater incidence of meconium staining, hypocalcemia, and hypomagnesemia [94].

Physicians may choose to induce labor in cases of IUGR out of fear of neonatal morbidity and later stillbirth. The Disproportionate Intrauterine Growth Intervention Trial At Term (DIGITAT) study looked at women with suspected IUGR at full term and found equal outcomes for induction of labor and expectant monitoring. However, while patients who prefer nonintervention can opt for expectant management with intensive maternal and fetal monitoring, the study investigators recommend induction in order to prevent possible neonatal morbidity [95].

The prenatal diagnosis of IUGR is essential for optimal perinatal management. Gestational age, extent of growth restriction, and oxygen supply of the fetus also impact the mode of delivery. For example, placental insufficiency may cause chronic or acute chronic fetal hypoxia with birth asphyxia and hypothermia [6]. While the body temperature in the neonate with IUGR may be initially elevated, subsequent heat loss is caused by the decreased (or even absent) layer of subcutaneous adipose tissue and the relatively large body surface area [96].

A diagnosis of IUGR can be confirmed through gestational assessment, anthropological measurements, and physical examination. These assessment tools can also help to classify the type of IUGR [5]. It should be noted that gestational age assessment may produce misleading results, because patients with IUGR generally have less subcutaneous adipose tissue, diminished breast tissue growth, incomplete formed cartilage of the ears, and underdeveloped genitalia. After an initial stabilization, a reflex examination can lead to a more accurate estimation of the gestational age because reflexes are not affected by IUGR [5]. An infant with IUGR may also appear hypertonic and anxious. The examination should carefully focus on typical signs of congenital infections (eg, petechias and rash, hepatosplenomegaly, cataracts, or chorioretinitis) and minor anomalies. Often there is an enlargement of the anterior fontanel [5]. Body weight, head circumference, and length at birth should be plotted on population-specific growth curves to determine if there is symmetric or asymmetric growth retardation [97].

References

1 Karlberg J, Albertsson-Wikland K. Growth in full-term small-for-gestational-age infants: from birth to final height. *Pediatr Res*. 1995;38:733-739.

2 Pallotto EK, Kilbride HW. Perinatal outcome and later implications of intrauterine growth restriction. *Clin Obstet Gynecol*. 2006;49:257-269.

3 Oro AS, Dixon SD. Perinatal cocaine and methamphetamine exposure: maternal and neonatal correlates. *J Pediatr*. 1987;111;571-578.

4 Gruenwald P. Abnormalities of placental vascularity in relation to intrauterine deprivation and retardation of fetal growth. Significance of avascular chorionic villi. *N Y State J Med*. 1961;6:1508-1513.

5 Yu VYH, Upadhyay A. Neonatal management of the growth-restricted infant. *Semin Fetal Neonatal Med*. 2004;9:403-409.

6 Halliday HL. Neonatal management and long-term sequelae. *Best Pract Res Clin Obstet Gynaecol*. 2009;23:871-880.

7 Romo A, Carceller R, Tobajas J. Intrauterine growth retardation (IUGR): epidemiology and etiology. *Pediatr Endocrinol Rev*. 2009;6(suppl 3):332-336.

8 Barker DJP. The developmental origins of adult disease. *J Am Coll Nutr*. 2004;23(6 suppl):588S-595S.

9 Holt RIG, Byrne CD. Intrauterine growth, the vascular system, and the metabolic syndrome. *Semin Vasc Med*. 2002;2:33-44.

10 Krikun G, Huang ST, Schatz F, Salafia C, Stocco C, Lockwood CJ. Thrombin activation of endometrial endothelial cells: a possible role in intrauterine growth restriction. *Thromb Haemost*. 2007;97:245-253.

11 Robertson MC, Murila F, Tong S, Baker LS, Yu VY, Wallace EM. Predicting perinatal outcome through changes in umbilical artery Doppler studies after antenatal corticosteroids in the growth-restricted fetus. *Obstet Gynecol*. 2009;113:636-640.

12 Li M, Huang SJ. Innate immunity, coagulation and placenta-related adverse pregnancy outcomes. *Thromb Res*. 2009;124:656-662.

13 Lao TT, Wong W-M. The neonatal implications of a high placental ratio in small-for-gestational age infants. *Placenta*. 1999;20:723-726.

14 Boers KE, Vijgen SMC, Bijlenga D, et al; on behalf of the DIGITAT Study Group. Induction versus expectant monitoring for intrauterine growth restriction at term: randomised equivalence trial (DIGITAT). *BMJ*. 2010;341:c7087.

15 Lazić-Mitrović T, Djukić M, Cutura N, et al. Transitory hypothermia as early prognostic factor in term newborns with intrauterine growth retardation. *Srp Arh Celok Lek*. 2010;138:604-608.

16 Bertino E, Occhi L, Fabris C. Intrauterine growth restriction: neonatal aspects. In: Buonocore G, Bracci R, Weindling M, eds. *Neonatology: A Practical Approach to Neonatal Diseases*. Milan, Italy: Springer-Verlag Italia; 2012:82-88.

17 Lal MK, Manktelow BN, Draper ES, Field DJ. Chronic lung disease of prematurity and intrauterine growth retardation: a population-based study. *Pediatrics*. 2003;111:483-487.

18 Rosenberg A. The IUGR newborn. *Semin Perinatol*. 2008;32:219-224.

19 Chinese Collaborative Study Group for Neonatal Respiratory Diseases. Treatment of severe meconium aspiration syndrome with porcine surfactant: a multicentre, randomized, controlled trial. *Acta Paediatrica*. 2005;94:896-902.

20 Vivian-Taylor J, Sheng J, Hadfield RM, Morris JM, Bowen JR, Roberts CL. Trends in obstetric practices and meconium aspiration syndrome: a population-based study. *BJOG*. 2011;118:1601-1607.

21 Curzi-Dascalova L, Peirano P, Christova E. Respiratory characteristics during sleep in healthy small-for-gestational age newborns. *Pediatrics*. 1996;97:554-559.

22 Biban P, Silvagni D. Early detection of neonatal depression and asphyxia. In: Buonocore G, Bracci R, Weindling M, eds. *Neonatology: A Practical Approach to Neonatal Diseases*. Milan, Italy: Springer-Verlag Italia; 2012:226-231.

23 Hankins GDV, Speer M. Defining the pathogenesis and pathophysiology of neonatal encephalopathy and cerebral palsy. *Obstet Gynecol*. 2003;102:628-636.

24 Richmond S, Wyllie J. European Resuscitation Council Guidelines for Resuscitation 2010. Section 7. Resuscitation of babies at birth. *Resuscitation*. 2010;81:1389-1399.

25 Crispi F, Hernandez-Andrade E, Pelsers MMAL, et al. Cardiac dysfunction and cell damage across clinical stages of severity in growth-restricted fetuses. *Am J Obstet Gynecol*. 2008;199:254.e1-254.e8.

26 Koklu E, Ozturk MA, Kurtoglu S, Akcakus M, Yikilmaz A, Gunes T. Aortic intima-media thickness, serum IGF-I, IGFBP-3, and leptin levels in intrauterine growth-restricted newborns of healthy mothers. *Pediatr Res*. 2007;62:704-709.

27 Jackson JA, Wailoo MP, Thompson JR, Petersen SA. Early physiological development of infants with intrauterine growth retardation. *Arch Dis Child Fetal Neonatal Ed*. 2004;89:F46-F50.

28 Robel-Tillig E, Knüpfer M, Vogtmann C. Cardiac adaptation in small for gestational age neonates after prenatal hemodynamic disturbances. *Early Hum Dev*. 2003;72:123-129.

29 Ream M, Ray AM, Chandra R, Chikaraishi DM. Early fetal hypoxia leads to growth restriction and myocardial thinning. *Am J Physiol Regul Integr Comp Physiol*. 2008;295:R583-R595.

30 Lim K, Zimanyi MA, Black MJ. Effect of maternal protein restriction during pregnancy and lactation on the number of cardiomyocytes in the postproliferative weanling rat heart. *Anat Rec (Hoboken)*. 2010;293:431-437.

31 Menendez-Castro C, Fahlbusch F, Cordasic N, et al. Early and late postnatal myocardial and vascular changes in a protein restriction rat model of intrauterine growth restriction. *PLoS One*. 2011;6:e20369.

32 Steurer MA, Berger TM. Massively elevated nucleated red blood cells and cerebral or pulmonary hemorrhage in severely growth-restricted infants–is there more than coincidence? *Neonatology*. 2008;94:314-319.

33 Gustafsson J. Neonatal energy substrate production. *Indian J Med Res*. 2009;130:618-623.

34 Diderholm B, Stridsberg M, Nordén-Lindeberg S, Gustafsson J. Decreased maternal lipolysis in intrauterine growth restriction in the third trimester. *BJOG*. 2006;113:159-164.

35 Diderholm B. Perinatal energy metabolism with reference to IUGR & SGA: studies in pregnant women & newborn infants. *Indian J Med Res*. 2009;130:612-617.

36 Schwartz R, Cornblath M, Kalhan SC. Hypoglycemia in the neonate. In: Stevenson DK, Sunshine P, Benitz WE, eds. *Fetal and Neonatal Brain Injury: Mechanisms, Management, and the Risks of Practice*. 3rd ed. Cambridge, UK: Cambridge University Press; 2003:553-570.

37 Montassir H, Maegaki Y, Ogura K. Associated factors in neonatal hypoglycemic brain injury. *Brain Dev*. 2009;31:649-656.

38 Narayan S, Aggarwal R, Deorari AK, Paul VK. Hypoglycemia in the newborn. *Indian J Pediatr*. 2001;68:963-965.

39 Mericq V. Prematurity and insulin sensitivity. *Horm Res*. 2006;65(suppl 3):131-136.

40 Özlü F, Týker F, Yüksel B. Neonatal diabetes mellitus. *Indian J Pediatr*. 2006;43:642-645.

41 Kush ML, Gortner L, Harman CR, Baschat AA. Sustained hematological consequences in the first week of neonatal life secondary to placental dysfunction. *Early Hum Dev*. 2006;82:67-72.

42 Mentzer WC, Glader BE. Erythrocyte disorders in infancy. In: Taeusch HW, Ballard RA, Gleason CA, eds. *Avery's Diseases of the Newborn*. 8th ed. Philadelphia, PA: Elsevier Saunders; 2005:1180-1215.

43 Cremer M, Weimann A, Schmalisch G, Hammer H, Bührer C, Dame C. Immature platelet values indicate impaired megakaryopoietic activity in neonatal early-onset thrombocytopenia. *Thromb Haemost*. 2010;103:1016-1021.

44 Sivakumar S, Bhat BV, Badhe BA. Effect of pregnancy induced hypertension on mothers and their babies. *Indian J Pediatr*. 2007;74:623-625.

45 Hohlfeld P, Forestier F, Kaplan C, Tissot J-D, Daffos F. Fetal thrombocytopenia: a retrospective survey of 5,194 fetal blood samplings. *Blood*. 1994;84:1851-1856.

46 Rivers A, Slayton WB. Congenital cytopenias and bone marrow failure syndromes. *Semin Perinatol*. 2009;33:20-28.

47 Maheshwari A, La Gamma EF. Fundamentals of feto-neonatal immunology and its clinical relevance. In: Buonocore G, Bracci R, Weindling M, eds. *Neonatology: A Practical Approach to Neonatal Diseases*. Milan, Italy: Springer-Verlag Italia; 2012:830-847.

48 Yang S-L, Lin C-C, River P, Moawad AH. Immunoglobulin concentrations in newborn infants associated with intrauterine growth retardation. *Obstet Gynecol*. 1983;62:561-564.

49 Özdemir OM, Ergin H, Şahiner T. Electrophysiological assessment of the brain function in term SGA infants. *Brain Res*. 2009;1270:33-38.

50 Malamitsi-Puchner A, Nikolaou KE, Economou E, et al. Intrauterine growth restriction and circulating neurotrophin levels at term. *Early Hum Dev*. 2007;83:465-469.

51 Wu YW, March WM, Croen LA, Grether JK, Escobar GJ, Newman TB. Perinatal stroke in children with motor impairment: a population-based study. *Pediatrics*. 2004;114:612-619.

52 Brandt I. Head circumference and brain development. Growth retardation during intrauterine malnutrition and catch-up growth mechanisms (author's transl). *Klin Wochenschr*. 1981;59:995-1007.

53 Saenger P, Czernichow P, Hughes I, Reiter EO. Small for gestational age: short stature and beyond. *Endocr Rev*. 2007;28:219-251.

54 Fança-Berthon P, Michel C, Pagniez A, et al. Intrauterine growth restriction alters postnatal colonic barrier maturation in rats. *Pediatr Res*. 2009;66:47-52.

55 Fança-Berthon P, Hoebler C, Mouzet E, David A, Michel C. Intrauterine growth restriction not only modifies the cecocolonic microbiota in neonatal rats but also affects its activity in young adult rats. *J Pediatr Gastroenterol Nutr*. 2010;51:402-413.

56 Tchirikov M, Kharkevich O, Steetskamp J, Beluga M, Strohner M. Treatment of growth-restricted human fetuses with amino acids and glucose supplementation through a chronic fetal intravascular perinatal port system. *Eur Surg Res*. 2010;45:45-49.

57 Erkkola M, Salmenhaara M, Kronberg-Kippilä C, et al. Determinants of breast-feeding in a Finnish birth cohort. *Public Health Nutr*. 2009;13:504-513.

58 Slykerman RF, Thompson JMD, Becroft DMO, et al. Breastfeeding and intelligence of preschool children. *Acta Paediatr*. 2005;94:832-837.

59 Agostoni C. Small-for-gestational-age infants need dietary quality more than quantity for their development: the role of human milk. *Acta Paediatr*. 2005;94:827-829.

60 Vaag A. Low birth weight and early weight gain in the metabolic syndrome: consequences for infant nutrition. *Int J Gynaecol Obstet*. 2009;104(suppl 1):S32-S34.

61 Kappeler L, De Magalhaes Filho C, Leneuve P, et al. Early postnatal nutrition determines somatotropic function in mice. *Endocrinology*. 2009;150:314-323.

62 Clemmons DR. Role of insulin-like growth factor binding proteins in controlling IGF actions. *Mol Cell Endocrinol*. 1998;140:19-24.

63 Gohlke BC, Fahnenstich H, Dame C, Albers N. Longitudinal data for intrauterine levels of fetal IGF-I and IGF-II. *Horm Res*. 2004;61:200-204.

64 Boyne MS, Thame M, Bennett FI, Osmond C, Miell JP, Forrester TE. The relationship among circulating insulin-like growth factor (IGF)-I, IGF-binding proteins-1 and -2, and birth anthropometry: a prospective study. *J Clin Endocrinol Metab*. 2003;88:1687-1691.

65 Holt RIG. Fetal programming of the growth hormone–insulin-like growth factor axis. *Trends Endocrinol Metab*. 2002;13:392-397.

66 Cianfarani S, Geremia C, Scott CD, Germani D. Growth, IGF system, and cortisol in children with intrauterine growth retardation: is catch-up growth affected by reprogramming of the hypothalamic-pituitary-adrenal axis? *Pediatr Res*. 2002;51:94-99.

67 Wollmann HA. Growth hormone and growth factors during perinatal life. *Horm Res*. 2000;53(suppl 1):50-54.

68 Diplas AI, Lambertini L, Lee M-J, et al. Differential expression of imprinted genes in normal and IUGR human placentas. *Epigenetics*. 2009;4:235-240.

69 Christians JK, Gruslin A. Altered levels of insulin-like growth factor binding protein proteases in preeclampsia and intrauterine growth restriction. *Prenat Diagn*. 2010;30:815-820.

70 Choi J-H, Kang M, Kim G-H, et al. Clinical and functional characteristics of a novel heterozygous mutation of the *IGF1R* gene and IGF1R haploinsufficiency due to terminal 15q26.2->qter deletion in patients with intrauterine growth retardation and postnatal catch-up growth failure. *J Clin Endocrinol Metab*. 2011;96:E130-E134.

71 Arends N, Johnston L, Hokken-Koelega A, et al. Polymorphism in the IGF-I gene: clinical relevance for short children born small for gestational age (SGA). *J Clin Endocrinol Metab*. 2002;87:2720-2724.

72 Fu Q, Yu X, Callaway CW, Lane RH, McKnight RA. Epigenetics: intrauterine growth retardation (IUGR) modifies the histone code along the rat hepatic IGF-1 gene. *FASEB J*. 2009;23:2438-2449.

73 Chard T. Insulin-like growth factors and their binding proteins in normal and abnormal human fetal growth. *Growth Regul*. 1994;4:91-100.

74 Lo H-C, Tsao L-Y, Hsu W-Y, Chen H-N, Yu W-K, Chi C-Y. Relation of cord serum levels of growth hormone, insulin-like growth factors, insulin-like growth factor binding proteins, leptin, and interleukin-6 with birth weight, birth length, and head circumference in term and preterm neonates. *Nutrition*. 2002;18:604-608.

75 Geary MPP, Pringle PJ, Rodeck CH, Kingdom JCP, Hindmarsh PC. Sexual dimorphism in the growth hormone and insulin-like growth factor axis at birth. *J Clin Endocrinol Metab*. 2003;88:3708-3714.

76 Vatten LJ, Nilsen ST, Ødegård RA, Romundstad PR, Austgulen R. Insulin-like growth factor I and leptin in umbilical cord plasma and infant birth size at term. *Pediatrics*. 2002;109:1131-1135.

77 Cance-Rouzaud A, Laborie S, Bieth E, et al. Growth hormone, insulin-like growth factor-I and insulin-like growth factor binding protein-3 are regulated differently in small-for-gestational-age and appropriate-for-gestational-age neonates. *Biol Neonate*. 1998;73:347-355.

78 Hübler A, Schlenvoigt D, Dost A, Schramm D, Schiedt B, Kauf E. Associations of the IGF/IGFBP axis and respiratory diseases in neonatal patients during the first 6 months of life. *Growth Horm IGF Res*. 2006;16:185-192.

79 Yang Y, Niu J, Guo L. The effects of antisense insulin-like growth factor-I receptor oligonucleotide on human cord blood lymphocytes. *J Mol Endocrinol*. 2002;28:207-212.

80 Bajoria R, Sooranna SR, Ward S, Hancock M. Placenta as a link between amino acids, insulin-IGF axis, and low birth weight: evidence from twin studies. *J Clin Endocrinol Metab*. 2002;87:308-315.

81 Kyriakakou M, Malamitsi-Puchner A, Mastorakos G, et al. The role of IGF-1 and ghrelin in the compensation of intrauterine growth restriction. *Reprod Sci*. 2009;16:1193-1200.

82 Shekhawat PS, Garland JS, Shivpuri C, et al. Neonatal cord blood leptin: its relationship to birth weight, body mass index, maternal diabetes, and steroids. *Pediatr Res*. 1998;43:338-343.

83 Christou H, Connors JM, Ziotopoulou M, et al. Cord blood leptin and insulin-like growth factor levels are independent predictors of fetal growth. *J Clin Endocrinol Metab*. 2001;86:935-938.

84 Hübler A, Schlenvoigt D, Dost A, Schramm D, Scheidt B, Kauf E. Associations of the IGF/IGFBP axis and respiratory diseases in neonatal patients during the first 6 months of life. *Growth Horm IGF Res*. 2006;16:185-192.

85 Woods KA, van Helvoirt M, Ong KKL, et al. The somatotropic axis in short children born small for gestational age: relation to insulin resistance. *Pediatr Res*. 2002;51:76-80.

86 Keselman A, Chiesa A, Malozowski S, Vieytes A, Heinrich JJ, de Papendieck LG. Abnormal responses to TRH in children born small for gestational age that failed to catch up. *Horm Res*. 2009;72:167-171.

87 Roje D, Tomas SZ, Prusac IK, Capkun V, Tadin I. Trophoblast apoptosis in human term placentas from pregnancies complicated with idiopathic intrauterine growth retardation. *J Matern Fetal Neonatal Med*. 2011;24:745-751.

88 Marconi AM, Ronzoni S, Vailati S, Bozzetti P, Morabito A, Battaglia FC. Neonatal morbidity and mortality in intrauterine growth restricted (IUGR) pregnancies is predicated upon prenatal diagnosis of clinical severity. *Reprod Sci*. 2009;16:373-379.

89 Marconi AM, Ronzoni S, Bozzetti P, Vailati S, Morabito A, Battaglia FC. Comparison of fetal and neonatal growth curves in detecting growth restriction. *Obstet Gynecol.* 2008;112:1227-1234.

90 Slykerman RF, Thompson JMD, Clark PM, et al. Determinants of developmental delay in infants aged 12 months. *Paediatr Perinat Epidemiol.* 2007;21:121-128.

91 Simmons RA, Flozak AS, Ogata ES. The effect of insulin and insulin-like growth factor-I on glucose transport in normal and small for gestational age fetal rats. *Endocrinology.* 1993;133:1361-1368.

92 Engineer N, Kumar S. Perinatal variables and neonatal outcomes in severely growth restricted preterm fetuses. *Acta Obstet Gynecol Scand.* 2010;89:1174-1181.

93 Torrance HL, Bloemen MCT, Mulder EJH, et al. Predictors of outcome at 2 years of age after early intrauterine growth restriction. *Ultrasound Obstet Gynecol.* 2010;36:171-177.

94 Crispi F, Bijnens B, Figueras F, et al. Fetal growth restriction results in remodeled and less efficient hearts in children. *Circulation.* 2010;121:2427-2436.

95 Bradley TJ, Potts JE, Lee SK, Potts MT, De Souza AM, Sandor GGS. Early changes in the biophysical properties of the aorta in pre-adolescent children born small for gestational age. *J Pediatr.* 2010;156:388-392.

96 Kotecha SJ, Watkins WJ, Heron J, Henderson J, Dunstan FD, Kotecha S. Spirometric lung function in school-age children: effect of intrauterine growth retardation and catch-up growth. *Am J Respir Crit Care Med.* 2010;181:969-974.

97 Tappy L. Adiposity in children born small for gestational age. *Int J Obes (Lond).* 2006;30(suppl 4):S36-S40.

Development of this book was supported by funding from Sandoz

Chapter 14

Endocrine regulation of fetal growth

Nordie Bilbao and Paul Saenger

Introduction

Substantial evidence in the past decade has linked changes in the in utero environment and nutrition to pubertal and adult diseases in later life. As early as 1962, JV Neel, an American population geneticist, proposed the concept of the 'thrifty genotype', which is described as metabolic characteristics that arise during famine to guarantee survival but which later become harmful during nutritional abundance (see Chapter 11) [1,2].

Nearly three decades later, in a study of 8000 adults in the UK, Barker et al [3] reported a correlation between low birth weight or weight at one year of life (which correlated with birth weight) and the prevalence of the metabolic syndrome, which includes type 2 diabetes mellitus, obesity, hypertension, dyslipidemia, and insulin resistance in adult life and can ultimately lead to the premature development of cardiovascular disease [3]. These reports have led to many studies examining the effects of adverse intrauterine environment on various physiological systems [1–3].

At the heart of this discussion is the concept of developmental plasticity, which can be defined as the phenomenon by which one genotype can give rise to a range of physiological or morphological states in response to different environmental conditions during development [4]. Implicit in this is the idea that there is a 'critical period' when a system is plastic and

S. Zabransky (ed.), *Caring for Children Born Small for Gestational Age*,
DOI: 10.1007/978-1-908517-90-6_14, © Springer Healthcare 2013

sensitive to the environment, followed by a loss of plasticity and a fixed functional capacity [4]. A reduction in nutrients required for optimal fetal growth reprograms the offspring via permanent structural and functional changes that, in the context of postnatal nutritional surfeit, predispose to disease [5].

The impact of being born small for gestational age (SGA) on the offspring is widespread and touches every physiological system, and this chapter will focus on endocrinopathies as consequences of fetal growth restriction. In childhood, infants born SGA are prone to neurological impairments, delayed cognitive development, and poor academic achievement [6–9]. As adults, they are at increased risk of developing a large number of complications which affect growth and puberty, such as changes in the insulin-like growth factor (IGF)/insulin system, changes in other hormones such as higher thyroid-stimulating hormone (TSH) levels, decreased adiponectin and follistatin, and increased fetal glucocorticoid

Consequences of fetal growth restriction

Effects on growth and puberty:

- born small for gestational age
- 90% catch-up in growth by 3 years of age; short stature persists in remainder
- common cause of short stature in adult population
- timing of puberty (gonadarche) is usually within normal limits for age and sex
- decreased fat mass at birth, accelerated gain in fat mass later in life

Resetting of IGF/insulin systems:

- circulating concentrations of IGF-1 are typically below average for age and sex; patients show mild-to-moderate growth hormone resistance
- indices of insulin sensitivity frequently indicate mild-to-moderate insulin resistance
- metabolic syndrome prevalence is increased

Changes in other hormones:

- mild hyperthyrotropinemia in absence of overt hypothyroidism
- decreased adiponectin and follistatin in children
- increased fetal/neonatal glucocorticoid exposure

Increased risk of adult disease:

- impaired academic achievement
- stroke
- type 2 diabetes mellitus
- heart failure
- obesity
- hypertension

Table 14.1 Consequences of fetal growth restriction. GH, growth hormone; IGF-1, insulin-like growth factor-1. Adapted with permission from Chernausek [10].

exposure (Table 14.1). In adulthood, there is then an increased risk of stroke, type 2 diabetes mellitus, heart failure, obesity, hypertension, obstructive pulmonary disease, renal insufficiency, impaired reproductive function, sensorineural hearing loss, and osteoporosis.

Glucose metabolism and obesity

Epidemiologic studies from countries as diverse as the US, Sweden, India, and South Africa have shown that adults that had a low birth weight have an increased prevalence of the metabolic syndrome [11]. For example, in a detailed prospective case-control study of birth weight and insulin resistance, singletons were assigned to the SGA group if their birth weight fell below the 10th percentile [12]. The comparable average for gestational age (AGA) group consisted of singletons with a birth weight between the 25th and 75th percentile. Both direct and indirect measurements revealed that insulin resistance was more prominent in the SGA group [12]. In another study, fasting insulin and glucose concentrations were significantly higher and values for the quantitative insulin sensitivity check index were significantly lower in the SGA group compared to the AGA group (Figure 14.1) [13–15]. Moreover, insulin sensitivity was 20% lower in 30% of the individuals born SGA compared with individuals born AGA when assessed by the hyperinsulinemic euglycemic clamp method [15]. This insulin resistance was independent of confounding factors such as body mass index (BMI), age, family history of diabetes or dyslipidemia, oral contraceptive use, and smoking.

Insulin resistance was already seen in childhood, which is much earlier than in cohorts studied by Barker, who were in their fifth or sixth decade [2]. In fact, insulin resistance was typically seen in the catch-up growth period of 0–2 years of age [16,17]. In a study by Soto et al, insulin resistance was found only in infants born SGA who achieved catch-up growth and not in infants who did not display catch-up growth or who were born AGA, suggesting that rapid catch-up growth can give rise to adverse metabolic outcomes early in life [16]. This phenomenon is further supported by a study in prepubertal children born SGA, which demonstrated that significant insulin resistance was found only in children with catch-up growth that resulted in an increased BMI [18].

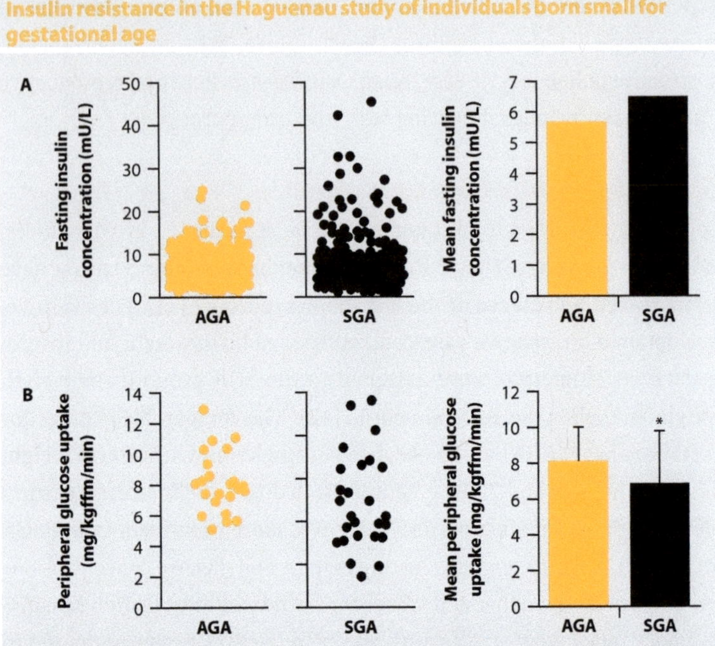

Figure 14.1 A and B Insulin resistance in the Haguenau study of individuals born small for gestational age. A, Fasting insulin concentrations in 734 adults born SGA and 689 born AGA; B, Peripheral glucose uptake during hyperinsulinemic clamps in 26 individuals born SGA and 25 born AGA. The *left-hand graphs* represent individual values and the *right-hand graphs* represent the mean values observed in the two groups. *Black circles and bars* = SGA; *open circles and bars* = AGA. AGA, average for gestational age; kgffm, kilograms fat-free mass; SGA, small for gestational age. *$P = 0.05$. Reproduced with permission from Lévy-Marchal and Czernichow [15].

Additionally, the concentrations of circulating leptin and adiponectin in individuals born SGA were lower than those found in AGA individuals [19]. Jacquet et al demonstrated a negative correlation between insulin resistance and adiponectin levels in infants born AGA and reduced adiponectin levels in SGA infants [20]. These observations were made in individuals born SGA and suggest that adipose tissue morphology or function is altered after a period of intrauterine growth restriction (IUGR) and highlights the critical contribution of adipose tissue in metabolic complications associated with reduced fetal growth. Thus, it is plausible that neonatal alterations in adipose tissue may program insulin resistance and related metabolic complications.

While the original Barker hypothesis postulated that poor intrauterine growth programs for insulin resistance in later life, a subsequent study by Eriksson et al found that children with the lowest birth weight and highest BMI at 11 years of age were at the greatest risk, not only for insulin resistance, but for subsequent development of type 2 diabetes mellitus [5].

In Germany, Reinehr et al examined the prevalence of metabolic syndrome in 804 overweight (BMI >90th percentile) children at an average age of 11 years, of whom 4% were born SGA [21]. In total, 40% of the overweight children born SGA had metabolic syndrome, compared with 17% of those born AGA [21]. Hypertension was increased five-fold in children born SGA and the prevalence of impaired glucose tolerance was more than double that observed in children born AGA [21].

Brufani et al in Italy showed that the metabolic deterioration in overweight or obese children born SGA is not only due to coincident insulin resistance, but also involves attenuated insulin secretion [22]. In a group of 257 children, of whom 44 were born SGA, the insulinogenic and disposition indices measured after oral glucose load indicated impairment of beta-cell function in the SGA group when compared with overweight children with a normal birth weight [22].

Leunissen et al in the Netherlands described the relationship between first-year growth and the prevalence of risk factors for cardiovascular and metabolic disease in a group of young adults (aged 18–24 years) born SGA [23]. The effect was greatest in the period from birth to 3 months of age; specifically, weight gain during the first 3 months of life was associated with reduced insulin sensitivity, lower high-density lipoprotein cholesterol, and higher serum triglycerides. These associations were present even when linear growth was factored in, suggesting that a rapid gain in adipose tissue was responsible. When the subjects were subdivided into fast and slow weight gainers over their first 3 months of life, those who rapidly gained weight had a higher body fat percentage, larger waist circumference, and lower insulin sensitivity as young adults [23].

Insulin sensitivity in intrauterine growth restriction

Studies of children with IUGR that have demonstrated impaired insulin sensitivity, even as early as the neonatal period and infancy, found no structural differences in the pancreas upon autopsy of deceased infants older than 32 weeks who were born AGA or SGA [24,25]. The percentage of beta cells found within the islets was identical in both groups [24,25].

Differential regulation of adipocytokines in the IUGR state may be predictive of adult disease. Most studies to date have reported lower leptin, lower adiponectin, and higher ghrelin levels in IUGR [19,26]. Visfatin may also be high, reflecting increased visceral fat deposits in IUGR [27].

Insulin resistance, an abnormal metabolic profile, high cortisol levels, raised plasma fibrinogen concentrations, and hypertension contribute to the risk of coronary heart disease and, thus, to increased morbidity and mortality [28,29].

These results demonstrate that early postnatal events in children born SGA have a profound impact on metabolic health as early as childhood and young adulthood and, as the Dutch data [23] and the updated follow-up studies suggest [10,30], much earlier than seen in Barkers original collective from the UK. This also illustrates that not only prenatal events lead to IUGR and SGA, but also postnatal events that occur in early infancy and childhood (ie, excessive weight gain in the first year of life) can impact on the frequency and risk of developing metabolic syndrome later in life.

Reversibility of metabolic programming

Vickers et al showed that neonatal administration of leptin into rats that were undernourished in utero reverses the metabolic phenotype of insulin resistance and obesity, suggesting that there appears to be an early postnatal window to reverse developmental programming [31]. Interestingly, relative undernutrition in early life has been associated with improved insulin sensitivity in adolescence [32]. One study investigated the relationship between relative undernutrition in infancy and the fasting concentrations of 32–33 split proinsulin at 13–16 years of age, and found that individuals fed ordinary formula (or better, breast milk) in infancy had lower fasting split proinsulin levels in adolescence than infants fed nutrient-enriched formula [33]. Fasting 32–33 split proinsulin levels were associated with weight gain in the first 2 weeks of life, independent of gestational age, birth weight, or other confounding factors [33].

This implies that programming can possibly be reversed or prevented by dietary modulation at a critical stage of postnatal development.

Growth and short stature

Catch-up growth

'Catch-up growth' is a term introduced by Prader et al to describe the increased growth velocity that occurs in children after a period of growth restriction when the cause of the growth restriction is removed [34,35]. Catch-up growth may also be defined as a growth velocity above the statistical limits of normality for age or maturity during a defined period of time. As a result of catch-up growth, final height is improved, although this recovery of adult stature is frequently incomplete.

Two principal models have been proposed to explain catch-up growth. The first model, proposed by Prader, postulates a central nervous system 'set-point' for an age that adjusts growth accordingly [35]. Today, more than 40 years have passed since the first publication of Prader's concept and yet the postulated central nervous system mechanism remains elusive. Fetal and juvenile growth is typically inhibited by IUGR, whereas postnatally, it can be inhibited by a growth hormone (GH) deficiency, hypothyroidism, or postnatal malnutrition. If these conditions resolve, the growth rate generally does not return to normal but briefly exceeds the normal rate for chronologic age [36].

The second model is based on recent studies by Baron and colleagues to elucidate a local endocrine concept governing catch-up growth, which proposes that local inhibition in a single growth plate is followed by local catch-up growth within the growth plate [37]. According to this persuasive model, growth-inhibiting conditions decrease the proliferation of growth plate stem cells, thus conserving their proliferative potential. This anatomic specificity suggests that the mechanism responsible for catch-up growth resides not in the central nervous system but rather within the growth plate [38].

Most children who are born SGA experience catch-up growth and will achieve a height that is greater than two standard deviations below average. In most infants born SGA, catch-up growth is completed by 2 years of age (for infants born prematurely and SGA, it may take longer to catch-up than full-term infants born SGA) [39–41]. In more than 80% of infants born SGA, catch-up growth in length occurs in the first 6 months of life [13]. Accelerated weight gain during infancy, even during the first weeks of life, can result in excess weight, insulin resistance, high leptin and cholesterol levels, and an elevated blood pressure even two decades later [42]. If rapid weight gain in infancy is indeed related to onset of disease later in life, physicians are faced with many challenges in overcoming deep-seated cultural stereotypes that a fat baby is a 'healthy' baby [42].

It is estimated that 90% of children born SGA eventually catch-up and maintain a height within the normal range [13]. Nonetheless, 10% remain short and represent a significant proportion of adults with short stature. The growth response of infants during their first months of life appears to be fundamental to the future health and stature of individuals born SGA, as most catch-up growth occurs in this relatively brief period.

Role of insulin-like glucose factor-1

Infants born SGA frequently exhibit increased concentrations of GH and low levels of IGF-1 and IGF-binding protein 3 (IGFBP3), suggesting that neonates born SGA are GH-insensitive [43–47]. However, normalization of the GH-IGF axis occurs early in postnatal life and most children born SGA go on to show normal responses to GH-stimulation tests and have normal levels of IGF-1 and IGFBP3 [47].

Polymorphisms of IGF-1 have been associated with pre- and postnatal growth retardation [48,49] and homozygous partial deletion of the gene encoding IGF-1 in humans results in severe impairment of growth [50]. The importance of IGF-1 is further underlined by the association of pre- and postnatal growth restriction with mutations of the *IGF-1R* gene [51]. Moreover, infants born SGA demonstrate reduced levels of IGFBP3, with consistently high levels of IGFBP1 and IGFBP2 [52].

Despite substantial evidence of abnormal levels of IGF-1 in these infants, there does not appear to be a firm link between IGF-related variables at birth and postnatal growth [43,44]. Cianfarani et al [53] have reported a correlation between catch-up growth and the IGF-1/IGFBP3 molar ratio in infancy and suggested that the affinity between IGF-BP3 and IGF-1 may be modulated by cation-dependent proteolytic enzymes that degrade

IGF-BP thereby increasing the levels and bioavailability of IGF-1 [53]. Postnatally, the IGF system is switched on, allowing catch-up growth in the majority of infants born SGA [51]. Furthermore, the alterations in IGF-1 levels observed in neonates born SGA appear to be transient [54].

In infants born SGA, low cord levels of IGF-1 normalize rapidly after birth (Figure 14.2) [12]. However, serum levels of IGF-1 remain significantly reduced in infants who fail to show catch-up growth by 2 years of age, suggesting mild GH resistance, whereas GH levels are normal [44,55]. In an observational case-controlled study, Verkauskiene et al analyzed the dynamics of IGF-1 and IGF-BP3 in a cohort of young adults born SGA and a cohort born AGA [56]. They found that serum IGF-1 concentrations and the IGF-1/IGF-BP3 ratio were lower in adults born SGA than in those born AGA [56]. This would suggest that any long-term abnormality of IGF-1 metabolism may be implicated in the association between IUGR and cardiovascular and metabolic disease in later life.

Growth hormone therapy

Variations in the GH receptor gene do not explain variability of the overall response to GH [57]. Therefore, determination of absence or presence

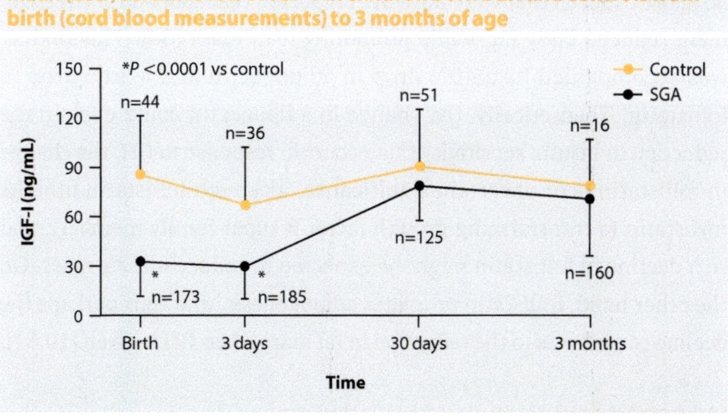

Figure 14.2 Mean (±SD) serum levels of IGF-1 in children born SGA and controls from birth (cord blood measurements) to 3 months of age. Levels of IGF-1 were significantly reduced in the cord blood of infants born SGA, but serum IGF-1 levels normalized rapidly after birth. IGF-1, insulin-like growth factor-1; SD, standard deviation; SGA, small for gestational age. Adapted with permission from Leger [12].

of the exon 3 deletion of GH receptor is not helpful. A recent genome-wide association study identified over 180 genes that are associated with stature [58]. Many of these affect the GH/IGF axis and potentially explain therapeutic responsiveness [10].

The efficacy of GH therapy in syndromic forms of short stature after IUGR has been the subject of much investigation. In general, the response to GH is not as good (eg, in patients with Silver-Russell syndrome or 3-M syndrome). The adult heights of these patients were, on average, significantly below their parental target heights [59–62].

GH treatment in children with short stature after IUGR is considered standard practice by many physicians worldwide, although questions remain concerning the safety and efficacy of such treatment. Short children born SGA represent a heterogeneous group of individuals in whom the short stature has multiple etiologies. As a consequence, response to GH and ultimate height achieved by treatment is highly variable. Prediction models unfortunately only explain about half of the response variability in the first year and a third of that in subsequent years [10,63]. Normalization of height is generally the primary justification for GH treatment [13,64].

Non-statural endpoints have also been examined. A recent study of 35 short children that were born SGA reported that short-term GH treatment reduced body fat, while promoting lean mass [64]. This finding was accompanied by a 40% drop in adiponectin and a 30% drop in follistatin. Theoretically, the change in adiponectin could explain the reduction in insulin sensitivity that occurs in response to GH; the change in follistatin is of uncertain significance, although follistatin inhibits myostatin (a transforming growth factor-B super-family member), and so a decline in follistatin might be expected to reduce muscle mass. On the other hand, follistatin promotes adipogenesis, and thus perhaps the decline contributes to the reduction in fat mass when GH is given [10,64].

Hypothalamic-pituitary-adrenal axis

Functioning of the hypothalamic-pituitary-adrenal axis (HPAA) may be permanently programmed during development [65]. Cianfarani et al reported that children born SGA who do not show catch-up growth have significantly higher fasting levels of plasma cortisol than children born SGA who achieved catch-up growth [13,66]. In addition, cortisol may limit IGF-BP3 proteolysis in the perinatal period, which minimizes the availability of circulating IGF and causing early growth restriction [13].

Hyperresponsiveness of the HPAA in children born SGA has been documented [13]. In a study of low-dose dexamethasone suppression followed by adrenocorticotropic hormone stimulation, an enhanced response of plasma and urinary cortisol was observed [67,68]. Tenhola et al observed high serum cortisol concentrations associated with high levels of epinephrine, low density lipoprotein, and total cholesterol in 12-year-old children born SGA, suggesting hyperresponsiveness of the HPAA [68]. Elevated corticotropin-releasing factor hormone levels have also been measured in infants with IUGR [69]. While these data also suggest the concept of early fetal programming, the underlying mechanisms for this HPAA hyperresponsiveness remain to be determined.

Thyroid

Reduced concentrations of circulating free T3 and free T4 thyroid hormones, together with a discreet rise in concentrations of TSH, have been reported in fetuses with IUGR [70]. Furthermore, a significant decrease in the expression of thyroid receptor isoforms in the human fetal nervous system has been documented in IUGR [71,72].

Effects on reproductive system

Premature pubarche and polycystic ovary syndrome

The sequence and tempo of puberty appear to be normal. A Dutch longitudinal study of children born SGA showed no difference for girls in timing of pubertal onset or in the tempo of puberty, including menarche [73,74]. Studies by de Zegher et al and Ibanez et al have hypothesized that the insulin resistance and dyslipidemia that follows SGA birth in girls yields a hyperandrogenic state, resulting in premature pubarche that is followed by polycystic ovary syndrome (PCOS) in adolescence [45,75]. Metformin may have the potential to prevent or delay manifestations of hyperandrogenism, including PCOS, and the timing of such treatment (eg, starting it before menarche) may be important [75].

However, the notion that low birth weight results in PCOS was challenged by Legro et al and the notion of an increase in premature adrenarche was also challenged by Dutch and French groups [74,76,77]. Legro studied 467 women with PCOS, their first degree relatives, and a group of unrelated controls and found that the distribution of birth weights in the affected women did not differ from US population norms, and there was no discernible relationship between birth weight and metabolic or reproductive abnormalities [76]. Birth weight was self-reported, but a validation study supported the veracity of the data. There then appears a conflict in the data between the relationship of birth weight and premature adrenarche and PCOS in later life. Indeed, no other group has been able to discern such a high prevalence of PCOS in adolescents with a history of low birth weight.

It may be that ethnicity plays a role and the data of Ibanez et al needs to be confirmed in other ethnicities and in larger cohorts. Preemptive therapy with metformin in girls with low birth weight and premature adrenarche has been advocated [10].

Reproductive tract abnormalities

There is a quartet of reproductive tract abnormalities (abnormal spermatogenesis, testicular cancer, cryptorchidism, and hypospadias) affecting males born SGA that has now assumed a syndromic designation – testicular dysgenesis syndrome [TDS] [78]. It has been proposed that TDS has a fetal origin [79] and low birth weight is a common risk factor for testicular cancer, hypospadias, and cryptorchidism [80]. For example, the contemporary, ongoing, prospective longitudinal Cambridge Birth Cohort Study reported a prevalence of 4.5% for cryptorchidism at birth and confirms the significant association with low birth weight for gestational age [13].

Effects on other organ systems

Being born SGA has been implicated in multiple unrelated conditions, including coronary heart disease, stroke, liver cirrhosis, respiratory infection, obstructive airway disease, and renal disease [81–86]. All of these conditions may have the commonality of occurring in a nutritionally-deficient environment.

Renal disease is increased in individuals born with low birth weight, perhaps due to a reduction in nephron number, with compensatory glomerular hypertrophy [85–87]. Even young adults born SGA with apparently normal renal function have been found to have microalbuminuria and reduced glomerular filtration rate [88]. Children born SGA with minimal change nephritis are at greater risk of a complicated and progressive course of renal disease [89,90].

Being born SGA may also be associated with impaired pulmonary development with a greater risk of bronchopulmonary dysplasia and chronic lung disease in the newborn [91]. Harding et al found that prenatal development of the brainstem or chemoreceptors may be affected by fetal hypoxia or hypoglycemia in infants born SGA [92]. They found that the air–blood barrier in the lungs was thicker and that consequently, the diffusion capacity for carbon monoxide in the lungs was lower in children born SGA. Furthermore, impaired fetal growth and adult obesity were reported to be risk factors for adult asthma [93]. Being born SGA has also been associated with an increased risk of mortality from cirrhosis of the liver [83].

There is increasing evidence that nutritional deficit in utero can lead to abnormal bone development and predispose to osteoporosis in later life [94]. Indeed, the bone mineral density adjusted for bone size of children born SGA has been shown to be significantly less than that of children born AGA, with children in the lowest quartile for height gain almost twice as likely to incur a hip fracture in later life than are children in the highest quartile [95,96]. In addition, bone maturation may show idiosyncratic variations in untreated children born SGA, particularly between 6 and 9 years of age [97]. This often leads to difficulties in bone age interpretation, and large inter- and intraindividual observer variation. However, it is not related to the advent of adrenarche and is not a consequence of GH therapy [97].

Neurodevelopmental outcomes

McCarton et al found that premature children born SGA had significantly lower cognitive scores at 1, 2, 3, and 6 years of age than premature children born AGA [98]. They concluded that premature infants born SGA are at greater risk of developmental impairment than equally premature infants born AGA [98].

A large UK-based study with a cohort of 14,189 infants showed that children born SGA (n=1064) had increased difficulties in academic and professional achievement compared to children born AGA [99]. However, those born SGA were no more likely to have emotional or social difficulties [99].

In a large landmark study of 254,426 Swedish males aged 18 years with short body length at birth, small head circumference at birth, and born pre-term were all found to have an increased risk of subnormal performance on psychological and intelligence tests [100]. The most important predictor of subnormal performance among individuals born SGA was the absence of catch-up growth in infancy [100].

Epigenetics: the missing link between intrauterine growth restriction and long-term health effects?

There is emerging evidence that epigenetic mechanisms are involved in fetal programming to either maintain health or develop disease as adults [10,101]. This concept is best elucidated by an animal model in rats where uterine blood flow was diminished and the offspring developed diabetes as adults due to reduced beta-cell mass [102]. This occurs because the expression of Pdx1 (a transcription factor involved in pancreatic islet development) was compromised as a result of specific alterations in DNA methylation and histone acetylation. These epigenetic changes induced by maternal–fetal environment changes are not necessarily immutable and can be reversed during critical development windows [103]. For example, the programming of diabetes in IUGR can be avoided by injections of a glucagon-like peptide analog (eg, Exendin-4) at birth, with subsequent restoration of beta cell mass [103].

References

1   Neel JV. Diabetes mellitus: a "thrifty" genotype rendered detrimental by "progress"? *Am J Hum Genet.* 1962;14:353-362.
2   Barker DJ. Adult consequences of fetal growth restriction. *Clin Obstet Gynecol.* 2006;49:270-283.
3   Barker DJ. The origins of the developmental origins theory. *J Intern Med.* 2007; 261:412-417.

4   Barker DJ, Winter PD, Osmond C, et al. Weight in infancy and death from ischemic heart disease. *Lancet.* 1989;2:577-580.

5   Eriksson JG, Osmond C, Kajantie E, et al. Patterns of growth among children who later develop type 2 diabetes or its risk factors. *Diabetologia.* 2006;49:2853-2858.

6   Low JA, Handley-Derry MH, Burke SO, et al Association of intrauterine fetal growth retardation and learning deficits at age 9 to 11 years. *Am J Obstet Gynecol.* 1992;167:1499-1505.

7   Taylor DJ, Howie PW. Fetal growth achievement and neurodevelopmental disability. *Br J Obstet Gynecol.* 1989;96:789-794.

8   Paz I, Gale R, Laor A, et al The cognitive outcome of full term small for gestational age infants at late adolescence. *Obstet Gynecol.* 1995;85:452-456.

9   Oyen N, Skjaerven R, Little RE, et al Fetal growth retardation in sudden infant death syndrome (SIDS) babies and their siblings. *Am J Epidemiol.* 1995;142:84-90.

10   Chernausek SD. Update: consequences of abnormal fetal growth. *J Clin Endocrinol Metab.* 2012;97:689-695.

11   Gluckman PD, Hanson MA. The developmental origins of health and disease: the breadth and importance of the concept. In: *Early Life Origins of Health and Disease.* New York, NY: Springer. 2006; 1-7.

12   Leger J, Levy-Marchal C, Bloch J, et al. Reduced final height and indications for insulin resistance in 20 year olds born small for gestational age: regional cohort study. *BMJ.* 1997;315:341-347.

13   Saenger P, Czernichow P, Hughes I, et al. Small for gestational age: short stature and beyond. *Endocrine Reviews.* 2007;28:219-251.

14   Jaquet D, Deghmoun S, Chevenne D, et al. Dynamic change in adiposity from fetal to postnatal life is involved in the metabolic syndrome associated with reduced fetal growth. *Diabetologia.* 2005;48:849-855.

15   Levy-Marchal C, Czernichow P. Small for gestational age and the metabolic syndrome: which mechanism is suggested by epidemiological and clinical studies? *Horm Res.* 2006;65 (suppl 3):123-130.

16   Soto N, Bazaes RA, Pena V, et al. Insulin sensitivity and secretion are related to catch-up growth in small-for-gestational-age infants at age 1 year: results from a prospective cohort. *J Clin Endocrinol Metab.* 2003;88:3645-3650.

17   Yajnik CS, Lubree HG, Rege SS, et al. Adiposity and hyperinsulinemia in Indians are present at birth. *J Clin Endocrinol Metab.* 2002;87:5575-5580.

18   Veening MA, Van Weissenbruch MM, Delemarre-Van De Waal HA. Glucose tolerance, insulin sensitivity, and insulin secretion in children born small for gestational age. *J Clin Endocrinol Metab.* 2002;87:4657-4661.

19   Siahanidou T, Mandyla H, Papassotiriou GP, Papassotiriou I, Chrousos G. Circulating levels of adiponectin in preterm infants. *Arch Dis Child Fetal Neonatal Ed.* 2007;92:F286-F290.

20   Jaquet D, Deghmoun S, Chevenne D, et al. Low serum adiponectin levels in subjects born small for gestational age: impact on insulin sensitivity. *Int J Obes (London).* 2006;30:83-87.

21   Reinehr T, Kleber M, Toschke AM. Small for gestational age status is associated with metabolic syndrome in overweight children. *Eur J Endocrinol.* 2009;160:579-584.

22   Brufani C, Grossi A, Fintini D, et al. Obese children with low birth demonstrate impaired β-cell funcion during oral glucose tolerance test. *J Clin Endocrinol Metab.* 2009;94:4448-4452.

23   Leunissen RW, Kerkhof GF, Stijnen T, et al. Timing and tempo of first-year rapid growth in relation to cardiovascular and metabolic risk profile in early adulthood. *JAMA.* 2009;301:2234-2242.

24   Leipala JA, Raivio KO, Sarnesto A, et al. Intrauterine growth restriction and postnatal steroid treatment effects on insulin sensitivity in preterm neonates. *J Pediatr.* 2002;14:473-476.

25   Beringue F, Bertrand B, Castelotti MC, et al. Endocrine pancreas development in growth-retarded human fetuses. *Diabetes.* 2002;53:385-391.

26   Kyriakakou M, Malamitsi-Puchner A, Militsi H et al. Leptin and adiponectin concentrations in intrauterine growth restricted and appropriate for gestational age fetuses, neonates, and their mothers. *Eur J Endocrinol.* 2008;158:343-348.

27   Briana DD, Milamitsi-Puchner A. Intrauterine growth restriction and adult disease: the role of adipocytokines. *Eur J Endocrinol.* 2009;160:337-347.

28   Fall CHD, Barker DJ, Osmond C, et al. Relation of infant feeding to adult serum cholesterol concentration and death from ischemic heart disease. *BMJ.* 1992;304:801-805.

29   Barker DJP, Meade TW, Fall CH, et al. Relation of fetal and infant growth to plasma fibrinogen and factor VII concentrations in adult life. *BMJ.* 1992;304:801-805.

30   Meas T, Deghmoun S, Alberti C, et al. Independent effects of weight gain and fetal programming on metabolic complications in adults born small for gestational age. *Diabetologia.* 2010;53:907-913.

31   Vickers MH, Gluckman PD, Coveny AH, et al. Neonatal leptin treatment reverses developmental programming. *Endocrinology.* 2005;146:4211-4216.

32   Singhal A, Fewtrell M, Cole TJ, et al. Low nutrient intake and early growth for later insulin resistance in adolescents born preterm. *Lancet.* 2003;361:1089-1097.

33   Hales CN, Barker DJ, Clark PM, et al. Fetal and infant growth and impaired glucose tolerance at age 64. *BMJ.* 1991;303:1019-1022.

34   Williams JPG. Catch-up growth. *J Embryol Exp Morphol.* 1981;65(suppl):89-101.

35   Prader A, Tanner JM, Von Harnack GA. Catch-up growth following illness or starvation. *J Pediatrics.* 1963;62:646-659.

36   Boersma B, Wit JM. Catch-up growth. *Endocr Rev.* 1997;18:646-661.

37   Lui J, Baron J. Mechanisms limiting body growth in mammals. *Endocr Rev.* 2011;32:422-440.

38   Gafni RI, Baron J. Catch-up growth: possible mechanisms. *Pediatr Nephrol.* 2000;14:616-619.

39   Hokken-Koelega AC, De Ridder MA, Lemmen RJ, et al Children born small for gestational age: do they catch up? *Pediatr Res.* 1995;38:267-271.

40   Ong KK, Ahmed ML, Emmett PM, et al. Association between postnatal catch-up growth and obesity in childhood: prospective cohort study. *BMJ.* 2000;320:967-971.

41   Albertsson-Wikland K, Karlberg J. Postnatal growth of children born small for gestational age. *Acta Paediatr Suppl.* 1997;423:193-195.

42   Gillman MW. Developmental origins of health and disease. *N Engl J Med.* 2005;353:1848-1850.

43   Cianfarani S, Germani D, Rossi P, et al. Intrauterine growth retardation: evidence for the activation of the insulin-like growth factor (IGF)-related growth-promoting machinery and the presence of a cation-independent IGF binding protein-3 proteolytic activity by two months of life. *Pediatr Res.* 1998;44:374-380.

44   Leger J, Noel M, Limal JM, et al. Growth factors and intrauterine growth retardation. II. Serum growth hormone, insulin-like growth factor (IGF) 1, and IGF-binding protein 3 levels in children with intrauterine growth retardation compared with normal control subjects: prospective study from birth to two years of age. Study group of IUGR. *Pediatr Res.* 1996;40:101-107.

45   de Zegher F, Kimpen J, Raus J, et al. Hypersomatotropism in the dysmature infant at term and preterm birth. *Biol Neonate.* 1990;58:188-191.

46   Deiber M, Chatelain P, Naville D, et al. Functional hypersomatotropism in small for gestational age (SGA) newborn infants. *J Clin Endocrinol Metab.* 1989;68:232-234.

47   Grunt JA, Howard CP, Daughaday WH. Comparison of growth and somatomedin C responses following growth hormone treatment in children with small-for-date short stature, significant idiopathic short stature and hypopituitarism. *Acta Endocrinol (Copenh).* 1984;106:168-174.

48   Arends N, Johnston L, Hokken-Koelega A, et al. Polymorphism in the IGF-1 gene: clinical relevance for short children born small for gestational age (SGA). *J Clin Endocrinol Metab.* 2002;87:2720.

49   Johnston LB, Dahlgren J, Leger J, et al. Association between insulin-like growth factor 1 (IGF-1) polymorphisms, circulating IGF-1, and pre- and postnatal growth in two European small for gestational age populations. *J Clin Endocrinol Metab.* 2003;88:2699-2705.

50   Woods KA, Camacho-Hubner C, Savage MO, et al. Intrauterine growth retardation and postnatal growth failure associated with deletion of the insulin-like growth factor 1 gene. *N Engl J Med.* 1996; 335:1363-1367.

51   Abuzzahab MJ, Schneider A, Goddard A, et al. IGF-1 receptor mutations resulting in intrauterine and postnatal growth retardation. *N Engl J Med.* 2003;349:2211-2222.

52   Giudice LC, de Zegher F, Gargosky SE, et al. Insulin-like growth factors and their binding proteins in the term and preterm human fetus and neonate with normal and extremes of intrauterine growth. *J Clin Endocrinol Metab.* 1995;80:1548-1555.

53   Cianfarani S, Geremia C, Scott CD, et al. Growth, IGF system, and cortisol in children with intrauterine growth retardation: is catch-up growth affected by reprogramming of the hypothalamic-pituitary-adrenal axis? *Pediatr Res.* 2002;51:94-99.

54   Cianfarani S, Maiorana A, Geremia C, et al. Blood glucose concentrations are reduced in children born small for gestational age (SGA), and thyroid-stimulating hormone levels are increased in SGA with blunted postnatal catch-up growth. *J Clin Endocrinol Metab.* 2003;88:2699-2705.

55   Constancia M, Hemberger M, Hughes J, et al. Placental-specific IGF-II is a major modulator of placental and fetal growth. *Nature.* 2002;417:945-948.

56   Verkauskiene R, Jaquet D, Deghmoun S, et al. Smallness for gestational age is associated with persistent change in insulin-like growth factor 1 (IGF-1) and the ratio of IGF1/IGF-binding protein-3 in adulthood. *J Clin Endocrinol Metab.* 2005;90:5672-5676.

57   Dorr HG, Bettendorf M, Hauffa BP, et al. Different relationships between the first two years on growth hormone treatment and the d3-growth hormone receptor polymorphism in short small-for-gestational-age (SGA) children. *Clin Endocrinol (Oxf).* 2011;75:656-660.

58   Lango AH, Estrada K, Lettre G, et al. Hundreds of variants clustered in genomic loci and biological pathways affect human height. *Nature.* 2010;467:832-838.

59   Huber C, Munnich A, Cormier-Daire V, et al. The 3M syndrome. *Best Pract Res Clin Endocrinol Metab.* 2011;25:143-151.

60   Hanson D, Murray PG, O'Sullivan J, et al. Exome sequencing identifies CCDC8 mutations in 3-M syndrome, suggesting that CCDC8 contributes in a pathway with CUL7 and OBSL1 to control human growth. *Am J Hum Genet.* 2011;89:148-153.

61   Ranke MB, Lindberg A. Height at start, first-year growth response and cause of shortness at birth are major determinants of adult height outcomes of short children born small for gestational age and Silver-Russell syndrome treated with growth hormone: analysis of data from KIGS. *Horm Res Pediatr.* 2010;74:259-266.

62   Toumba M, Albanese A, Azcona C, et al. Effect of long-term growth hormone treatment on final height of children with Russell-Silver syndrome. *Horm Res Pediatr.* 2010;74:212-217.

63   Ranke MB, Lindberg A. Prediction models for short children born small for gestational age (SGA) covering the total growth phase. Analyses based on data from KIGS (Pfizer International Growth Database). *BMC Med Inform Decis Mak.* 2011;11:38.

64   Ibanez L, Lopez-Bermejo A, Díaz M, et al. Growth hormone therapy in short children born small for gestational age: effects on abdominal fat partitioning and circulating follistatin and high-molecular-weight adiponectin. *J Clin Endocrinol Metab.* 2010;95:2234-2239.

65   Levine S. Maternal and environmental influences on the adrenocortical response to stress in weanling rats. *Science.* 1967;156:258-260.

66   Cianfarani S, Ladaki C, Geremia C. Hormonal regulation of postnatal growth in children born small for gestational age. *Horm Res.* 2006;65(suppl 3):70-74.

67   Reynolds RM, Walker BR, Syddall HE, et al. Altered control of cortisol secretion in adult men with low birth weight and cardiovascular risk factors. *J Clin Endocrinol Metab.* 2001;86:245-250.

68   Tenhola S, Martikainen A, Rahiala E, et al. Increased adrenocortical and adrenomedullary hormonal activity in 12-year-old children born small for gestational age. *J Pediatr.* 2002;141:477-482.

69   Ibanez L, Potau N, Marcos MV, et al. Corticotropin-releasing hormone: a potent androgen secretagogue in girls with hyperandrogenism after precocious pubarche. *J Clin Endocrinol Metab.* 1999;84:4602-4606.

70 Kilby MD, Verhaeg J, Gittoes N, et al. Circulating thyroid hormone concentrations and placental thyroid hormone receptor expression in normal human pregnancy and pregnancy complicated by intrauterine growth restriction (IUGR). *J Clin Endocrinol Metab.* 1998;83:2964-2971.

71 Kilby MD, Gittoes N, McCabe C, et al. Expression of thyroid receptor isoforms in the human fetal central nervous system and the effects of intrauterine growth restriction. *Clin Endocrinol (Oxf).* 2000;53:469-477.

72 de Kort SW, Willemsen RH, van der Kaay DC, et al. Thyroid function in short children born small-for-gestational age (SGA) before and during GH treatment. *Clin Endocrinol (Oxf).* 2008;69:318-322.

73 Hernandez MI, Martinez A, Capurro T, et al. Comparison of clinical, ultrasonographic, and biochemical differences at the beginning of puberty in healthy girls born either small for gestational age or appropriate for gestational age: preliminary results. *J Clin Endocrinol Metab.* 2006;91:3377-3381.

74 Veening MA, Van Weissenbruch MM, Roord JJ, et al. Pubertal development in children born small for gestational age. *J Pediatr Endocrinol Metab.* 2004;17:1497-1505.

75 Ibanez L, Lopez-Bermejo A, Diaz M, et al. Early metformin therapy (age 8–12 years) in girls with precocious pubarche to reduce hirsutism, androgen excess, and oligomenorrhea in adolescence. *J Clin Endocrinol Metab.* 2011;96:E1262-E1267.

76 Legro RS, Roller RL, Dodson WC, et al. Associations of birthweight and gestational age with reproductive and metabolic phenotypes in women with polycystic ovarian syndrome and their first-degree relatives. *J Clin Endocrinol Metab.* 2010;95:789-799.

77 Jaquet D, Leger J, Chevenne D, et al. Intrauterine growth retardation predisposes to insulin resistance but not to hyperandrogenism in young women. *J Clin Endocrinol Metab.* 1999;84:3945-3949.

78 Skakkebaek NE. Testicular dysgenesis syndrome: new epidemiological evidence. *Int J Androl.* 2004;27:189-191.

79 Bay K, Asklund C, Skakkebaek NE, Andersson AM. Testicular dysgenesis syndrome: possible role of endocrine disrupters. *Best Pract Res Clin Endocrinol Metab.* 2006;20:77-90.

80 Main KM, Jensen RB, Asklund C, Hoi-Hansen CE, Skakkebaek NE. Low birth weight and male reproductive function. *Horm Res.* 2006;65(suppl 3):116-122.

81 Barker DJ. *Mothers, babies, and disease later in life.* Second edn. London: Elsevier Health Sciences; 1998.

82 Martyn C, Barker D, Osmond C. Mother's pelvic size, fetal growth and death from stroke in men. *Lancet.* 1996;348:1264-1268.

83 Andersen A-M, Ostler M. Birth dimensions, parental mortality, and mortality in early adult age: a cohort study of Danish men born in 1953. *Int J Epidemiol.* 2004;33:92-99.

84 Barker DJ, Godfrey KM, Fall C, et al. Relation of birth weight and childhood respiratory infection to adult lung function and death from chronic obstructive airways disease. *BMJ.* 1991;303:671-675.

85 Lackland DT, Bendall HE, Osmond C, et al. Low birth weights contribute to high rates of early-onset chronic renal failure in the Southeastern United States. *Arch Intern Med.* 2000;160:1472-1476.

86 Hoy WE, Rees M, Kile E, et al. A new dimension to the Barker hypothesis: low birthweight and susceptibility to renal disease. *Kidney Int.* 1999;56:1072-1077.

87 Zandi-Nejad K, Luyckx VA, Brenner BM. Adult hypertension and kidney disease: the role of fetal programming. *Hypertension.* 2006;47:502-508.

88 Keijzer-Veen MG, Schrevel M, Finken MJ, et al; Dutch POPS-19 Collaborative Study Group. Microalbuminuria and lower glomerular filtration rate at young adult age in subjects born very premature and after intrauterine growth retardation. *J Am Soc Nephrol.* 2005;16:2762-2768.

89 Sheu JN, Chen JH. Minimal change nephrotic syndrome in children with intrauterine growth retardation. *Am J Kidney Dis.* 2001;37:909-914.

90 Na YW, Yang HJ, Choi JH, et al. Effect of intrauterine growth retardation on the progression of nephrotic syndrome. *Am J Nephrol.* 2002;22:463-467.

91 Sharma P, McKay K, Rosenkrantz TS, et al. Comparisons of mortality and pre-discharge respiratory outcomes in small-for-gestational-age and appropriate-for-gestational-age premature infants. *BMC Pediatr.* 2004;4:9.

92 Harding R, Tester M, Moss T, et al. Effects of intra-uterine growth restriction on the control of breathing and lung development after birth. *Clin Exp Pharmacol Physiol.* 2000;27:114-119.

93 Cole TJ. Secular trends in growth. *Proc Nutr Soc.* 2000;59:317-324.

94 Tobias JH, Cooper C. PTH/PTHrP activity and the programming of skeletal development in utero. *J Bone Miner Res.* 2004;19:177-182.

95 Arends NJ, Boonstra VH, Mulder PG, et al. GH treatment and its effect on bone mineral density, bone maturation and growth in short children born small for gestational age: 3-year results of a randomized, controlled GH trial. *Clin Endocrinol (Oxf).* 2003;59:779-787.

96 Cooper C, Eriksson JG, Forsen T, et al. Maternal height, childhood growth and risk of hip fracture in later life: a longitudinal study. *Osteoporos Int.* 2001;12:623-629.

97 Sas T, de Waal W, Mulder P, et al. Growth hormone treatment in children with short stature born small for gestational age: 5-year results of a randomized, double-blind, dose-response trial. *J Clin Endocrinol Metab.* 1999;84:3064-3070.

98 McCarton CM, Wallace IF, Divon M, et al. Cognitive and neurologic development of the premature, small for gestational age infant through age 6: comparison by birth weight and gestational age. *Pediatrics.* 1996;98:1167-1178.

99 Strauss RS. Adult functional outcome of those born small for gestational age: twenty-six-year follow-up of the 1970 British Birth Cohort. *JAMA.* 2000;283:625-632.

100 Lundgren EM, Cnattingius S, Jonsson B, et al. Intellectual and psychological performance in males born small for gestational age with and without catch-up growth. *Pediatr Res.* 2001;50:91-96.

101 Sebert S, Sharkey D, Budge H, et al. The early programming of metabolic health: is epigenetic setting the missing link? *Am J Clin Nutr.* 2011;94:1953S-1958S.

102 Park JH, Stoffers DA, Nicholls RD, et al. Development of type 2 diabetes following intrauterine growth retardation in rats is associated with progressive epigenetic silencing of Pdx1. *J Clin Invest.* 2008;118:2316-2324.

103 Pinney SE, Jaeckle Santos LJ, Han Y, et al. Exendin-4 increases histone acetylase activity and reverses epigenetic modifications that silence Pdx1 in the intrauterine growth retarded rat. *Diabetologia.* 2011;54:2606-2614.

Development of this book was supported by funding from Sandoz

Chapter 15

Growth hormone treatment

Roland Schweizer and David D Martin

Introduction

Approximately 8–10% of children born small for gestational age (SGA) do not show catch-up growth by the age of 2 years and older [1,2], with approximately 10% of all children born SGA still below the third percentile at the age of 8 years [3]. These children later have a reduced adult height [4]. For these children, short stature is an approved indication for recombinant human growth hormone (GH) treatment.

Requirements of the regulatory authorities for growth hormone treatment

Table 15.1 shows the differences in requirements for GH treatment in short children born SGA in the US and the EU. The main difference is that the recommended GH dose in the EU is approximately half the dose approved in the US (however, both dosages are above the substitution dose range). In the US, GH treatment is approved from the age of 2 years onwards, whereas in the EU, treatment is not approved for children under the age of 4 years. Distance to mid-parental height plays a role in the EU but not in the US, where idiopathic short stature is also an approved indication for GH treatment.

In the EU, it is recommended that treatment should be discontinued after the first year if it is ineffective; the criteria for differentiating between effective and ineffective treatment is a minimum increase of

S. Zabransky (ed.), *Caring for Children Born Small for Gestational Age*,
DOI: 10.1007/978-1-908517-90-6_15, © Springer Healthcare 2013

	US	EU
Requirements for growth hormone treatment of short children born small for gestational age in the US and EU		
Height	<Third percentile	<–2.5 SDS
Recommended GH dose	68 µg/kg/day	35 µg/kg/day
Age at start of treatment	>2 years	>4 years
Growth	No catch-up growth	HV ≤50th percentile of HV charts
Distance to mid-parental height	No limitations	>–1 SDS

Table 15.1 Requirements for growth hormone treatment of short children born small for gestational age in the US and EU. GH, growth hormone; HV, height velocity; IGF-1, insulin-like growth factor 1; IGFBP-3, insulin-like growth factor-binding protein 3; SDS, standard deviation score.

height velocity (HV) standard deviation score (SDS) of one standard deviation (SD). This very conservative recommendation equates to an increase in HV of about 1.5 cm in the first year.

Prognostically more favorable for a significant increase in adult height is an average growth velocity in the first year that exceeds the 97th percentile of age-appropriate rate charts (ie, HV>+1.88 SDS), corresponding to an increase in growth rate by more than 2 cm in the first year of treatment. This goal is reached in about 80–85% of children born SGA and has been proposed as a more appropriate cut-off for assessing the effectiveness of GH treatment [5].

Growth during growth hormone treatment

The safety and efficacy of GH treatment for children born SGA has been evaluated in a number of randomized, open-label, controlled clinical trials [6,7] In the pioneering trials in this area, patients (age range of 2–8 years) were observed for 12 months before being randomized to receive either somatropin as a daily subcutaneous injection (usually involving two different dosing regimens per study: 0.24 mg/kg/week and 0.48 mg/kg/week, corresponding to 34 µg/kg/day and 68 µg/kg/day) or no treatment for the first 24 months [6,7]. After 24 months, all patients received somatropin. In a study by de Zegher et al, patients who received any dose of somatropin showed significant increases in growth during the first 24 months when compared with patients who received no treatment [6]. Children receiving 0.48 mg/kg/week demonstrated a significantly larger increase in height SDS when compared with children treated with

0.24 mg/kg/week (34 µg/kg/day). Both of these doses resulted in a slower, but nevertheless increased, rate of growth between 24–72 months. After 6 years, the height increase was significantly greater in the higher dosage group. However, a study by Sas et al did not show a dose-dependent difference in height increase in the two dosage groups [7]. This difference is perhaps explained by the fact that in the Sas study group, patients who showed an impaired GH secretion were included, whereas the latter was an exclusion criterion in the de Zegher study [6,7].

Adult height data available from the Sas et al study show that 85% of patients treated with somatropin reached an adult height within the normal range [7,8]. The total height gain in both dosage groups was almost two SDs (Figure 15.1). A Swedish study [9] reported that children born SGA who started GH therapy at least 2 years before the onset of

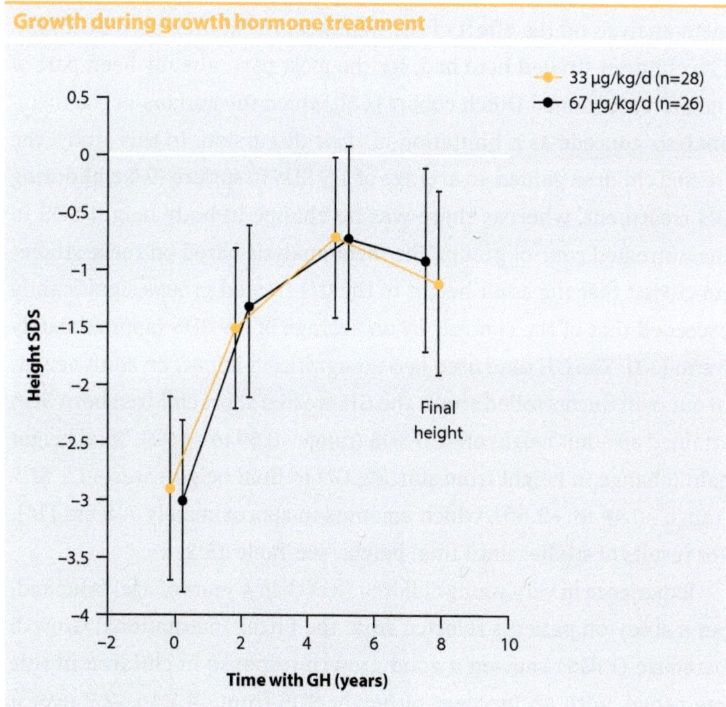

Figure 15.1 Growth during growth hormone treatment. Two dosage groups until final height (n=54). GH, growth hormone; SDS, standard deviation score. Adapted with permission from van Pareren et al [8].

puberty gained a mean adult height SDS of +1.7 (corresponding to a 12 cm increase in adult height), compared with pretreatment predictions. By contrast, children who started GH therapy at a later age gained a mean adult height SDS of +0.9 (corresponding to a 6 cm increase in adult height) [9].

Similarly, studies in which children started treatment at a mean age of 7.8 years estimated that the gains in adult height were approximately +2 SDS [8]. However, it must be noted that height predictions in short stature tend to underestimate adult height and they tend to do so more between bone ages of 4–10 years [10]. A French study showed that no significant improvement in adult height was achieved when compared to an untreated control cohort where GH treatment was started late (ie, around puberty); the gain in height was only 0.6 SDS (approximately 4 cm) [11].

A further trial, part of a Dutch study [12], has been included in a meta-analysis on the effect of GH treatment in children born SGA [13]. The children studied here had, for the most part, already been part of the aforementioned Dutch cohort [12], which the authors of the meta-analysis concede as a limitation in their discussion. In this study, the treated children gained an average of 1.5 SDS in stature (9.4 cm) during GH treatment, whereas there was no change in body height SDS in the untreated control group. The meta-analysis based on these studies concluded that the adult height of the GH-treated groups significantly exceeded that of the controls by an average of 0.9 SDS (approximately 7 cm) [13]. The GH dose used had no significant impact on adult height. In our own uncontrolled study, the GH-treated short children born SGA attained an adult height of –2.0 SDS (range –0.59 to –4.92). Total height gain (change in height from starting GH to final height) was +1.1 SDS (range –0.49 to +2.56), which amounts to approximately 7–8 cm [14]. For results of studies until final height, see Table 15.2.

Experience in very young children (less than 4 years of age) is limited, but a study on patients selected from the Pfizer International Growth Database (KIGS) showed a good growth response in children in this age range, with an increase of height SDS from –4.2 to –2.7 over a 2-year treatment period [20]. Serious adverse events were not reported. The mean height SDS gain for chronological age in children treated for

24 months was 2.10, while it was 1.43 SDS in those treated only during the last 12 months. In both groups, children under 4 years of age had the greatest gain in growth velocity. No significant acceleration of bone age or side effects related to treatment was seen.

A multicenter, controlled, randomized, open clinical trial of GH in 2- to 5-year-old short children born SGA reported an increase in mean height by 2.1 SDS in children treated for 24 months, and 1.4 SDS in those observed for 12 months and then treated for 12 months [21]. No treatment-related side effects and no significant acceleration of bone age were reported. When continuous GH treatment ended after 3 years, the gain in height was lost again after 5 years of growth without GH treatment in most patients. To identify patients able to retain their height gain during the off-treatment period, patients were divided in two subgroups of children: those who lost less than 0.5 height SDS during the 3-year follow-up, and those who lost more than 0.5 height SDS. In the study, 20 out of 62 children retained their height SDS during the follow-up period with no significant catch-down in growth 3 years after treatment. These 20 children were older and had a more advanced bone age at the start of the GH treatment. A majority of these children went into puberty during the first 3 years of follow-up (60% versus 30%) in comparison with the catch-down group. Other parameters were similar in both subgroups included height and weight at birth, height velocity, and height SDS at the start of GH treatment. Most of the children in the subgroup who did not catch down had entered puberty after 5 years and had gone through Tanner pubertal stages 3–5, whereas only 65% of the children with catch-down growth had reached puberty. There was no significant difference in time of onset of puberty between the two subgroups [22].

Whether treatment should be continuous or stopped after reaching a normal height remains controversial, especially since a study by de Zegher et al showed that a height increase of 2.5 SD during 2 years of GH treatment was followed by a decrease of 0.3–0.4 SD during the first and second year after GH withdrawal [23]. Subsequently, when stature was not extremely short at the start (eg, height SDS of –2.7), no further GH treatment was given and the adjusted height was stabilized around

Summary of studies reporting final height data in growth hormone-treated short children born small for gestational age

Author	Treatment yes/no	Number of patients	Age at start of treatment	GH dose (µg/kg/d)
RCTs				
van Pareren et al, 2003	Yes	28	7.9	33
	Yes	26	8.2	67
	No	15	7.8	0
Carel et al, 2003	Yes	102	12.7	67
	No	47	12.8	0
Dahlgren and Wikland, 2005	Yes	36	8.9	33
	Yes	41	12.3	33
	No	34	8.3	0
van Dijk et at, 2007	Yes	37	8.5	33 to 67
	No	25	7.8	0
No RCTs				
Ranke and Lindberg, 1996	Yes	16	12.7	33
Coutant et al, 1998	Yes	70	10.3	19.8
	No	40	Not reported	0
Zucchini et al, 2001	Yes	29	10.9	33
	No	20	10.7	0
Rosilio et al, 2005	Yes	20	9.6	67
Bannink et al, 2007	Yes	26	7.5	33
	Yes	20	7.9	67
Schweizer et al, 2007	Yes	27	8.95	54

Table 15.2 Summary of studies reporting final height data in growth hormone-treated short children born small for gestational age. Data adapted from Maiorana and Cianfarani, et al [13–20].

–1.0 SDS; when stature was very short at the start (eg, height SDS of –3.3), a second course of GH treatment (66 mg/kg/day) was initiated either 2 or 3 years after initial GH withdrawal. This second course was associated with renewed catch-up growth and also resulted in a mean adjusted height of –1.0 SDS [24]. The discontinuation period was not as long as that employed in the study by Fjellestad-Paulsen et al [22].

Predictive factors for response during growth hormone treatment

As in all indications for GH therapy, children born SGA with the greatest parental height-/adjusted height-deficit responded best to GH therapy [8,9]. Studies also suggest that the younger the child at the start of GH therapy, the quicker the initial GH response [8,9,11]. A further predictor

Duration of GH (years)	Height at start of GH SDS	Adult height SDS	Height gain SDS	Final height (cm) boys/girls
7.9	−2.9	−1.1	1.8	169.3/160.1
7.5	−3	−0.9	2.1	173.7/159.2
0	−2.6	−2.3	0.3	Not reported
2.7	−3.2	−2.1	1.1	159/147
0	Not reported	−3.2		162/151
8.5	−3.1	−1.2	1.9	Not reported
5.5	−2.5	−1.6	0.9	Not reported
0	−2.2	−2	0.2	Not reported
7.3	−2.9	−1.4	1.5	Not reported
0	−2.6	−2.6	0	Not reported
4.3	−1.7	−1.7	1	Not reported
4.6	−2.9	−2	0.9	Not reported
0	−2.8	−2.2	0.6	Not reported
3 to 7	−2.3	−1.8	0.5	Not reported
0	−2	−1.9	0.1	Not reported
2+2 off ±4	−2.6	−2	0.6	161.2/152.5
8.5	−3.1	−1.5	1.6	Not reported
7.9	−3.1	−1.2	1.9	Not reported
5.5	−3.2	−2.1	1.1	162.6/157.4

of growth response to GH is the d3-GH receptor polymorphism. Patients with the *d3/d3* variant respond significantly better to GH than patients with the *d3/fl* or *fl/fl* variant [24].

Another attempt to predict growth response to somatropin was presented by Ranke et al [25]. They developed a so-called 'prediction model' with the parameters of age at start, weight SDS at start, GH dose, and mid-parental height SDS to predict growth in the first 3 years of GH treatment [25] (and also until final height [26]). These models explain approximately 50% of the variability of growth response to GH.

It can be concluded that the start of GH treatment should be early, and clearly before puberty, to achieve best results in terms of adult height. Also, GH works best if given continuously. The effect on growth is dose- dependent in the first years of GH treatment but this effect has not been confirmed with regards to adult height. Whether GH treatment during puberty contributes to adult height, whether GH doses need to be increased during puberty, or whether GH can be stopped altogether in mid puberty is still unclear. Several factors (age, height, d3-GH receptor polymorphism) are valuable for predicting growth response.

Combination of growth hormone and gonadotropin-releasing hormone agonist treatment

Gonadotropin-releasing hormone (GnRH) agonists are used for the treatment of central precocious puberty, and they effectively stop the premature acceleration of skeletal maturity and elicit a significant improvement in adult height in this indication [27]. Prescribing GnRH agonists at early-to-normal onset of puberty, and thus at a much later stage of childhood growth, resulted in no significant gain in adult height in most studies [27]. Hence, an international panel of experts recently came to the conclusion that additional GnRH agonist treatment in short children born SGA who are undergoing GH treatment is not recommended unless the respective children have precocious puberty [27].

In the only randomized controlled study to date to examine the adult height of short children born SGA following treatment with a GnRH agonist and GH, both drugs were co-administered from the start of treatment: this design therefore does not allow for a separate analysis of the effect of the GnRH agonist [28]. In daily practice, however, additional GnRH agonist treatment to slow bone maturation in short SGA children with early onset of puberty is not uncommon. There is an urgent need for further research in this area because early puberty in short SGA children can abrogate the gains in height achieved with GH treatment.

Side effects

No significant side effects have been associated with GH treatment in short SGA children. A study by van Dijk et al reported that, at 6.5 years after discontinuation of long-term GH treatment, common metabolic parameters (such as insulin sensitivity and body mass index) were equivalent for GH-treated and untreated young adults with SGA [12].

The most serious and most frequently observed (albeit rare) adverse reactions during treatment with somatropin include [12]:

- glucose intolerance, including impaired glucose tolerance/ impaired fasting glucose, as well as (often unmasking latent) diabetes mellitus;
- intracranial hypertension, due to water retention;
- slipped capital femoral epiphysis;
- progression of pre-existing scoliosis;
- unmasking of latent central hypothyroidism;
- injection site reactions, rashes, and lipoatrophy; and
- generalized hypersensitivity reactions.

In an additional study of 273 pediatric patients born SGA and treated with GH, the following clinically significant events were reported [29]:

- mild transient hyperglycemia;
- benign intracranial hypertension;
- precocious puberty;
- jaw prominence;
- aggravation of preexisting scoliosis;
- injection site reactions; and
- self-limited progression of pigmented nevi.

Anti-GH antibodies have not been detected in any patients treated with GH.

The growth hormone–insulin-like growth factor 1 axis

The European Medicines Agency (EMA) recommended that insulin-like growth factor 1 (IGF-1) levels should not exceed the normal range during GH treatment, since there is concern that long term high IGF-1 levels can increase the risk for certain tumors (eg, breast cancer, prostate cancer) later in life. A 2001 study showed that IGF-1 levels in approximately 2.3% of prepubertal children and 11% in pubertal children born with a GH deficiency exceeded the 95th centile of the reference values for their age group during GH treatment [30]. The recommendation is that if a high level is measured, it should be repeated and if it is again above the normal range, the GH dose should be reduced.

Results from an ongoing study by Carel et al on the safety of GH treatments [31] suggest that patients treated with high doses of GH (>50 µg/kg/day) have an increased risk of mortality later in life (unpublished data from the Santé Adulte GH Enfant [SAGhE] study). This study is controversial because study design issues but the EMA recommends that doses exceeding 50 µg/kg/day should be avoided [31]. The issues and recommendations for GH treatment in children born SGA are summarized in Simon et al [32].

Changes in psychosocial features and body composition

Changes in psychosocial features

In addition to growth acceleration and gain in adult height, further effects of GH treatment have been studied and described. In an uncontrolled Dutch study [33], changes in intelligence and psychosocial functions of SGA children with GH treatment were measured and positive changes in IQ, behavior, and self-awareness were observed. These findings are encouraging, but require independent confirmation by additional controlled studies.

Changes in muscle, fatty tissue, and bone

Short children born SGA are characteristically slender and underweight. Compared to non-SGA peers, they have a severely reduced muscle mass and decreased fat mass. These findings come from studies that have examined the body composition of short SGA children in the following body parts with the following methods: upper arm with conventional anthropometric measurement methods [34], thigh with magnetic resonance imaging [35], upper arm and femur with peripheral quantitative computed tomography (pQCT) [36], or total body by dual energy X-ray absorptiometry (DXA) [35]. During GH treatment, short children born SGA showed a significant increase in muscle mass and a significant decrease in fat mass compared to untreated controls [37]. The increase in muscle mass was associated with an increase in muscle strength (Figure 15.2) [36].

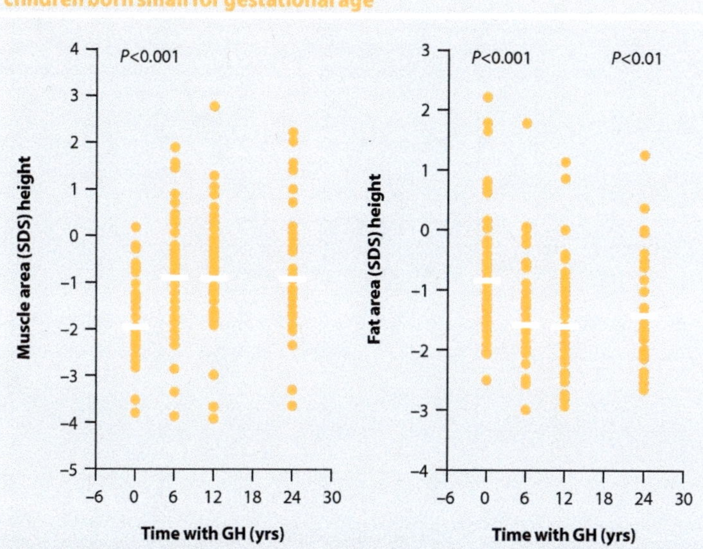

Figure 15.2 Changes of muscle and fat during growth hormone treatment in short children born small for gestational age. GH, growth hormone; SDS, standard deviation score. Modified with permission from Schweizer et al [36].

The reduced muscle mass and the short stature in children born SGA leads to a different bone structure when compared to non-SGA peers that is partially normalized through GH treatment. Bone mineral density (measured by DXA) is lower in short children born SGA compared with controls and increases significantly during GH treatment [38]. This effect is mainly due to height gain, because the bone mineral density assessed with DXA in prepubertal children largely depends on stature. But even after correction for body height and using a pQCT method that can represent the structure of bones more exactly, a bone structure with reduced bone strength index is more likely to be found in short children born SGA. GH treatment leads to an increase in bone area and cortical thickness (following an initial decrease in cortical bone density), which nevertheless results in an increase in bone strength index after 2 years of treatment (Figure 15.3) [39]. The effect of GH on bone age was described by Sas et al [40]. They showed a slight acceleration of about

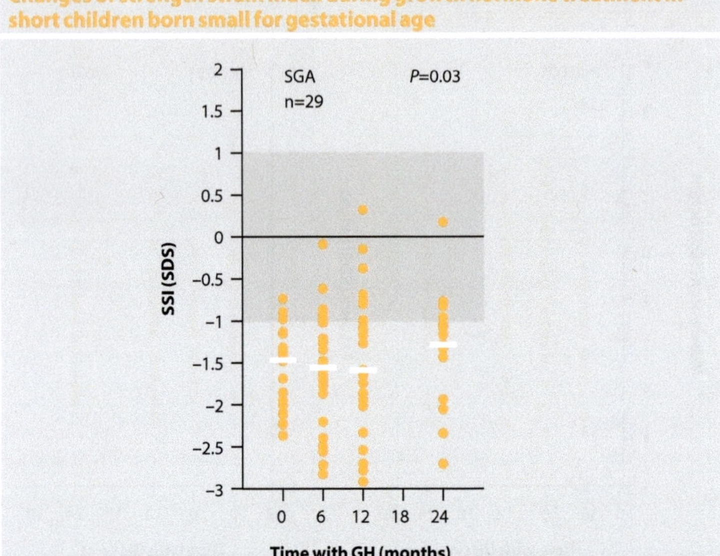

Figure 15.3 Changes of strength strain index during growth hormone treatment in short children born small for gestational age. GH, growth hormone; SGA, small for gestational age; SDS, standard deviation score; SSI, strength strain index. Modified with permission from Schweizer et al [36].

1.2–1.4 bone years per human year in the first 4 years of GH-treatment. Bone age acceleration is also observed in children born SGA not treated with GH. Therefore, the impact of the GH-induced acceleration on adult height remains controversial [41].

Changes in carbohydrate and lipid metabolism and blood pressure

On average, short children born SGA have a slightly increased insulin secretion compared with controls of similar age. During GH treatment, insulin secretion further increases, as would be expected [42]. There is a parallel decrease in insulin sensitivity which can be partially, but not fully, offset by the increase in muscle mass and decrease in fat mass [43]. Half a year after termination of GH treatment, insulin secretion was found to return to baseline levels [8] and to remain normal 6 years after GH treatment [12].

The serum levels of cholesterol – high density lipoprotein (HDL) cholesterol and low density lipoprotein (LDL) cholesterol – are normal in most SGA children, although LDL cholesterol levels can decrease significantly during GH treatment [7]. Children with initially increased cholesterol often show a normalization of their cholesterol levels under GH treatment (unpublished data from University Children's Hospital Tübingen). The blood pressure of many children born SGA can be slightly increased and returns to normal levels during GH treatment [7].

These observations are especially interesting in the context of reports from epidemiological studies that low birth weight is associated with an increased risk for developing a metabolic syndrome (insulin resistance, lipid increase, blood pressure increase) later in life [44,45]. Meanwhile, most experts assume that the main cause for metabolic disruptions later in life is not low birth weight itself, but the combination of low birth weight with rapid weight gain in the first few years of life.

It seems plausible that the aforementioned described changes in metabolism and body composition during GH treatment do not increase the risk for metabolic syndrome. A follow-up of SGA patients after GH treatment even found a reduction of risk factors for metabolic syndrome compared to untreated SGA children [12].

Summary

GH is approved for the treatment of short stature in children born SGA and leads to an increase in height during childhood as well as an increase in adult height (mean of approximately 7 cm). The question as to what dose should be given or which parameters the dose should be titrated to has not yet been definitively answered. The effect on growth is dose dependent in the first years of GH treatment but this effect is not shown thereafter or with regards to adult height. The dose should probably not be below 35 µg/kg/day, and GH doses exceeding 50 µg/kg/day should be avoided. Treatment should start before puberty and continue until the end of growth since a disruption can lead to loss of the gained height.

No definitive recommendation can be given with regards to the use of GnRH agonists to slow bone maturation, unless patients show signs of puberty before the age of 7 years, and further studies are needed.

To avoid potential late adverse effects the IGF-1 levels should be controlled regularly and the GH dose titrated to keep IGF-1 levels within the normal range. Furthermore, glucose metabolism should be checked regularly by determination of fasting insulin and blood glucose (Table 15.3). Besides increased growth, GH leads to an increase in the ratio of muscle mass to fat mass and appears to have a positive effect on the blood lipid profile and on blood pressure. The changes in glucose metabolism due to increased insulin levels are reversible upon cessation of GH treatment.

Minimum recommendations for regular controls during growth hormone treatment in short children born small for gestational age

Recommended controls	Time span
Height, weight	Twice a year (quarterly in the first 6 months)
IGF-1, IGFBP-3	Twice a year (quarterly in the first 6 months)
Fasting glucose, insulin, C-peptide	Once a year
Blood pressure	Once a year
X-ray of left hand for bone age	Once a year

Table 15.3 Minimum recommendations for regular controls during growth hormone treatment in short children born small for gestational age. IGF-1, insulin-like growth factor 1; IGFBP-3, insulin-like growth factor-binding protein 3.

References

1   Albertsson-Wikland K, Karlberg J. Natural growth in children born small for gestational age with and without catch-up growth. *Acta Paediatr Suppl.* 1994;399:64-70.
2   Hokken-Koelega AC, De Ridder MA, Lemmen RJ, et al. Children born small for gestational age: do they catch up? *Pediatr Res.* 1995;38:267-271.
3   Karlberg J, Albertsson-Wikland K. Growth in full-term small-for-gestational-age infants: from birth to final height. *Pediatr Res.* 1995;38:733-739.
4   Roede MJ, van Wieringen JC. Growth diagrams 1980: Netherlands third nation-wide survey. *Tijdschrift voor Sociale Gezondheidszorg.* 1985;63(suppl):1-34.
5   Ranke MB, Lindberg A; KIGS International Board. Height at start, first-year growth response and cause of shortness at birth are major determinants of adult height outcomes of short children born small for gestational age and Silver-Russell syndrome treated with growth hormone: analysis of data from KIGS. *Horm Res Paediatr.* 2010;74:259-266.
6   de Zegher F, Albertsson-Wikland K, Wollmann HA, et al. Growth hormone treatment of short children born small for gestational age: growth responses with continuous and discontinuous regimens over 6 years. *J Clin Endocrinol Metab.* 2000;85:2816-2821.
7   Sas TC, Gerver WJ, De Bruin R, et al. Body proportions during 6 years of GH treatment in children with short stature born small for gestational age participating in a randomised, double-blind, dose-response trial. *Clin Endocrinol (Oxf).* 2000;53:675-681.

8 Van Pareren Y, Mulder P, Houdijk M, Jansen M, Reeser M, Hokken-Koelega A. Adult height after long-term, continuous growth hormone (GH) treatment in short children born small for gestational age: results of a randomized, double-blind, dose-response GH trial. *J Clin Endocrinol Metab.* 2003;88:3584-3590.

9 Dahlgren J, Wikland KA; Swedish Study Group for Growth Hormone Treatment. Final height in short children born small for gestational age treated with growth hormone. *Pediatr Res.* 2005;57:216-222.

10 Martin DD, Jenni O, Ranke M, Thodberg HH, Binder G. The relationship between bone age and stature: implications for the paediatrician. *Horm Res Paediatr.* 2011;76(suppl 2):214.

11 Carel JC, Chatelain P, Rochiccioli P, Chaussain JL. Improvement in adult height after growth hormone treatment in adolescents with short stature born small for gestational age: results of a randomized controlled study. *J Clin.Endocrinol Metab.* 2003;88:1587-1593.

12 van Dijk M, Bannink EM, van Pareren YK, Mulder PG, Hokken-Koelega AC. Risk factors for diabetes mellitus type 2 and metabolic syndrome are comparable for previously growth hormone-treated young adults born small for gestational age (SGA) and untreated short SGA controls. *J Clin Endocrinol Metab.* 2007;92:160-165.

13 Maiorana A, Cianfarani S. Impact of growth hormone therapy on adult height of children born small for gestational age. *Pediatrics.* 2009;124:e519-e531.

14 Schweizer R, Martin D, Haase M, Ranke MB. Final height of short children born small for gestational age (SGA) treated with growth hormone (GH) in a single centre. *Horm Res.* 2007;68(suppl 1):209.

15 Ranke MB, Lindberg A. Growth hormone treatment of short children born small for gestational age or with Silver-Russell syndrome: results from KIGS (Kabi International Growth Study), including the first report on final height. *Acta Paediatr Suppl.* 1996;417:18-26.

16 Coutant R, Carel JC, Letrait M, et al. Short stature associated with intrauterine growth retardation: final height of untreated and growth hormone-treated children. *J Clin Endocrinol Metab.* 1998;83:1070-1074.

17 Zucchini S, Cacciari E, Balsamo A, et al. Final height of short subjects of low birth weight with and without growth hormone treatment. *Arch Dis Child.* 2001;84:340-343.

18 Rosilio M, Carel JC, Ecosse E, Chaussainon JL. Adult height of prepubertal short children born small for gestational age treated with GH. *Eur J Endocrinol.* 2005;152:835-843.

19 Bannink EM, van Doorn J, Mulder PG, Hokken-Koelega AC. Free/dissociable insulin-like growth factor (IGF)-I, not total IGF-1, correlates with growth response during growth hormone treatment in children born small for gestational age. *J Clin Endocrinol Metab.* 2007;92:2992-3000.

20 Boguszewski MCS, Lindberg A, Wollmann HA. Two years growth response to growth hormone (GH) treatment in very young children born small for gestational age (SGA) - data from KIGS. *Horm Res Paediatr.* 2010;74(suppl 3):155.

21 Argente J, Gracia R, Ibáñez L, et al; for the Spanish SGA Working Group. Improvement in growth after two years of growth hormone therapy in very young children born small for gestational age and without spontaneous catch-up growth: results of a multicenter, controlled, randomized, open clinical trial. *J Clin Endocrinol Metab.* 2007;92:3095-3101.

22 Fjellestad-Paulsen A, Simon D, Czernichow P. Short children born small for gestational age and treated with growth hormone for three years have an important catch-down five years after discontinuation of treatment. *J Clin Endocrinol Metab.* 2004;89:1234-1239.

23 de Zegher F, Du Caju MV, Heinrichs C, et al. Early, discontinuous, high dose growth hormone treatment to normalize height and weight of short children born small for gestational age: results over 6 years. *J Clin Endocrinol Metab.* 1999;84:1558-1561.

24 Binder G, Baur F, Schweizer R, Ranke MB. The d3-growth hormone (GH) receptor polymorphism is associated with increased responsiveness to GH in Turner syndrome and short small-for-gestational-age children. *J Clin Endocrinol Metab.* 2006;91:659-664.

25 Ranke MB, Lindberg A, Cowell CT, et al; for the KIGS International Board. Prediction of response to growth hormone treatment in short children born small for gestational age: analysis of data from KIGS (Pharmacia International Growth Database). *J Clin Endocrinol Metab*. 2003;88:125-131.

26 Ranke MB, Lindberg A; for the KIGS International Board. Prediction models for short children born small for gestational age (SGA) covering the total growth phase. Analyses based on data from KIGS (Pfizer International Growth Database). *BMC Med Inform Decis Mak*. 2011;11:38.

27 Carel JC, Eugster EA, Rogol A, et al. Consensus statement on the use of gonadotropin-releasing hormone analogs in children. *Pediatrics*. 2009;123:e752-e762.

28 van Gool SA, Kamp GA, Visser-van Balen H, et al. Final height outcome after three years of growth hormone and gonadotropin-releasing hormone agonist treatment in short adolescents with relatively early puberty. *J Clin Endocrinol Metab*. 2007;92:1402-1408.

29 Food and Drug Administration. Draft package insert for Genotropin (NDA 20-280/S-031). FDA Website. www.accessdata.fda.gov/drugsatfda_docs/label/2001/20280s31lbl.pdf. Accessed February 20, 2013.

30 Ranke MB, Schweizer R, Elmlinger MW, et al. Relevance of IGF-1, IGFBP-3, and IGFBP-2 measurements during GH treatment of GH-deficient and non-GH-deficient children and adolescents. *Horm Res*. 2001;55:115-124.

31 European Medicines Agency. "Update on somatropin-containing medicines." EMA website. www.ema.europa.eu/ema/index.jsp?curl=pages/news_and_events/news/2010/12/news_detail_001167.jsp&mid=WC0b01ac058004d5c1&murl=menus/news_and_events/news_and_events.jsp. Accessed February 20, 2013.

32 Simon D, Leger J, Carel JC. Optimal use of growth hormone therapy for maximizing adult height in children born small for gestational age. *Best Pract Res Clin Endocrinol Metab*. 2008;22:525-537.

33 van Pareren YK, Duivenvoorden HJ, Slijper FS, Koot HM, Hokken-Koelega AC. Intelligence and psychosocial functioning during long-term growth hormone therapy in children born small for gestational age. *J Clin Endocrinol Metab*. 2004;89:5295-5302.

34 Hediger ML, Overpeck MD, Kuczmarski RJ, McGlynn A, Maurer KR, Davis WW. Muscularity and fatness of infants and young children born small- or large-for-gestational-age. *Pediatrics*. 1998;102:E60.

35 Leger J, Garel C, Fjellestad-Paulsen A, Hassan M, Czernichow P. Human growth hormone treatment of short-stature children born small for gestational age: effect on muscle and adipose tissue mass during a 3-year treatment period and after 1 year's withdrawal. *J Clin Endocrinol Metab*. 1998;83:3512-3516.

36 Schweizer R, Martin DD, Schönau E, Ranke MB. Muscle function improves during growth hormone therapy in short children born small for gestational age: results of a peripheral quantitative computed tomography study on body composition. *J Clin Endocrinol Metab*. 2008;93:2978-2983.

37 Willemsen RH, Arends NJT, Bakker-van Waarde WM, et al. Long-term effects of growth hormone on body composition and bone mineral density in short children born small-for-gestational-age: six-year follow-up of a randomized controlled GH trail. *Clinical Endocrinology*. 2007;67:485-492.

38 Arends NJT, Boonstra VH, Mulder PGH, et al. GH treatment and its effect on bone mineral density, bone maturation and growth in short children born small for gestational age: 3-year results of a randomized, controlled GH trial. *Clinical Endocrinology*. 2003;59:779-787.

39 Schweizer R, Martin DD, Haase M, et al. Similar effects of long-term exogenous growth hormone (GH) on bone and muscle parameters: A pQCT study of GH-deficient and small-for-gestational-age (SGA) children. *Bone*. 2007;41:875-881.

40 Sas T, de Waal W, Mulder P, et al. Growth hormone treatment in children with short stature born small for gestational age: 5-year results of a randomized, double-blind, dose-response trial. *J Clin Endocrinol Metab*. 1999;84:3064-3070.

41 Martin DD, Wit JM, Hochberg Z, et al. The use of bone age in clinical practice – part one. *Horm Res Paediatr*. 2011;76:1-9.

42 Sas T, Mulder P, Aanstoot HJ, et al. Carbohydrate metabolism during long-term growth hormone treatment in children with short stature born small for gestational age. *Clin Endocrinol (Oxf)*. 2001;54:243-251.

43 Martin DD, Schweizer R, Schönau E, Binder G, Ranke MB. Growth hormone-induced increases in skeletal muscle mass alleviates the associated insulin resistance in short children born small for gestational age, but not with growth hormone deficiency. *Horm Res*. 2009;72:38-45.

44 Barker DJ, Hales CN, Fall CH, Osmond C, Phipps K, Clark PM. Type 2 (non-insulin-dependent) diabetes mellitus, hypertension and hyperlipidaemia (syndrome X): relation to reduced fetal growth. *Diabetologia*. 1993;36:62-67.

45 Lévy-Marchal C, Czernichow P. Small for gestational age and the metabolic syndrome: which mechanism is suggested by epidemiological and clinical studies? *Horm Res*. 2006;65:123-130.

Development of this book was supported by funding from Sandoz

Chapter 16

Renal function
Jörg Dötsch

Introduction

It has been shown that there is a correlation between low birth weight and adverse cardiovascular and renal outcomes [1]. This relationship can become evident as early as childhood and may include arterial hypertension, glomerular disease, and renal failure; these conditions are often ascribed to a phenomenon called 'fetal programming.' Other conditions potentially leading to an adverse renal outcome caused by fetal programming are maternal diabetes mellitus, preeclampsia, maternal hypertension, excessive salt intake, and glucocorticoid use during pregnancy. There are numerous underlying mechanisms involved in fetal programming of renal disease including:

- reduced nephron number via diminished nephrogenesis;
- renal alterations (eg, via the intrarenal renal renin–angiotensin aldosterone system); and
- non-renal alternations (eg, changes in endothelial function).

Additionally, it seems likely that the outcome of fetal programming is influenced postnatally [2].

Low birth weight and renal function

Low birth weight has been found to be associated with an increase in arterial blood pressure in later life. A recent meta-analysis showed a drop of approximately 1 mmHg systolic blood pressure per kilogram of birth

S. Zabransky (ed.), *Caring for Children Born Small for Gestational Age*,
DOI: 10.1007/978-1-908517-90-6_16, © Springer Healthcare 2013

weight [3]. Additionally, as shown in recent studies, end-stage renal failure has an increased prevalence in adults who were born small for gestational age (SGA) [4,5]. However, the following fundamental questions need to be addressed in more detail and require further elucidation:

- Is low birth weight a primary risk factor for renal dysfunction in later life?
- Is epidemiological evidence showing an increased risk of later renal dysfunction in low birth-weight infants robust?

Ultimately, further investigation is needed to reveal crucial underlying mechanisms and to delineate the role of the postnatal period in fetal programming of renal diseases.

Causes of fetal programming

Low birth weight is only one possible cause leading to fetal programming of renal disease. Another hypothesis is an 'overload' of nutrients in utero. This can either be observed on a general basis (eg, maternal obesity) or on a more specific basis (eg, maternal diabetes mellitus). Both conditions may cause infants to be born with a higher than average birth weight and have a subsequent predisposition for metabolic syndrome. This observation can be explained by the lower incidence of extreme variants, as well as by the more subtle phenotype outcomes in the offspring themselves [6].

The more heterogeneous group of programming events leading to fetal programming of renal disease includes maternal stress, preeclampsia, maternal hypertension, glucocorticoid use, and excessive salt intake. Regardless of the origin, there is increasing data suggesting that the postnatal environment not only modifies intrauterine growth but may induce postnatal programming, even after a normal pregnancy [2]. This is due to the fact that critical windows for programming are not necessarily 'closed' with birth but may persist into infancy and even childhood. Therefore, both prenatal and postnatal situations need to be considered in the context of programming of renal function.

Perinatal programming and energy deficiency
Epidemiological and experimental evidence

A relatively low birth weight has been associated with many subsequent health problems. Over the last decade, various epidemiological studies have tried to prove the association between lower birth weight and elevated blood pressure later in life. For example, a 2002 meta-analysis examined the impact of study size and investigators on the severity of hypertension. The authors found that studies with fewer participants showed a more pronounced inverse association between birth weight and blood pressure [7]. However, in larger studies ($n>3000$), the authors still found a systolic blood pressure decrease of 0.6 mmHg per kg of birth weight [7]. Even when an adjustment for present weight was omitted, the calculated blood pressure reduction reached 0.4 mmHg/kg.

These observations may indicate that low birth weight is a risk factor for later blood pressure elevation. However, an epidemiological linkage of birth weight and elevated arterial blood pressure later in life does not sufficiently address the issue of perinatal programming of hypertension. Nevertheless, perinatal programming of hypertension should be considered when screening for and treating complex metabolic and cardiovascular diseases in later life due to the pathogenic link between excess body weight, blood pressure elevation, diabetes, and metabolic syndrome with low birth weight.

In 2000, Lackland et al reported that low birth weight was associated with early onset end-stage renal failure in US residents from a variety of ethnic backgrounds [8]. Within the study of patients ($n=1230$) with end-stage renal disease (ESRD), the odds ratio (OR) for renal failure was 1.4 (95% confidence interval [CI], 1.1–1.8) for the entire group, including patients with diabetes mellitus and hypertension. More recently, Li et al reported that men who self-reported having a relatively low or a relatively high birth weight were more likely to display evidence of chronic kidney disease (CKD) when screened using estimated glomerular filtration rate (GFR) [9]. A U-shaped association between birth weight and CKD in men was observed; compared with men whose birth weight was 3000–3999 g, those whose birth weight was <2500 g were 1.65 times more likely to develop CKD (95% CI, 1.24–2.20), whilst those whose birth weight was >4500 g were 1.41 times more likely to develop CKD (95% CI, 1.06–1.88) [9].

Focusing on ESRD as a clinical endpoint, a large population-based cohort study of children born in Norway between 1967 and 2004 found that children with a birth weight below the 10th percentile (classified as SGA) had a higher risk of end-stage renal failure than those who were not born SGA (relative risk 1.5; 95% CI, 1.2–1.9) [5]. Furthermore, when compared to controls, the development of ESRD in children born SGA seemed to be more common before 14 years of age than after [5]. As patients under the age of 14 years are unlikely to have factors predisposing for chronic renal failure (eg, diabetes mellitus and hypertension), the reason for higher incidence of ESRD under the age of 14, and whether it is related to congenital malformation, remains unclear. While this study was able to show an association between birth weight and ESRD, not all studies have been able to demonstrate altered renal function in SGA children [10].

In a meta-analysis by White et al that included 32 studies, 16 studies reported a significant association between low birth weight and risk of CKD, while 16 did not observe a correlation [11]. The combination of weighted estimates from the 18 studies for which risk estimates were available (n=46,249; total of 2,183,317 subjects from the record linkage study) gave an overall OR of 1.73 (95% CI, 1.44–2.08). Combined ORs were consistent in magnitude and direction for risks of albuminuria (OR=1.81; 95% CI, 1.19–2.77), ESRD (OR=1.58; 95% CI, 1.33–1.88), and low estimated GFR (OR=1.79; 95% CI, 1.31–2.45) [11]. An increased prevalence of albuminuria in children born SGA (even as early as 18 months of age) was shown in a more recent study [12].

Glomerular disease in childhood and relation to birth weight

Idiopathic or minimal lesion nephrotic syndrome in childhood is usually associated with a good prognosis and an initial complete response to glucocorticoids with resolution of proteinuria in about 90% of patients [13]. Retrospective clinical studies have reported that children with a history of low birth weight who develop idiopathic nephrotic syndrome have a higher incidence of relapses and steroid dependence [14,15]. Other recent studies have confirmed a more severe course and a higher rate of steroid resistance in children with nephrotic syndrome that were born SGA [16,17]. However, the underlying mechanisms linking low birth weight and glomerular disease have not yet been delineated.

Data reported in the 1990s indicate that up to 30% of patients with immunoglobulin A (IgA) nephropathy (or Berger's disease) presenting in childhood eventually develop end-stage renal failure [18]. A retrospective study of 62 children with IgA nephropathy reported three times as many sclerotic glomeruli among children with IgA nephropathy who were born SGA compared with those who had an average birth weight [19]. However, more recent data linking birth weight with progression of Henoch-Schönlein purpura nephritis, an IgA-mediated systemic vasculitic disorder, does not suggest a substantial influence of birth weight but rather indicates that postnatal catch-up growth subsequent to low birth weight might play a pivotal role on progression of renal disease [20].

Intrauterine growth restriction and later morbidity: animal models

Most data originating from human studies are based on epidemiological associations. Although epidemiological methods minimize confounding factors as much as possible, such studies are associative and thus cannot prove definitive causal relationships. Studies on laboratory animals have been useful in elucidating a causal relationship between an initial programming event such as intrauterine growth restriction (IUGR) and later morbidity. Protein restriction in laboratory animals has been the most widely used method for demonstrating how IUGR affects the cardiovascular system and the kidney [21–23]. In such studies, pregnant rats are fed an isocaloric, protein-restricted diet, varying from 10–40% of normal protein intake. This model mimics protein restriction, which is thought to be a frequent cause for IUGR in developing countries.

Animal models can be used to examine both causal relationships and mechanisms. For example, the protein-restricted model was employed to examine susceptibility to acquired renal diseases. Plank et al studied male IUGR offspring of protein-restricted mothers and observed that these offspring subsequently had increased susceptibility to a more severe and potentially chronic course of acute mesangioproliferative glomerulonephritis when this condition was induced by an injection of anti-Thy-1.1 antibody [24]. Similar observations were made for arterial hypertension [25].

One interesting question recently addressed in the rat model is whether the impairment in nephrogenesis is passed on to further generations. Harrison and Langeley-Evans have shown that there is in fact intergenerational programming of impaired nephrogenesis and hypertension in the second generation [26]. The use of animal models in studying mechanisms of fetal programming are reviewed further by Langley-Evans and Nuyt [27,28].

Mechanisms contributing to fetal programming

Nephron number

Nephron number has been acknowledged as a determinant of susceptibility to renal disease and possibly the development of hypertension in both animal and human studies [29–35]. During nephrogenesis, both intrinsic and extrinsic factors 'program' an individual's nephron number, ultimately resulting in what has been named 'nephron endowment' [35]. Following the completion of nephrogenesis no further nephrons are formed, and aging or renal injury decreases nephron number.

The hypothesis was confirmed by Keller et al who showed an inverse relationship of glomerular count and blood pressure in previously healthy accident victims by renal autopsy [33]. For this study, kidney size was used as approximation for nephron number, and it was found that in children affected by IUGR, kidney size was reduced [33]. A recent study shows that twin infants born prematurely and SGA with a birth weight below the third percentile are unable to achieve catch-up growth in kidney length in the first 24 months of life [36]. In a retrospective cohort study (n=206), 36% of patients with a single functioning kidney showed hypertension, albuminuria, or a need for renoprotective medication at the median age of 9.5 years [37]. However, the hypothesis falls short of explaining why patients with unilateral renal agenesis do not suffer from hypertension in later life [38].

Renin-angiotensin-aldosterone system

A number of vasoactive systems that contribute to nephrogenesis seem to be altered in response to a change in the intrauterine milieu. An important indicator of changes in the prenatal environment that might lead to fetal programming of renal disease is thought to be an alteration in the renin-angiotensin-aldosterone system (RAAS) [39].

Experimental models of fetal programming have shown an increased renal renin expression in adult rats subsequent to IUGR due to maternal protein restriction during gestation. [39–41]. In neonatal rats born to protein-restricted dams, there was a suppression of the RAAS [21]. More recently, it was reported that the adrenal expression of the angiotensin II type-1b receptor in rats with IUGR is increased [41]. This is probably due to an epigenetic mechanism, as the authors observed that the proximal promoter of the angiotensin II type-1b receptor gene was hypomethylated, which facilitates heightened transcriptional activity. In humans, there is only one angiotensin II type-1 receptor, rendering it unclear whether these findings would apply to humans. However, increased salt sensitivity was reported to be present in children with low birth weight, which might indicate a higher aldosterone activity or a change in angiotensin II type-1 receptor expression or affinity [42]. These results indicate that RAAS is primarily suppressed after IUGR before it becomes hyperactive later in life, which ultimately might contribute to hypertension and renal disease.

Another renal alteration that has been reported in models of maternal protein restriction is a deregulation of the activity of 11β-hydroxysteroid dehydrogenase [11βHSD]. This enzyme, present in the cells of the distal renal tubule, converts active cortisol into inactive cortisone [43]. Under physiological circumstances, this reaction protects the mineralocorticoid receptor from stimulation by cortisol. In the IUGR rat model, renal 11βHSD expression is reduced, allowing for increased mineralocorticoid activity [44]. Interestingly, a reduction of 11βHSD has been reported in the placenta of human pregnancies complicated by IUGR [45,46]. These observations imply that maternal cortisol, which is usually inactivated by the placental 11βHSD type 2, can be passed to the fetus. As a consequence, cortisol may lead to growth restriction and potentially to a programming of renal 11βHSD deregulation in the unborn child [43,44,47].

Extrarenal tissue

In addition to renal mechanisms, programming of extrarenal tissue has been investigated with regard to potential roles in increasing the risk of future renal and vascular disease. For example, the endothelium and its interaction with vascular smooth muscle cells via multiple signaling systems (eg, renal nitric oxide system) may contribute to the likelihood of future arterial hypertension, and renal and vascular disease [48–51; Figure 16.1 and Figure 16.2]. Apart from functional changes at the vessel site, there is evidence that impaired vascular structure is encountered in IUGR. For instance, lower elastin content has already been shown in the aorta of rats with IUGR [52]. In addition, a rarefication of arterioles and capillaries is seen in former low-birth-weight infants at young adulthood [53]. However, these changes might be secondary due to the functional impairment of vascular regulation and hypertension. Newer studies show vascular and myocardial changes that are already present at birth in a protein restriction model of IUGR [54]. In line with these experimental results, infants born with a low birth weight show an increased intima-media thickness at birth [55].

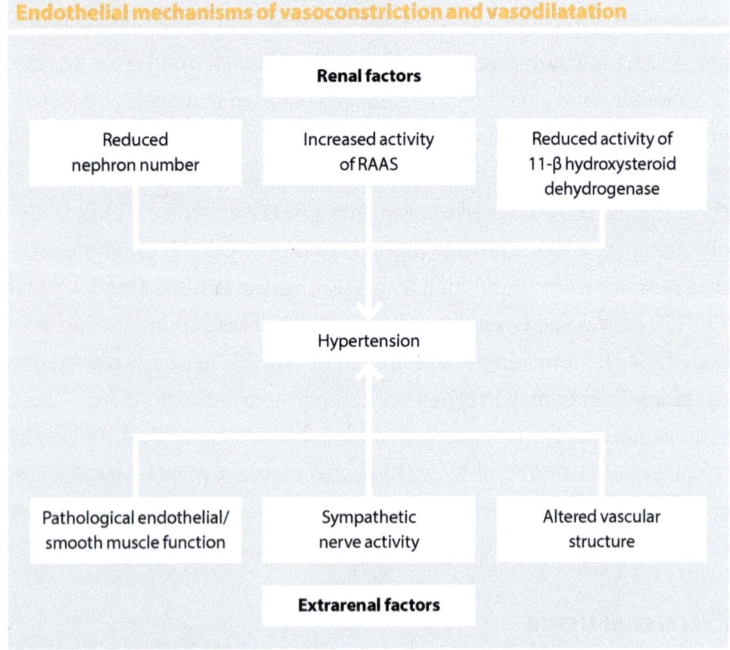

Figure 16.1 Endothelial mechanisms of vasoconstriction and vasodilatation.
RAAS, renin-angiotensin-aldosterone system.

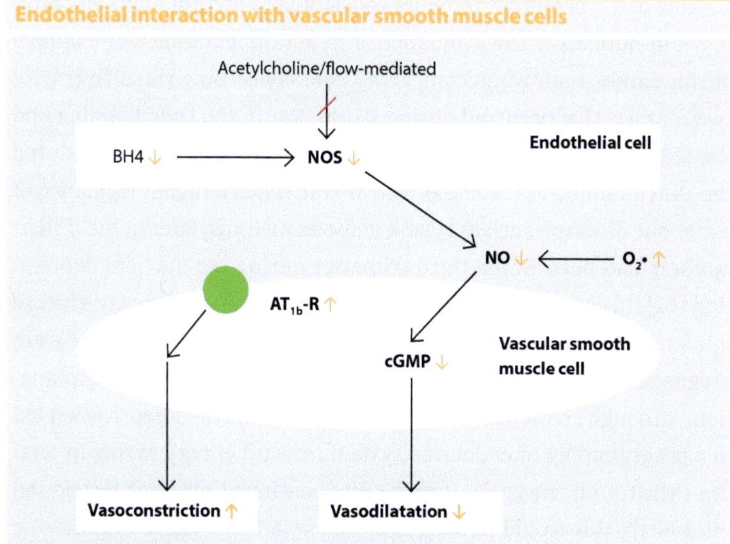

Figure 16.2 Endothelial interaction with vascular smooth muscle cells. AT_{1b}-R, angiotensin receptor subtype 1b; BH4, tetrahydrobiopterin; cGMP, cyclic guanosine monophosphate; NO, nitric acid; NOS, nitric acid synthase; O_2•, oxygen free radicals.

Another extrarenal mechanism that has been considered in the context of fetal programming of kidney disease is increased sympathetic nerve activity, as there is a relation between birth weight and basal heart rate in adulthood [56]. The hypothesis that increased sympathetic nerve activity is a consequence of a challenging intrauterine environment is supported by animal data reporting that denervation of renal sympathetic nerve supply leads to normalization of blood pressure in IUGR rats [57]. Such a mechanism is important for renal function, as sympathetic nerve activity regulates intrarenal renin synthesis and salt retention.

Postnatal modification

In animal studies, early postnatal and periodic supplementation with fish oil, a low sodium diet, angiotensin-converting enzyme inhibitors, the superoxide dismutase mimetic tempol, or immunosuppression with mycophenolate mofetil have been shown to counterbalance adverse fetal programming of arterial hypertension [58–60].

One of the potential strategies considered to prevent morbidity after IUGR in humans is the avoidance of hyperalimentation. An example of this can be seen when comparing data concerning the offspring of two famines that occurred during World War II: the Dutch famine and the Siege of Leningrad [61,62]. The offspring of women who endured the Dutch famine at the end of World War II had a higher incidence of metabolic diseases, such as type 2 diabetes mellitus, later in life if their mothers had been in the third trimester during the nutrient depriva-tion [61]. In contrast, there was no increase in the incidence of glucose intolerance or type 2 diabetes among offspring whose mothers were pregnant during the siege of Leningrad [62]. The traditional explana-tion, although challenged, is that intrauterine nutrient deprivation led to a programming of endocrine systems toward energy saving in fetal life ('thrifty phenotype'). If there was continued nutrient restriction after birth, this would be well tolerated by a baby whose intrauterine environment was similarly deprived (as in the Leningrad offspring). In contrast, rapid reconstitution of energy supplies and, therefore relative surplus of energy, as was the case with offspring of the Dutch famine, would lead to deposition of adipose tissue, predisposing to pathological glucose tolerance. Details concerning this so-called 'match–mismatch' phenomenon are summarized in a recent review by Gluckman et al (see Figure 12.2) [63].

There is considerable evidence that rapid increase in caloric and protein intake postnatally plays an important pathophysiological role in developmental origins of disease [64]. Low birth weight and pre-mature infants grow at different rates and rapid catch-up growth may not be beneficial and may even be associated with high blood pressure [65,66]. Given such reports, the International Societies of Pediatric Endocrinology and the Growth Hormone Research Society presently discourage nutrient-enriched diets for low birth-weight infants [64].

Whether these observations are of importance for renal function as well is not yet known and might be subject for future studies. In the previously discussed retrospective study of 62 children with idiopathic nephrotic syndrome, the authors looked at the course of the disease and related it to birth weight and weight gain in the first 24 months of life [16].

In this study, an association between the extent of postnatal catch-up growth and the severity of disease was not observed. More recently, Alejandre Alcázar et al showed that postnatal hyperalimentation leads to a dysregulated signaling of neuropeptide Y in renal tissue. The data demonstrate that factors in the early postnatal environment exert important changes in the tubular function [67]. Most interestingly, this was shown in animals with no former IUGR.

Perinatal programming

Energy surplus

The classical nutritional 'surplus' situation for a fetus is poorly controlled maternal diabetes mellitus. The pathophysiological context is quite well established: high maternal glucose concentrations are freely passed to the fetus via the placenta. This leads to beta cell stimulation and an excess in insulin secretion in the fetus. Hyperinsulinism not only leads to an increased cellular uptake of glucose in the macrosomic phenotype, but also to a stimulation of cerebral insulin receptors that modify energy expenditure and 'program' the hypothalamic regulation of appetite and energy expenditure later in life.

Human data on the fetal programming of arterial hypertension and renal function during maternal diabetes is very scarce. A recent study has addressed the changes in GFR and blood pressure in 19 non-diabetic offspring of mothers with type 1 diabetes and in 18 non-diabetic offspring of fathers with type 1 diabetes aged 18–41 years [5]. Under basal conditions, GFR, mean arterial pressure, and renal vascular resistances were similar between the two groups [5]. Only stimulation with amino acid infusions showed that GFR and effective renal plasma flow increased less in offspring of type 1 diabetic mothers than in control subjects. Additionally, mean arterial pressure and renal vascular resistances declined less in offspring from mothers with diabetes than in control subjects [5]. The authors conclude that maternal diabetes may lead to a reduced number of nephrons undergoing hyperfiltration and predispose offspring to glomerular and vascular disease [5]. The strength of this study is that it examined renal function with state-of-the-art in vivo methods and controlled for genetic variables by having offspring of diabetic fathers as the control group.

Until now, however, there are no human studies that have measured nephron number in the offspring of diabetic mothers.

In male rat offspring, maternal diabetes had a long-term effect on vascular reactivity and renal function [68]. Exposure to maternal diabetes induces salt-sensitive hypertension and impairs renal function in adult rat offspring [69]. More recently, Chen et al demonstrated that the intrarenal renin-angiotensin and the transforming-growth-factor beta system might play a role in the perinatal programming of hypertension and renal injury [70]. A previous article from the same group also demonstrated a role for the NF-κB pathway in impaired nephrogenesis in the offspring of diabetic rats [71]. The effect of maternal diabetes can, at least in animal models, be enhanced by simultaneous sodium chloride overload [72].

A more complex situation of energy overload of the fetus is maternal obesity. This leads to hyperinsulinism and hyperleptinism in mothers and their fetuses. In addition, a number of partially proinflammatory adipokines are increased in the maternal circulation. It is quite likely that these alterations may influence the fetus and its renal development. However, data to support this notion is scarce.

There are some data on the effect of early postnatal overfeeding on renal function. Boubred et al have shown that postnatal hyperalimentation increases nephron number but impairs renal development by causing glomerulosclerosis [73]. In conclusion, nutrient surplus is at least as important for perinatal programming as nutrient deficiency.

Other causes

Excessive salt intake

Salt overload is an important risk factor for renal disease in postnatal life. Therefore, the hypothesis that an increased salt intake during pregnancy leads to renal impairment via fetal programming has been tested in animal models [74]. As expected, changes in the function of RAAS were observed after increased salt exposure during fetal life. The combination of prenatal and postnatal salt overload resulted in a more prominent phenotype with regard to the reduction of GFR and an increase in renal protein excretion [74]. In this context, a developmental window may exist which allows postnatal reprogramming of hypertension.

Interestingly, in another animal model, mild overexposure to salt lead to a more rapid excretion of oral salt in the offspring [75]. However, when the salt exposure of the pregnant animal exceeded potential physiological intakes, the beneficial adaption of salt excretion was lost.

Glucocorticoids

Pregnant women often have to take glucocorticoids for a variety of reasons: to prevent respiratory distress syndrome and enhance pulmonary maturation in the fetus, to treat immunological diseases, or to avoid rejection after organ transplantation. Whether this leads to fetal programming in humans remains controversial.

There are data from animal studies showing an adverse effect of glucocorticoids on renal development. For example, it has been shown that dexamethasone treatment of mice during mid-gestation reduces nephron number and leads to an increased expression of bone morphogenetic protein 4 and transforming growth factor beta in the fetus [76]. However, a 15–20 day course of dexamethasone had no effect on blood pressure in the offspring of rats [77]. Therefore, unlike the effect of glucocorticoids on the programming of the metabolic syndrome, no conclusive data for the effect of glucocorticoids on renal function are available [78].

Maternal hypertension and preeclampsia

Up to 9.1% of all pregnancies are complicated by maternal hypertension. Preeclampsia, defined as a pregnancy-specific syndrome with blood pressure elevation and albuminuria after gestational week 20, is diagnosed in 1.4–4.0% of all pregnancies [79]. Tenhola et al demonstrated blood pressure elevation by the age of 12 in study participants born to mothers with preeclampsia [80].

Additionally, in a large cohort of the Avon longitudinal study of parents and children, offspring of women with preeclampsia presented elevation of systolic and diastolic blood pressure [81]. Gestational hypertension of the mothers increased systolic blood pressure and diastolic blood pressure at that age. Interestingly, in none of the cohorts the offspring showed vascular alterations or metabolic derangements. The authors concluded that this might be indicative for a non-metabolic 'shared mother–offspring risk factor' [81]. A second analysis of the same study excluded familial adiposity as the sole explanation for the development of blood pressure elevation in the offspring of hypertensive mothers. Nevertheless, the high rate of IUGR in the offspring of women with preeclampsia may cause a different, and perhaps more complex, pathogenic pathway in this population [82]. Although the association between a hypertensive prenatal environment and early blood pressure elevation during youth seems likely, additional data on the mediating mechanism is still needed.

It also seems likely that the outcomes of fetal programming may be influenced postnatally, for example, by the nutritional factors during critical vulnerable developmental periods (Figure 16.3). Thus, it is important to consider how much alimentation and salt intake should be provided during a neonatal intensive care unit stay, or whether, in some circumstances, it should be avoided altogether.

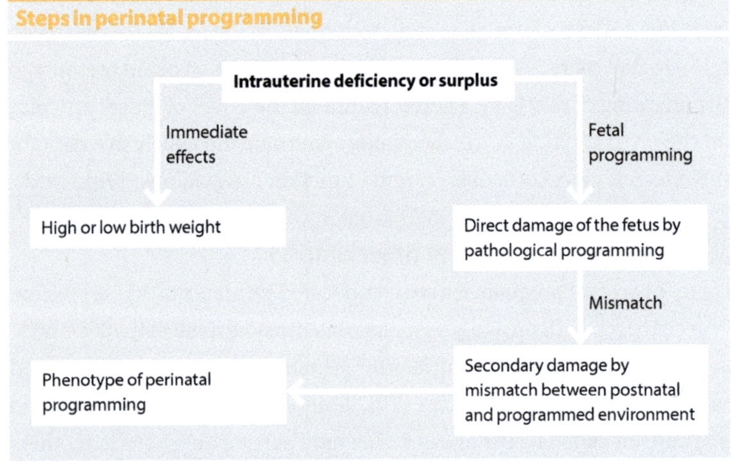

Figure 16.3 Steps in perinatal programming.

References

1   Reyes L, Mānalich R. Long-term consequences of low birth weight. *Kidney Intl Suppl.* 2005;(suppl):S107-S111.

2   Dötsch J, Plank C, Amann K, Ingelfinger J. The implications of fetal programming of glomerular number and renal function. *J Mol Med (Berl).* 2009;87:841-848.

3   Gamborg M, Byberg L, Rasmussen F, et al. Birth weight and systolic blood pressure in adolescence and adulthood: meta-regression analysis of sex- and age-specific results from 20 Nordic studies. *Am J Epidemiol.* 2007;166:634-645.

4 Lackland DT, Egan BM, Fan ZJ, Syddall HE. Low birth weight contributes to the excess prevalence of end-stage renal disease in African Americans. *J Clin Hypertens [Greenwich]*. 2001;3:29-31.

5 Vikse BE, Irgens LM, Leivestad T, Hallan S, Iversen BM. Low birth weight increases risk for end-stage renal disease. *J Am Soc Nephrol*. 2008;19:151-157.

6 Abi Khalil C, Travert F, Fetita S, et al. Fetal exposure to maternal type 1 diabetes is associated with renal dysfunction at adult age. *Diabetes*. 2010;59:2631-2636.

7 Huxley R, Neil A, Collins R. Unravelling the fetal origins hypothesis: is there really an inverse association between birthweight and subsequent blood pressure? *Lancet*. 2002;360:659-665.

8 Lackland DT, Bendall HE, Osmond C, Egan BM, Barker DJ. Low birth weights contribute to high rates of early-onset chronic renal failure in the Southeastern United States. *Arch Intern Med*. 2000;160:1472-1476.

9 Li S, Chen SC, Shlipak M, et al; Kidney Early Evaluation Program Investigators. Low birth weight is associated with chronic kidney disease only in men. *Kidney Int*. 2008;73:637-642.

10 Franco MC, Nishida SK, Sesso R. GFR estimated from cystatin C versus creatinine in children born small for gestational age. *Am J Kidney Dis*. 2008;51:925-932.

11 White SL, Perkovic V, Cass A, et al. Is low birth weight an antecedent of CKD in later life? A systematic review of observational studies. *Am J Kidney Dis*. 2009;54:248-261.

12 Zanardo V, Fanelli T, Weiner G, et al. Intrauterine growth restriction is associated with persistent aortic wall thickening and glomerular proteinuria during infancy. *Kidney Int*. 2011;80:119-123.

13 Dötsch J, Dittrich K, Plank C, Rascher W. Is tacrolimus for childhood steroid-dependent nephrotic syndrome better than ciclosporin A? *Nephrol. Dial Transplant*. 2006;21:1761-1763.

14 Sheu JN, Chen JH. Minimal change nephrotic syndrome in children with intrauterine growth retardation. *Am J Kidney Dis*. 2001;37:909-914.

15 Zidar N, Avgustin Cavic M, Kenda RB, Ferluga D. Unfavorable course of minimal change nephrotic syndrome in children with intrauterine growth retardation. *Kidney Int*. 1998;54:1320-1323.

16 Plank C, Östreicher I, Dittrich K, et al. Low birth-weight, but not postnatal weight gain aggravates the course of nephrotic syndrome in children. *Pediatr Nephrol*. 2007;22:1881-1889.

17 Teeninga N, Schreuder MF, Bökenkamp A, Delemarre-van de Waal HA, van Wijk JA. Influence of low birth weight on minimal change nephrotic syndrome in children, including a meta-analysis. *Nephrol Dial Transplant*. 2008;23:1615-1620.

18 Goldstein AR, White RH, Akuse R, Chantler C. Long-term follow-up of childhood Henoch-Schönlein nephritis. *Lancet*. 1992;339:280-282.

19 Zidar N, Cavić MA, Kenda RB, Koselj M, Ferluga D. Effect of intrauterine growth retardation on the clinical course and prognosis of IgA glomerulonephritis in children. *Nephron*. 1998;79:28-32.

20 Plank C, Vasilache I, Dittrich K, Dötsch J. Early weight gain and outcome in Henoch-Schönlein nephritis. *Klin Padiatr*. 2010;222:455-459.

21 Woods LL, Ingelfinger JR, Nyengaard JR, Rasch R. Maternal protein restriction suppresses the newborn renin-angiotensin system and programs adult hypertension in rats. *Pediatr Res*. 2001;49:460-467.

22 Elmes MJ, Gardner DS, Langley-Evans SC. Fetal exposure to a maternal low-protein diet is associated with altered left ventricular pressure response to ischaemia-reperfusion injury. *Br J Nutr*. 2007;98:93-100.

23 Plank C, Östreicher I, Hartner A, et al. Intrauterine growth retardation aggravates the course of acute mesangioproliferative glomerulonephritis in the rat. *Kidney Int*. 2006;70:1974-1982.

24 Plank C, Nüsken KD, Menendez-Castro C, et al. Intrauterine growth restriction following ligation of the uterine arteries leads to more severe glomerulosclerosis after mesangioproliferative glomerulonephritis in the offspring. *Am J Nephrol*. 2010;32:287-295.

25 Vehaskari VM, Aviles DH, Manning J. Prenatal programming of adult hypertension in the rat. *Kidney Int*. 2001;59:238-245.

26 Harrison M, Langley-Evans SC. Intergenerational programming of impaired nephrogenesis and hypertension in rats following maternal protein restriction during pregnancy. *Br J Nutr*. 2009;101:1020-1030.

27 Langley-Evans SC. Nutritional programming of disease: unravelling the mechanism. *J Anat.* 2009;215:36-51.

28 Nuyt AM. Mechanisms underlying developmental programming of elevated blood pressure and vascular dysfunction: evidence from human studies and experimental animal models. *Clin Sci (Lond).* 2008;114:1-17.

29 Brenner BM, Mackenzie HS. Nephron mass as a risk factor for progression of renal disease. *Kidney Int Suppl.* 1997;63:S124-S127.

30 Hoy WE, Bertram JF, Denton RD, Zimanyi M, Samuel T, Hughson MD. Nephron number, glomerular volume, renal disease and hypertension. *Curr Opin Nephrol Hypertens.* 2008;17:258-265.

31 Woods LL, Weeks DA, Rasch R. Programming of adult blood pressure by maternal protein restriction: role of nephrogenesis. *Kidney Int.* 2004;65:1339-1348.

32 Brenner BM, Garcia DL, Anderson S. Glomeruli and blood pressure: Less of one, more of the other? *Am J Hypertens.* 1988;1:335-347.

33 Keller G, Zimmer G, Mall G, Ritz E, Amann K. Nephron number in patients with primary hypertension. *N Engl J Med.* 2003;348:101-108.

34 Hughson MD, Douglas-Denton R, Bertram JF, Hoy WE. Hypertension, glomerular number, and birth weight in African Americans and white subjects in the southeastern United States. *Kidney Int.* 2006;69:671-678.

35 Kuure S, Vuolteenaho R, Vainio S. Kidney morphogenesis: cellular and molecular regulation. *Mech Dev.* 2000;92:31-45.

36 Giapros V, Drougia A, Hotoura E, Argyropoulou M, Papadopoulou F, Andronikou S. Kidney growth in twin children born small for gestational age. *Nephrol Dial Transplant.* 2010;25:3548-3554.

37 Westland R, Schreuder MF, Bökenkamp A, Spreeuwenberg MD, van Wijk JA. Renal injury in children with a solitary functioning kidney--the KIMONO study. *Nephrol Dial Transplant.* 2011;26:1533-1541.

38 Fotino S. The solitary kidney: a model of chronic hyperfiltration in humans. *Am J Kidney Dis.* 1989;13:88-98.

39 Langley-Evans SC, Sherman RC, Welham SJ, Nwagwu MO, Gardner DS, Jackson AA. Intrauterine programming of hypertension: the role of the renin-angiotensin system. *Biochem Soc Trans.* 1999;27:88-93.

40 Sahajpal V, Ashton N. Renal function and angiotensin AT1 receptor expression in young rats following intrauterine exposure to a maternal low-protein diet. *Clin Sci (Lond).* 2003;104:607-614.

41 Bogdarina I, Welham S, King PJ, Burns SP, Clark AJ. Epigenetic modification of the renin-angiotensin system in the fetal programming of hypertension. *Circ Res.* 2007;100:520-526.

42 Simonetti GD, Raio L, Surbek D, Nelle M, Frey FJ, Mohaupt MG. Salt sensitivity of children with low birth weight. *Hypertension.* 2008;52:625-630.

43 Seckl JR, Meaney MJ. Glucocorticoid programming. *Ann NY Acad Sci.* 2004;1032:63-84.

44 Bertram C, Trowern AR, Copin N, Jackson AA, Whorwood CB. The maternal diet during pregnancy programs altered expression of the glucocorticoid receptor and type 2 11beta-hydroxysteroid dehydrogenase: potential molecular mechanisms underlying the programming of hypertension in utero. *Endocrinology.* 2001;142:2841-2853.

45 Schoof E, Girstl M, Frobenius W, et al. Decreased gene expression of 11beta-hydroxysteroid dehydogenase type 2 and 15-hydrodroxyprostaglandin dehydrogenase in human placenta of patients with preeclampsia. *J. Clin. Endocrinol Metabol.* 2001;86:1313-1317.

46 Struwe E, Berzl GM, Schild RL, et al. Simultaneously reduced gene expression of cortisol-activating and cortisol-inactivating enzymes in placentas of small-for-gestational-age neonates. *Am J Obstet Gynecol.* 2007;197:43.e1-6.

47 Ostreicher I, Almeida JR, Campean V, et al. Changes in 11beta-hydroxysteroid dehydrogenase type 2 expression in a low-protein rat model of intrauterine growth restriction. *Nephrol Dial Transplant.* 2010;25:3195-3203.

48 Martin H, Gazelius B, Norman M. Impaired acetylcholine-induced vascular relaxation in low birth weight infants: implications for adult hypertension? *Pediatr Res*. 2000;47:457-462.

49 Franco MC, Christofalo DM, Sawaya AL, Ajzen SA, Sesso R. Effects of low birth weight in 8- to 13-year-old children: implications in endothelial function and uric acid levels. *Hypertension*. 2006;48:45-50.

50 Martin H, Hu J, Gennser G, Norman M. Impaired endothelial function and increased carotid stiffness in 9-year-old children with low birth weight. *Circulation*. 2000;102:2739-2744.

51 Nuyt AM. Mechanisms underlying developmental programming of elevated blood pressure and vascular dysfunction: evidence from human studies and experimental animal models. *Clin. Sci. (Lond)*. 2008;114:1-17.

52 Berry CL, Looker T. An alteration in the chemical structure of the aortic wall induced by a finite period of growth inhibition. *J Anat*. 1973;114:83-94.

53 Hellström A, Dahlgren J, Marsál K, Ley D. Abnormal retinal vascular morphology in young adults following intrauterine growth restriction. *Pediatrics*. 2004;113:e77-80.

54 Menendez-Castro C, Fahlbusch F, Cordasic N, et al. Early and late postnatal myocardial and vascular changes in a protein restriction rat model of intrauterine growth restriction. *PLoS One*. 2011;6:e20369.

55 Skilton MR, Evans N, Griffiths KA, Harmer JA, Celermajer DS. Aortic wall thickness in newborns with intrauterine growth restriction. *Lancet*. 2005;365:1484-1486.

56 Phillips DI, Barker DJ. Association between low birth weight and high resting pulse in adult life: is the sympathetic nervous system involved in programming the insulin resistance syndrome? *Diabet Med*. 1997;14:673-677.

57 Alexander BT, Hendon AE, Ferril G, Dwyer TM. Renal denervation abolishes hypertension in low-birth-weight offspring from pregnant rats with reduced uterine perfusion. *Hypertension*. 2005;45:754-758.

58 Gregório BM, Souza-Mello V, Mandarim-de-Lacerda CA, Aguila MB. Maternal fish oil supplementation benefits programmed offspring from rat dams fed low-protein diet. *Am J Obstet Gynecol*. 2008;199: 82.e1-7.

59 Manning J, Vehaskari VM. Postnatal modulation of prenatally programmed hypertension by dietary Na and ACE inhibition. *Am J Physiol Regul Integr Comp Physiol*. 2005;288:R80-84.

60 Stewart T, Jung FF, Manning J, Vehaskari VM. Kidney immune cell infiltration and oxidative stress contribute to prenatally programmed hypertension. *Kidney Int*. 2005;68:2180-2188.

61 Ravelli AC, van der Meulen JH, Michels RP, et al. Glucose tolerance in adults after prenatal exposure to famine. *Lancet*. 1998;351:173-177.

62 Stanner SA, Yudkin JS. Fetal programming and the Leningrad Siege study. *Twin Res*. 2001;4:287-292.

63 Gluckman PD, Hanson MA, Cooper C, Thornburg KL. Effect of in utero and early-life conditions on adult health and disease. *N Engl J Med*. 2008;359:61-73.

64 Clayton PE, Cianfarani S, Czernichow P, Johannsson G, Rapaport R, Rogol A. Management of the child born small for gestational age through to adulthood: a consensus statement of the International Societies of Pediatric Endocrinology and the Growth Hormone Research Society. *J Clin Endocrinol Metab*. 2007;92:804-810.

65 Singhal A, Cole TJ, Fewtrell M, et al. Promotion of faster weight gain in infants born small for gestational age: is there an adverse effect on later blood pressure? *Circulation*. 2007;115:213-220.

66 Ben-Shlomo Y, McCarthy A, Hughes R, Tilling K, Davies D, Smith DG. Immediate postnatal growth is associated with blood pressure in young adulthood: the Barry Caerphilly Growth Study. *Hypertension*. 2008;52:638-644.

67 Alejandre Alcázar MA, Boehler E, Amann K, et al. Persistent changes within the intrinsic ey-associated NPY system and tubular function by litter size reduction. *Nephrol Dial Transplant*. 2011;26:2453-2465.

68 Rocha SO, Gomes GN, Forti AL, et al. Long-term effects of maternal diabetes on vascular reactivity and renal function in rat male offspring. *Pediatr Res*. 2005;58:1274-1279.

69 Nehiri T, Duong Van Huyen JP, Viltard M, et al. Exposure to maternal diabetes induces salt-sensitive hypertension and impairs renal function in adult rat offspring. *Diabetes.* 2008;57:2167-2175.

70 Chen YW, Chenier I, Tran S, Scotcher M, Chang SY, Zhang SL. Maternal diabetes programs hypertension and kidney injury in offspring. *Pediatr Nephrol.* 2010;25:1319-1329.

71 Tran S, Chen YW, Chenier I, et al. Maternal diabetes modulates renal morphogenesis in offspring. *J Am Soc Nephrol.* 2008;19:943-952.

72 Rocco L, Gil FZ, da Fonseca Pletiskaitz TM, de Fátima Cavanal M, Gomes GN. Effect of sodium overload on renal function of offspring from diabetic mothers. *Pediatr Nephrol.* 2008;23:2053-2060.

73 Boubred F, Buffat C, Feuerstein JM, et al. Effects of early postnatal hypernutrition on nephron number and long-term renal function and structure in rats. *Am J Physiol Renal Physiol.* 2007;293:F1944-F1949.

74 Cardoso HD, Cabral EV, Vieira-Filho LD, Vieyra A, Paixão AD. Fetal development and renal function in adult rats prenatally subjected to sodium overload. *Pediatr Nephrol.* 2009;24:1959-1965.

75 Chadwick MA, Vercoe PE, Williams IH, Revell DK. Dietary exposure of pregnant ewes to salt dictates how their offspring respond to salt. *Physiol Behav.* 2009;97:437-445.

76 Dickinson H, Walker DW, Wintour EM, Moritz K. Maternal dexamethasone treatment at midgestation reduces nephron number and alters renal gene expression in the fetal spiny mouse. *Am J Physiol Regul Integr Comp Physiol.* 2007;292:R453-R461.

77 Woods LL, Weeks DA. Prenatal programming of adult blood pressure: role of maternal corticosteroids. *Am J Physiol Regul Integr Comp Physiol.* 2005;289:R955-R962.

78 Fetita LS, Sobngwi E, Serradas P, Calvo F, Gautier JF. Consequences of fetal exposure to maternal diabetes in offspring. *J Clin Endocrinol Metab.* 2006;91:3718-3724.

79 Roberts CL, Ford JB, Algert CS, et al. Population-based trends in pregnancy hypertension and pre-eclampsia: an international comparative study. *BMJ Open.* 2011;1:e000101.

80 Tenhola S, Rahiala E, Halonen P, Vanninen E, Voutilainen R. Maternal preeclampsia predicts elevated blood pressure in 12-year-old children: evaluation by ambulatory blood pressure monitoring. *Pediatr Res.* 2006;59:320-324.

81 Lawlor DA, Macdonald-Wallis C, Fraser A, et al. Cardiovascular biomarkers and vascular function during childhood in the offspring of mothers with hypertensive disorders of pregnancy: findings from the Avon Longitudinal Study of Parents and Children. *Eur Heart J.* 2012;33:335-345.

82 Geelhoed JJ, Fraser A, Tilling K, et al. Preeclampsia and gestational hypertension are associated with childhood blood pressure independently of family adiposity measures: the Avon Longitudinal Study of Parents and Children. *Circulation.* 2010;122:1192-1199.

Development of this book was supported by funding from Sandoz

Chapter 17

Pancreatic development

Patricia Vuguin and Paul Saenger

Introduction

Fetal undernutrition and low birth weight have been identified as risk factors for increased incidence of cardiovascular disease, type 2 diabetes mellitus, and precursors such as dyslipidemia, impaired glucose tolerance, and vascular endothelial dysfunction [1]. An unfavorable fetal environment can also lead to inappropriate development of the endocrine pancreas [2–5]. As such, type 2 diabetes and the metabolic syndrome represent examples of human diseases in which an altered intrauterine environment contributes to disease pathogenesis.

The underlying molecular mechanisms responsible for these pathologies have been poorly defined. It has been suggested that cellular mechanisms such as mitochondrial dysregulation leading to oxidative damage, as well as molecular mechanisms such as epigenetic changes (including alteration of DNA methylation), may contribute to pathogenesis [6]. These changes could permanently alter pancreatic development, damaging the pancreatic beta cells and resulting in a population of insulin-secreting cells that may not be able to meet metabolic demand and oxidative stress later in life. While beta cell dysfunction has been considered to be the pathogenesis that leads to type 2 diabetes, decreased beta-cell mass also seems to play a major role in disease susceptibility. Therefore, the identification of factors that influence differentiation of endocrine cells (with special emphasis on beta cell development) has important implications in the treatment of diabetes.

S. Zabransky (ed.), *Caring for Children Born Small for Gestational Age*, 227
DOI: 10.1007/978-1-908517-90-6_17, © Springer Healthcare 2013

The development of the endocrine pancreas is regulated by several cell and matrix interactions that generate a diverse array of intracellular signals, which in turn determine the progression of a multipotent progenitor to a mature endocrine cell [8–10]. This process involves interactions between the endothelial, epithelial, and mesenchymal cells, followed by coordinated signaling that contributes to the maintenance of the differentiated endocrine cell phenotype. Pancreatic development has been shown to be conserved among species (eg, rodents, sheep, humans) and the mouse model has been a well-established tool for understanding pancreatic development. The following chapter will discuss our current knowledge of the stages of pancreatic development and will compare the animal models of fetal programming of adult disease that have an associated pancreatic phenotype.

Overview of pancreatic morphogenesis

The mammalian pancreas is a gland composed of exocrine and endocrine cells that produces digestive enzymes and hormones. Enzymes are produced by cells of the exocrine portion, while hormones are synthesized by cells clustered in the islets of Langerhans [11]. The islet is comprised of beta cells that secrete insulin, alpha cells that secrete glucagon, delta cells that secrete somatostatin, epsilon cells that secrete ghrelin, and pancreatic polypeptide-producing (PP) cells that secrete pancreatic polypeptide [12,13]. These endocrine cells play a central role in glucose homeostasis. Insulin released from beta cells after a meal promotes the uptake of glucose into target organs, such as skeletal muscle. The action of insulin is counterbalanced by glucagon, a hormone produced by alpha cells that acts on the liver to stimulate glycogenolysis and gluconeogenesis [14]. Somatostatin suppresses the release of pancreatic hormones. The organogenesis of the mammalian pancreas is a complex and highly coordinated process [15,16].

Endocrine cell differentiation

The extrinsic signals that specifically promote endocrine cell differentiation are not clearly defined. The pancreatic buds contain undifferentiated precursor cells that are specified towards the endocrine or exocrine lineages.

All the cells that derive from the endoderm (endocrine, exocrine, and ductal cells) have been shown to express duodenal homeobox factor-1 (Pdx1) [17]. From E-9.5 to E-12.5, the majority of endocrine cells formed are glucagon cells. Subsequently, during the so-called 'secondary transition,' endocrine cells differentiate in exponentially increasing numbers with insulin cells predominating [15]. The cascade of transcription factors or intrinsic signals important for pancreas development can be grouped according to their expression pattern [18,19]:

- transcription factors found in early non-hormone progenitor cells;
- transcription factors found in cells that produce each of the endocrine hormones; and
- transcription factors found in a specific hormone-producing cell type.

Early non-hormone progenitor cells

Several signals and transcription factors are necessary for the maintenance of early progenitors. The Notch signaling pathway, a highly conserved cell signaling system, is critical for the decision between endocrine and progenitor/exocrine fates in the developing pancreas [20]. In conjunction with the Notch pathway, the sex-determining region Y-box 9 protein (or Sox9) maintains the progenitor state [21]. A member of the transforming growth factor-beta superfamily, bone morphogenetic protein 4, also promotes the proliferation of the progenitor cells [22]. In addition, a pair of opposing transcription factors, pancreas-specific transcription factor 1a (Ptf1a) and neurogenin-3 (Ngn3), act as the first fate-determining factors in the branching of pancreatic progenitors into the endocrine or exocrine pancreas [23]. Expression of Ptf1a, a transcriptional activator, gives rise to the exocrine cells, while Ngn3, a basic helix-loop-helix (bHLH) transcription factor, drives pancreatic precursors towards an endocrine cell fate [24–28]. During the differentiation of islet cells, Ngn3 regulates the cell cycle; its down-regulation allows the mature islet cell population to expand [29]. Cyclin-dependent kinase 4, member of the Ser/Thr protein kinase family, and its downstream transcription factor, the retinoblastoma-associated protein 1 (E2f1) regulate activation of Ngn3, increasing the pool of endocrine precursors [30]. Downstream of Ngn3 is the regulatory factor X,6 (Rfx6) which has been shown to play a crucial role in the development, maturation, and function of endocrine cell lines [31].

Hormone-producing endocrine precursors

The homeobox protein NK-2 homolog B (or Nkx2.2) belongs to the natural killed (NK) class of homeodomain-encoding genes and its expression is initiated at E-9.5 in the dorsal epithelium, becoming progressively restricted to alpha, beta, and PP-cell subtypes [32]. Nkx6.1, an additional member of the NK family, is also detectable at E-9.5 in both pancreatic buds, becoming specifically restricted to beta cells [33–35].

The second level of branching is directed by another pair of opposing transcription factors 'Pax4-Arx' [23]. Aristaless-related homeobox or Arx appears to specify the alpha-cell fate, whereas paired box 4 or Pax4 first allows the commitment towards a beta/delta-cell fate by repressing Arx and subsequently induces precursor cells towards a beta-cell fate through the inhibition of the delta-cell destiny [18,36]. Pax4, a member of the paired-box family of transcription factors, is expressed around E-9.5 in both of the pancreatic buds and becomes progressively restricted to beta cells until E-15 [36,37]. It has been shown that both Pax4 and Arx require the activity of Nkx2.2. In addition, Nkx2.2 and Pax4 control Arx gene activity in committed beta-cell precursors [38,39].

Specific hormone-producing cell type

Beta cell lineages

It has been proposed that there may be two separate beta-cell lineages: 'first wave' or protodifferentiated beta cells that usually coexpress glucagon and appear at E-10.5; and the 'mature' or second transition beta cells that appear at E-13.5 and persist during adulthood [40].

Protodifferentiated cells

Protodifferentiated cells are multi-hormonal cells, co-expressing glucagon and insulin [34,41]. Although early studies contested the existence of these cells [42], this point has now been confirmed repeatedly [43–50]. Double- and triple-staining studies of early pancreatic buds show that the vast majority of the co-expressing glucagon-insulin cells are negative for Pdx1, Nkx6.1 [34], or Pax4 [36], suggesting that these cells derive from a different progenitor cell. They usually appear in clusters surrounded by alpha cells and express activin [50]. Furthermore, there is some evidence that the co-expressing glucagon-insulin cells can proliferate [41], which may contribute to a pull towards either alpha or beta cells.

Mature cells

Mature cells arise directly from a non-hormone protodifferentiated epithelial cell that expresses the facilitative glucose transporter 2 (GLUT2) as well as Pdx1 [40,51–53]. In mature organized insulin cells, Pdx1 (which transactivates the insulin gene among others) is involved in glucose sensing and metabolism [40,54,55]. GLUT2 and glucokinase (GK) play key roles in glucose sensing and are the initial activating event in the pathway for glucose-stimulated insulin secretion [56]. The eukaryotic translation initiation factor 2-alpha kinase 3 (EIF2AK3 or PERK) expression during fetal life is also required for the differentiation of beta cells and development of normal islet architecture [57].

Other important transcription factors include neurogenic differentiation (NeuroD), a basic helix-loop-helix transcription factor involved in promoting cell cycle exit [8]; and v-maf musculoaponeurotic fibrosarcoma oncogene homolog avian (MafA), which activate insulin transcription by binding to the insulin promoter [58]. MafA also plays a crucial role in beta cell maintenance [58]. In addition, MafA interacts with Pdx1 and NeuroD to activate insulin transcription [59].

Alpha cell lineages

Alpha cells share major similarities with beta cells [60]. Recently it has been demonstrated that alpha cells can transdifferentiate into beta cells [61–63]. Thus, it is important to understand how alpha cells develop. Following the development of the endocrine progenitor, a third pair of opposing transcription factors (Arx and forkhead box A2 [FOXA2]) will direct the development of alpha cells. Arx and FOXA2 are implicated in the initial or terminal differentiation of alpha cells. In addition, forkhead box A1, paired box 6 (Pax6), brain4 (Brn4) and islet-1 (Isl-1) are involved in the preproglucagon transcription and maintenance of alpha-cell function [64,65].

MicroRNAs (approx 20 nt) are posttranscriptional regulators that are integrated into an RNA-induced silencing complex to repress translation, leading to gene silencing [66]. These small noncoding RNAs are important during development of the pancreas and the fetal pancreas expresses at least 125 of them. During development, microRNAs are important in regulating ductal, exocrine, and endocrine development, particularly beta-cell neogenesis [67]. An overview of specific hormone-producing cells is depicted in Figure 17.1.

Human pancreatic development

The pancreas is first apparent at 25-to-26 day gestational age (dGA) and develops as a ventral and dorsal outgrowth [68]. These outgrowths elongate into a loose mesenchymal bed [69], which plays an important role in cell fate differentiation [70]. By 35th dGA, the ventral pancreatic bud begins to rotate, and eventually comes into contact and fuses with the dorsal bud during the 6th week of gestational age (wGA) [71–77]. By 9th–11th wGA, the mesenchymal tissue contains scattered hormone-negative Ngn3-positive endocrine cells [70] which have been found to be associated with the ductal epithelium [78]. The critical window of differentiation of endocrine cells in humans is from the 9th to the 23rd wGA [70]. Glucagon cells are the first cells that appear (7th wGA) [79] followed by insulin, somatostatin and PP cells (8th–10th wGA) [74]. Peak proliferation of glucagon cells occurs at 20th wGA, followed by insulin and somatostatin cells at 23rd wGA [70]. Islets are seen as early as 11th wGA, and vascularized structures appear by 20th–23rd wGA [70,80].

Adult islets have two populations of cells: larger cells with dense cytoplasm that constitute the majority of the islet population, and distinctly smaller cells [81]. Mutation of several transcription factors mentioned above have been found to be associated with maturity onset diabetes of the young, an autosomal disease characterized by early onset (<25 years of age) of a non-ketotic diabetes mellitus secondary to a major defect in pancreatic beta-cell function. Despite the similarity to rodents, human

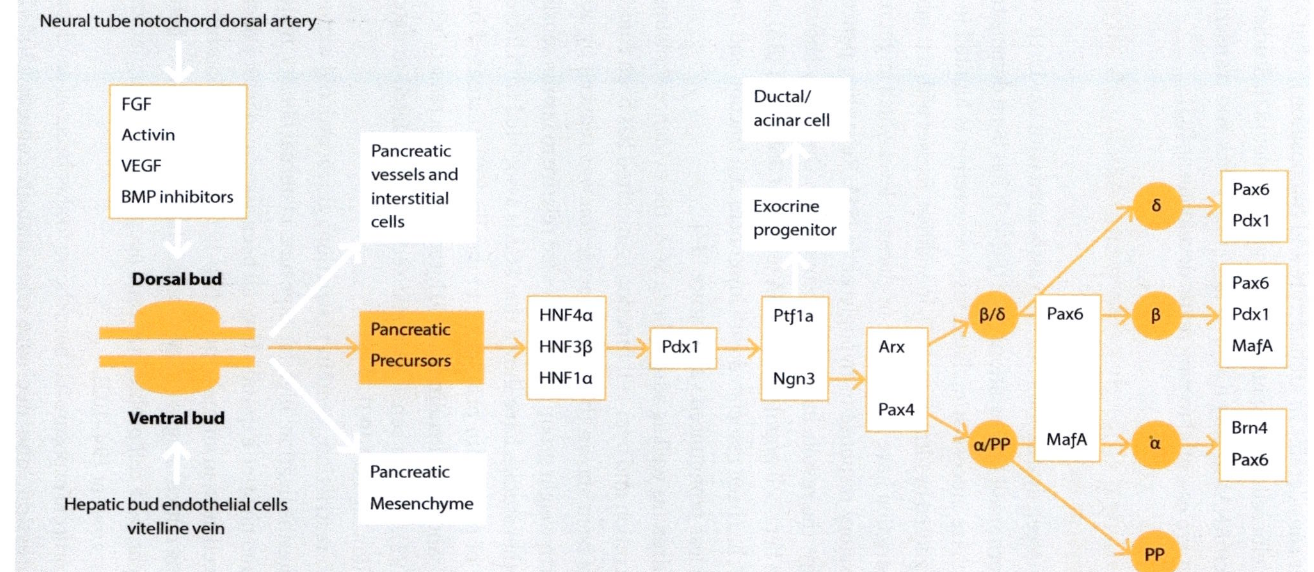

Figure 17.1 Specific hormone-producing cells. Arx, aristaless-related homeodomain protein; BMP, bone morphogenetic protein; Brn4, brain-specific POU-box 4; FGF, fibroblast growth factor; HNF, hepatocyte nuclear factor; MaF, musculoaponeurotic fibrosarcoma oncogene homolog; Ngn3, neurogenin 3; Pax, Paired box gene; Pdx1, pancreatic and duodenal homeobox 1; Ptf1a, pancreas transcription factor 1a; VEGF, vascular endothelial growth factor.

islets differ considerably in architecture and composition in that alpha, beta, and delta cells are dispersed throughout the islet [82]. Studies have shown microRNAs to play a role in targeting genes and transcription factors that are essential to pancreatic development [83].

Programming of endocrine pancreas by an altered intrauterine milieu

Human beta-cell dysfunction has been associated with low birth weight or being born small for gestational age (SGA). It has been demonstrated that first-phase glucose-stimulated insulin secretion is blunted in SGA fetuses diagnosed by ultrasound [84]. In addition, fetuses with intrauterine growth restriction have an increase in glucagon level which might reflect a compensatory response to hypoglycemia [85]. Regarding pancreatic morphology, the results have been inconclusive. One study showed no changes in beta-cell population in SGA fetuses at 36th wGA [86], while severe SGA has been associated with lower beta-cell fraction and smaller islets with less pronounced vasculature [87].

In children (as well as adults) born SGA, the evidence showing that insulin secretion and beta-cell function is impaired has been contradictory. It has been shown that insulin secretion was reduced by 30% in the low birth weight group when expressed relative to insulin sensitivity [88,89]. Other studies have shown that SGA is associated with increased efficiency of proinsulin processing to insulin [90], increased insulin resistance, and hyperinsulinemia [91], rather than decreased beta-cell capacity [92]. Insulin sensitivity and secretion is related to catch-up growth following SGA [93].

Caloric restriction, protein restriction, glucocorticoid exposure, bilateral uterine ligation, high fat exposure, maternal obesity, maternal diabetes, and nicotine exposure have all been associated with a decrease in insulin cell mass in animal models [94–102]. Most of the interventions done during critical stages of development have shown to alter beta cell development, beta cell proliferation and apoptosis, islet vascularization, and insulin content [94–102].

Glucocorticoid exposure has been shown to alter beta cell development, Pdx1 expression, and decrease islet insulin content [103–107].

Protein restriction decreases pancreatic weight, islet size, insulin cell proliferation, and islet vasculature, increases apoptosis and Pdx1 expression, and alters mitochondrial gene expression [108–115]. Interestingly, this phenomenon is transmitted over three consecutive generations [116]. In addition, taurine supplementation seems to restore the changes in the fetal pancreas [117]. Caloric restriction has also been associated with impaired beta-cell differentiation, reduced pancreatic weight, insulin content, islet density, and beta-cell mass [111,117–119]. Additional decline in beta-cell mass and insulin content are evident if the caloric restriction is sustained during the newborn period [118,120,121].

Bilateral uterine ligation has been associated with a decrease in beta-cell proliferation, reduced vascular density, and absent first-phase insulin secretion [122–124]. Pdx1 expression is decreased upon changes in methylation of the *Pdx1* gene along with deacetylation of histone H3 and H4 [123]. There is also alteration in cytosine methylation in 1400 loci at conserved intergenic regions near genes related to vascularization, beta-cell proliferation, insulin secretion, and cell death before the development of diabetes [125]. Interestingly, brief treatment with exendin-4, a GLP-1 agonist, during the newborn period restores chromatin structure, preserving Pdx1 transcription [126]. Interestingly, if the uterine artery ligation is conducted earlier during development, beta-cell mass is prematurely reduced [127].

The effects of the exposure to high fat in utero seem to depend on the balance and composition of dietary nutrients [56,128,129]. One study examining a high-fat diet reported decreased beta-cell volume, reduced and altered Pdx1 localization, as well as reduced GLUT2 expression [129,130]. In contrast, in a different high-fat diet composition, there was an increase in the numbers of large islets and a significant increase in the total pancreatic beta-cell mass during the newborn period [131].

In contrast to what is known regarding the effect of an altered intrauterine milieu on beta-cell development and function, little is known about the effect of an altered intrauterine environment on glucagon/glucagon cell development and function. High fat exposure in utero has been associated with alpha cell hypertrophy and hyperplasia, resulting in an increase in alpha-cell volume and number in the newborn period [128].

Conclusion

Regulation of insulin and glucagon cell differentiation and maturation is a process that, in utero, depends on precisely timed expression of transcription factors. These initiate and promote pancreas development and can be regulated by many intrinsic (hormones, growth factors) as well as extrinsic signals associated with the intrauterine environment. Thus, alterations in this environment may alter the signals that specifically promote endocrine cell differentiation. Until now, our understanding of the pancreatic phenotype associated with fetal programming of adult disease is limited. Because the ontogeny of alpha- and beta-cell development in rodents is similar to what has been observed in the human, our knowledge based on the outcomes of the animal studies will help clarify the mechanism of alpha- and beta-cell dysfunction found in subjects born SGA.

References

1   Barker D, Hales C, Fall C, Osmond C, Phipps K, Clark P. Type 2 (non-insulin-dependent) diabetes mellitus, hypertension and hyperlipidemia (syndrome X): relation to reduced fetal growth. *Diabetologia*. 1993;36:62-67.

2   Remacle C, Dumortier O, Bol V, et al. Intrauterine programming of the endocrine pancreas. *Diabetes Obes Metab*. 2007;9 (suppl 2):196-209.

3   Vuguin PM. Animal models for small for gestational age and fetal programming of adult disease. *Horm Res*. 2007;68:113-123.

4   Vuguin P. Animal models for assessing the consequences of intrauterine growth restriction on subsequent glucose metabolism of the offspring: a review. *J Matern Fetal Neonatal Med*. 2002;11:254-257.

5   Schwitzgebel VM, Somm E, Klee P. Modeling intrauterine growth retardation in rodents: Impact on pancreas development and glucose homeostasis. *Mol Cell Endocrinol*. 2009;304:78-83.

6   Simmons RA. Developmental origins of beta-cell failure in type 2 diabetes: the role of epigenetic mechanisms. *Pediatr Res*. 2007;61:64R-67R.

7   Donath MY, Halban PA. Decreased beta-cell mass in diabetes: significance, mechanisms and therapeutic implications. *Diabetologia*. 2004;47:581-589.

8   Jensen J. Gene regulatory factors in pancreatic development. *Dev Dynamics*. 2004;229:176-200.

9   Ranjan AK, Joglekar MV, Hardikar AA. Endothelial cells in pancreatic islet development and function. *Islets*. 2009;1:2-9.

10 Lin CL, Vuguin PM. Determinants of pancreatic islet development in mice and men: a focus on the role of transcription factors. *Horm Res Paediatr*. 2012;77:205-213.

11 Bosco D, Armanet M, Morel P, et al. Unique arrangement of alpha- and beta-cells in human islets of Langerhans. *Diabetes*. 2010;59:1202-1210.

12 Murtaugh LC. Pancreas and beta-cell development: from the actual to the possible. *Development*. 2007;134:427-438.

13 Gromada J, Franklin I, Wollheim CB. Alpha cells of the endocrine pancreas: 35 years of research but the enigma remains. *Endocr Rev*. 28:84-116

14 Aronoff SL, Berkowitz K, Shreiner B, Want L. Glucose metabolism and regulation: beyond insulin and glucagon. *Diabetes Spectrum*. 2004;17:183-190.

15 Pictet R, Rutter WJ. Development of the embryonic pancreas. In: Steiner DF, Frenkel N, eds. *Handbook of Physiology*. Washington, DC. American Physiological Society; 1972:25-66.

16 Gittes GK. Developmental biology of the pancreas: a comprehensive review. *Dev Biol*. 2009;326:4-35.

17 Gu G, Dubauskaite J, Melton DA. Direct evidence for the pancreatic lineage: NGN3+ cells are islet progenitors and are distinct from duct progenitors. *Development*. 2002;129:2447-2457.

18 Collombat P, Mansouri A, Hecksher-Sorensen J, et al. Opposing actions of Arx and Pax4 in endocrine pancreas development. *Genes Dev*. 2003;17:2591-2603.

19 Wilson ME, Scheel D, German MS. Gene expression cascades in pancreatic development. *Mech Dev*. 2003;120:65-80.

20 Apelqvist A, Li H, Sommer L, et al. Notch signaling controls pancreatic cell differentiation. *Nature*. 1999;400:877-881.

21 Seymour PA, Freude KK, Tran MN, et al. SOX9 is required for maintenance of the pancreatic progenitor cell pool. *Proc Natl Acad Sci USA*. 2007;104:1865-1870.

22 Hua H, Zhang YQ, Dabernat S, et al. BMP4 regulates pancreatic progenitor cell expansion through Id2. *J Biol Chem*. 2006;281:13574-13580.

23 Zhou JX, Brusch L, Huang S. Predicting pancreas cell fate decisions and reprogramming with a hierarchical multi-attractor model. *PLoS One*. 2011;6:e14752.

24 Gradwohl G, Dierich A, LeMeur M, Guillemot F. neurogenin3 is required for the development of the four endocrine cell lineages of the pancreas. *Proc Natl Acad Sci USA*. 2000;97:1607-1611.

25 Jensen J, Heller RS, Funder-Nielsen T, et al. Independent development of pancreatic alpha and beta-cells from neurogenin3-expressing precursors: a role for notch pathway in repression of premature differentiation. *Diabetes*. 2000;49:163-176.

26 Rukstalis JM, Habener JF. Neurogenin3: a master regulator of pancreatic islet differentiation and regeneration. *Islets*. 2009;1:177-184.

27 Mellitzer G, Bonné S, Luco RF, et al. IA1 is NGN3-dependent and essential for differentiation of the endocrine pancreas. *EMBO J*. 2006;25:1344-1352.

28 Kawaguchi Y, Cooper B, Gannon M, Ray M, MacDonald RJ, Wright CV. The role of the transcriptional regulator Ptf1a in converting intestinal to pancreatic progenitors. *Nat Genet*. 2002;32:128-134.

29 Miyatsuka T, Kosaka Y, Kim H, German MS. Neurogenin3 inhibits proliferation in endocrine progenitors by inducing Cdkn1a. *Proc Natl Acad Sci USA*. 2011;108:185-190.

30 Kim SY, Rane SG. The Cdk4-E2f1 pathway regulates early pancreas development by targeting Pdx1+ progenitors and Ngn3+ endocrine precursors. *Development*. 2011;138:1903-1912.

31 Smith SB, Qu HQ, Taleb N, et al. Rfx6 directs islet formation and insulin production in mice and humans. *Nature*. 2010;463:775-780.

32 Sussel L, Kalamaras J, Hartigan-O'Connor DJ, et al. Mice lacking the homeodomain transcription factor Nkx2.2 have diabetes due to arrested differentiation of pancreatic beta cells. *Development*. 1998;125:2213-2221.

33 Pedersen JK, Nelson SB, Jorgensen MC, et al. Endodermal expression of Nkx6 genes depends differentially on Pdx1. *Dev Biol*. 2005;288:487-501.

34 Oster A, Jensen J, Edlund H, Larsson LI. Homeobox gene product Nkx 6.1 immunoreactivity in nuclei of endocrine cells of rat and mouse stomach. *J Histochem Cytochem*. 1998;46:717-721.

35 Sander M, Sussel L, Conners J, et al. Homeobox gene Nkx6.1 lies downstream of Nkx2.2 in the major pathway of beta-cell formation in the pancreas. *Development*. 2000;127:5533-5540.

36 Sosa-Pineda B. The gene Pax4 is an essential regulator of pancreatic beta-cell development. *Mol Cells*. 2004;18:289-294.

37 Smith SB, Ee HC, Conners JR, German MS. Paired-homeodomain transcription factor PAX4 acts as a transcriptional repressor in early pancreatic development. *Mol Cell Biol*. 1999;19:8272-8280.

38   Kordowich S, Collombat P, Mansouri A, Serup P. Arx and Nkx2.2 compound deficiency redirects pancreatic alpha- and beta-cell differentiation to a somatostatin/ghrelin co-expressing cell lineage. *BMC Dev Biol.* 2011;11:52.

39   Sander M, Paydar S, Ericson J, et al. Ventral neural patterning by Nkx homeobox genes: Nkx6.1 controls somatic motor neuron and ventral interneuron fates. *Genes Dev.* 2000;14:2134-2139.

40   Pang K, Mukonoweshuro C, Wong GG. Beta cells arise from glucose transporter type 2 (Glut2)-expressing epithelial cells of the developing rat pancreas. *Proc Natl Acad Sci USA.* 1994;91:9559-9563.

41   Jackerott M, Oster A, Larsson LI. PYY in developing murine islet cells: comparisons to development of islet hormones, NPY, and BrdU incorporation. *J Histochem Cytochem.* 1996;44:809-817.

42   Herrera PL, Huarte J, Sanvito F, Meda P, Orci L, Vassalli JD. Embryogenesis of the murine endocrine pancreas; early expression of the pancreatic polypeptide gene. *Development.* 1991;113:1257-1265.

43   Vuguin PM, Kedees MH, Cui L, et al. Ablation of the glucagon receptor gene increases fetal lethality and produces alterations in islet development and maturation. *Endocrinology.* 2006;147:3995-4006.

44   De Krijger R, Aanstoot HJ, Kranenburg G, Reinhard M, Visser WJ, Bruining GJ. The midgestational human fetal pancreas contains cells coexpressing islet hormones. *Dev Biol.* 1992;153:368-375.

45   Guz Y, Montminy MR, Stein R, et al. Expression of murine STF-1, a putative insulin gene transcription factor, in beta cells of pancreas, duodenal epithelium and pancreatic exocrine and endocrine progenitors during ontogeny. *Development.* 1995;121:11-18.

46   Larsson. L, Hougaard DM. Coexpression of islet hormones and messenger mRNAs in the human fetal pancreas. *Endocrine.* 1994;2:759-765.

47   Teitelman G, Alpert S, Polak JM, Martinez A, Hanahan D. Precursor cells of mouse endocrine pancreas coexpress insulin, glucagon and the neuronal proteins tyrosine hydroxylase and neuropeptide Y, but not pancreatic polypeptide. *Development.* 1993;118:1031-1039.

48   Lukinius A, Ericsson JL, Grimelius L, Korsgren O. Ultrastructural studies of the ontogeny of fetal human and porcine endocrine pancreas, with special reference to colocalization of the four major islet hormones. *Dev Biol.* 1992;153:376-385.

49   Lukinius A, Wilander E, Eriksson B, Oberg K. A chromogranin peptide is co-stored with insulin in the human pancreatic islet B-cell granules. *Histochem J.* 1992;24:679-684.

50   Furukawa M, Eto Y, Kojima I. Expression of immunoreactive activin A in fetal rat pancreas. *Endocr J.* 1995;42:63-68.

51   Jonsson J, Carlsson L, Edlund T, Edlund H. Insulin-promoter-factor 1 is required for pancreas development in mice. *Nature.* 1994;371:606-609.

52   Offield MF, Jetton TL, Labosky PA, et al. PDX-1 is required for pancreatic outgrowth and differentiation of the rostral duodenum. *Development.* 1996;122:983-995.

53   Scharfmann R, Czernichow P. Differentiation and growth of pancreatic beta cells. *Diabetes Metab.* 1996;22:223-228.

54   Nishimura W, Kondo T, Salameh T, et al. A switch from MafB to MafA expression accompanies differentiation to pancreatic beta-cells. *Dev Biol.* 2006;293:526-539.

55   Kaneto H, Miyatsuka T, Kawamori D, et al. PDX-1 and MafA play a crucial role in pancreatic beta-cell differentiation and maintenance of mature beta-cell function. *Endocr J.* 2008;55:235-252.

56   Cerf ME. High fat diet modulation of glucose sensing in the beta-cell. *Med Sci Monit.* 2007;13:RA12-17.

57   Zhang W, Feng D, Li Y, Iida K, McGrath B, Cavener DR. PERK EIF2AK3 control of pancreatic beta cell differentiation and proliferation is required for postnatal glucose homeostasis. *Cell Metab.* 2006;4:491-497.

58   Kataoka K, Han SI, Shioda S, Hirai M, Nishizawa M, Handa H. MafA is a glucose-regulated and pancreatic beta-cell-specific transcriptional activator for the insulin gene. *J Biol Chem*. 2002;49903-49910.

59   Aramata S, Han SI, Kataoka K. Roles and regulation of transcription factor MafA in islet beta-cells. *Endocr J*. 2007;54:659-666.

60   Wang J, Webb G, Cao Y, Steiner DF. Contrasting patterns of expression of transcription factors in pancreatic alpha and beta cells. *Proc Natl Acad Sci USA*. 2003;100:12660-12665.

61   Lu J, Herrera PL, Carreira C, et al. Alpha cell-specific Men1 ablation triggers the transdifferentiation of glucagon-expressing cells and insulinoma development. *Gastroenterology*. 2010;138:1954-1965.

62   Thorel F, Népote V, Avril I, et al. Conversion of adult pancreatic alpha-cells to beta-cells after extreme beta-cell loss. *Nature*. 2010; 464:1149-1154.

63   Sangan CB, Tosh D. A new paradigm in cell therapy for diabetes: turning pancreatic alpha-cells into beta-cells. *Bioessays*. 2010;32:881-884.

64   Bramswig NC, Kaestner KH. Transcriptional regulation of α-cell differentiation. *Diabetes Obes Metab*. 2011;13 (suppl 1):13-20.

65   Gosmain Y, Marthinet E, Cheyssac C, et al. Pax6 controls the expression of critical genes involved in pancreatic α cell differentiation and function. *J Biol Chem*. 2010;285:33381-33393.

66   Ambros V. The functions of animal microRNAs. *Nature*. 2004;431:350-355.

67   Lynn FC, Skewes-Cox P, Kosaka Y, McManus MT, Harfe BD, German MS. MicroRNA expression is required for pancreatic islet cell genesis in the mouse. *Diabetes*. 2007;56:2938-2945.

68   Piper K, Ball SG, Turnpenny LW, Brickwood S, Wilson DI, Hanley NA. Beta-cell differentiation during human development does not rely on nestin-positive precursors: implications for stem cell-derived replacement therapy. *Diabetologia*. 2002;45:1045-1047.

69   Piper K, Brickwood S, Turnpenny LW, et al. Beta cell differentiation during early human pancreas development. *J Endocrinol*. 2004;181:11-23.

70   Sarkar SA, Kobberup S, Wong R, et al. Global gene expression profiling and histochemical analysis of the developing human fetal pancreas. *Diabetologia*. 2008;51:285-297.

71   Falin LI. The development and cytodifferentiation of the islets of Langerhans in human embryos and foetuses. *Acta Anat (Basel)*. 1967;68:147-168.

72   Orci L, Perrelet A, Like AA. Fenestrae in the rough endoplasmic reticulum of the exocrine pancreatic cells. *J Cell Biol*. 1972;55:245-249.

73   Like AA, Orci L. Embryogenesis of the human pancreatic islets: a light and electron microscopic study. *Diabetes*. 1972;21 (2 suppl):511-534.

74   Stefan Y, Grasso S, Perrelet A, Orci L. A quantitative immunofluorescent study of the endocrine cell populations in the developing human pancreas. *Diabetes*. 1983;32:293-301.

75   Clark A, Grant AM. Quantitative morphology of endocrine cells in human fetal pancreas. *Diabetologia*. 1983;25:31-35.

76   Fukayama M, Ogawa M, Hayashi Y, Koike M. Development of human pancreas. Immunohistochemical study of fetal pancreatic secretory proteins. *Differentiation*. 1986;31:127-133.

77   Bocian-Sobkowska J, Zabel M, Woźniak W, Surdyk-Zasada J. Prenatal development of the human pancreatic islets. Immunocytochemical identification of insulin-, glucagon-, somatostatin- and pancreatic polypeptide-containing cells. *Folia Histochem Cytobiol*. 1997;35:151-154.

78   Meier JJ, Köhler CU, Alkhatib B, et al. Beta-cell development and turnover during prenatal life in humans. *Eur J Endocrinol*. 2010;162:559-568.

79   Assan R, Boillot J. Pancreatic glucagon and glucagon-like material in tissues and plasma from human fetuses 6–26 weeks old. *Pathol Biol (Paris)*. 1973;21:149-155.

80   Jeon J, Correa-Medina M, Ricordi C, Edlund H, Diez JA. Endocrine cell clustering during human pancreas development. *J Histochem Cytochem*. 2009;57:811-824.

81   Chiang MK, Melton DA. Single-cell transcript analysis of pancreas development. *Dev Cell*. 2003;4:383-393.

82 Brissova M, Fowler MJ, Nicholson WE, et al. Assessment of human pancreatic islet architecture and composition by laser scanning confocal microscopy. *J Histochem Cytochem.* 2005;53:1087-1097.

83 Rosero S, Bravo-Egana V, Jiang Z, et al. MicroRNA signature of the human developing pancreas. *BMC Genomics.* 2010;11:509.

84 Nicolini U, Hubinont C, Santolaya J, Fisk NM, Rodeck CH. Effects of fetal intravenous glucose challenge in normal and growth retarded fetuses. *Horm Metab Res.* 1990;22:426-430.

85 Hubinont C, Nicolini U, Fisk NM, Tannirandorn Y, Rodeck CH. Endocrine pancreatic function in growth-retarded fetuses. *Obstet Gynecol.* 1991;77:541-544.

86 Béringue F, Blondeau B, Castellotti MC, Bréant B, Czernichow P, Polak M. Endocrine pancreas development in growth-retarded human fetuses. *Diabetes.* 2002;51:385-391.

87 Van Assche FA, De Prins F, Aerts L, Verjans M. The endocrine pancreas in small-for-dates infants. *Br J Obstet Gynaecol.* 1977;84:751-753.

88 Jensen CB, Storgaard H, Dela F, Holst JJ, Madsbad S, Vaag AA. Early differential defects of insulin secretion and action in 19-year-old caucasian men who had low birth weight. *Diabetes.* 2002;51:1271-1280.

89 Li C, Johnson MS, Goran MI. Effects of low birth weight on insulin resistance syndrome in caucasian and African-American children. *Diabetes Care.* 2001;24:2035-2042.

90 Crowther NJ, Trusler J, Cameron N, Toman M, Gray IP. Relation between weight gain and beta-cell secretory activity and non-esterified fatty acid production in 7-year-old African children: results from the Birth to Ten study. *Diabetologia.* 2000;43:978-985.

91 Flanagan DE, Moore VM, Godsland IF, Cockington RA, Robinson JS, Phillips DI. Fetal growth and the physiological control of glucose tolerance in adults: a minimal model analysis. *Am J Physiol Endocrinol Metab.* 2000;278:E700-E706.

92 Veening MA, van Weissenbruch MM, Heine RJ, Delemarre-van de Waal HA. Beta-cell capacity and insulin sensitivity in prepubertal children born small for gestational age: influence of body size during childhood. *Diabetes.* 2003;52:1756-1760.

93 Soto N, Bazaes RA, Peña V, et al. Insulin sensitivity and secretion are related to catch-up growth in small-for-gestational-age infants at age 1 year: results from a prospective cohort. *J Clin Endocrinol Metab.* 2003;88:3645-3650.

94 Dumortier O, Blondeau B, Duvillie B, Reusens B, Breant B, Remacle C. Different mechanisms operating during different critical time-windows reduce rat fetal beta cell mass due to a maternal low-protein or low-energy diet. *Diabetologia.* 2007;50:2495-2503.

95 Garofano A, Czernichow P, Breant B. In utero undernutrition impairs rat beta-cell development. *Diabetologia.* 1997;40:1231-1234.

96 Blondeau B, Garofano A, Czernichow P, Breant B. Age-dependent inability of the endocrine pancreas to adapt to pregnancy: a long-term consequence of perinatal malnutrition in the rat. *Endocrinology.* 1999;140:4208-4213.

97 Lim JS, Lee JA, Hwang JS, Shin CH, Yang SW. Non-catch-up growth in intrauterine growth-retarded rats showed glucose intolerance and increased expression of PDX-1 mRNA. *Pediatr Int.* 2011;53:181-186.

98 Garofano A, Czernichow P, Breant B. Postnatal somatic growth and insulin contents in moderate or severe intrauterine growth retardation in the rat. *Biol Neonate.* 1998;73:89-98.

99 Nyirenda MJ, Lindsay RS, Kenyon CJ, Burchell A, Seckl JR. Glucocorticoid exposure in late gestation permanently programs rat hepatic phosphoenolpyruvate carboxykinase and glucocorticoid receptor expression and causes glucose intolerance in adult offspring. *J Clin Invest.* 1998;101:2174-2181.

100 Petrik J, Reusens B, Arany E, et al. A low protein diet alters the balance of islet cell replication and apoptosis in the fetal and neonatal rat and is associated with a reduced pancreatic expression of insulin-like growth factor-II. *Endocrinology.* 1999;140:4861-4873.

101 Park JH, Stoffers DA, Nicholls RD, Simmons RA. Development of type 2 diabetes following intrauterine growth retardation in rats is associated with progressive epigenetic silencing of Pdx1. *J Clin Invest.* 2008;118:2316-2324.

102 Thompson RF, Fazzari MJ, Niu H, Barzilai N, Simmons RA, Greally JM. Experimental intrauterine growth restriction induces alterations in DNA methylation and gene expression in pancreatic islets of rats. *J Biol Chem.* 2010;285:15111-15118.

103 Srinivasan M, Katewa SD, Palaniyappan A, Pandya JD, Patel MS. Maternal high-fat diet consumption results in fetal malprogramming predisposing to the onset of metabolic syndrome-like phenotype in adulthood. *Am J Physiol Endocrinol Metab.* 2006;291:E792-E799.

104 Matthews LC, Hanley NA. The stress of starvation: glucocorticoid restraint of beta cell development. *Diabetologia.* 2011;54:223-226.

105 Shen CN, Seckl JR, Slack JM, Tosh D. Glucocorticoids suppress beta-cell development and induce hepatic metaplasia in embryonic pancreas. *Biochem J.* 2003;375(Pt 1):41-50.

106 Valtat B, Dupuis C, Zenaty D, et al. Genetic evidence of the programming of beta cell mass and function by glucocorticoids in mice. *Diabetologia.* 2011;54:350-359.

107 Gesina E, Blondeau B, Milet A, et al. Glucocorticoid signalling affects pancreatic development through both direct and indirect effects. *Diabetologia.* 2006;49:2939-2947.

108 Gesina E, Tronche F, Herrera P, et al. Dissecting the role of glucocorticoids on pancreas development. *Diabetes.* 2004;53:2322-2329.

109 Snoeck A, Remacle C, Reusens B, Hoet JJ. Effect of a low protein diet during pregnancy on the fetal rat endocrine pancreas. *Biol Neonate.* 1990;57:107-118.

110 Dahri S, Snoeck A, Reusens-Billen B, Remacle C, Hoet JJ. Islet function in offspring of mothers on low-protein diet during gestation. *Diabetes.* 1991;40:115-120.

111 Dumortier O, Blondeau B, Duvillié B, Reusens B, Bréant B, Remacle C. Different mechanisms operating during different critical time-windows reduce rat fetal beta cell mass due to a maternal low-protein or low-energy diet. *Diabetologia.* 2007;50:2495-2503.

112 Reusens B, Sparre T, Kalbe L, et al. The intrauterine metabolic environment modulates the gene expression pattern in fetal rat islets: prevention by maternal taurine supplementation. *Diabetologia.* 2008;51:836-845.

113 Boujendar S, Reusens B, Merezak S, et al. Taurine supplementation to a low protein diet during foetal and early postnatal life restores a normal proliferation and apoptosis of rat pancreatic islets. *Diabetologia.* 2002;45:856-866.

114 Lim JS, Lee JA, Hwang JS, Shin CH, Yang SW. Non-catch-up growth in intrauterine growth-retarded rats showed glucose intolerance and increased expression of PDX-1 mRNA. *Pediatr Int.* 2011;53:181-186.

115 Lee YY, Lee HJ, Lee SS, et al. Taurine supplementation restored the changes in pancreatic islet mitochondria in the fetal protein-malnourished rat. *Br J Nutr.* 2011;106:1198-1206.

116 Frantz ED, Aguila MB, Pinheiro-Mulder Ada R, Mandarim-de-Lacerda CA. Transgenerational endocrine pancreatic adaptation in mice from maternal protein restriction in utero. *Mech Ageing Dev.* 2011;132:110-116.

117 Garofano A, Czernichow P, Bréant B. In utero undernutrition impairs rat beta-cell development. *Diabetologia.* 1997;40:1231-1234.

118 Garofano A, Czernichow P, Bréant B. Postnatal somatic growth and insulin contents in moderate or severe intrauterine growth retardation in the rat. *Biol Neonate.* 1998;73:89-98.

119 Matveyenko AV, Singh I, Shin BC, Georgia S, Devaskar SU. Differential effects of prenatal and postnatal nutritional environment on ß-cell mass development and turnover in male and female rats. *Endocrinology.* 2010;151:5647-5656.

120 Blondeau B, Garofano A, Czernichow P, Bréant B. Age-dependent inability of the endocrine pancreas to adapt to pregnancy: a long-term consequence of perinatal malnutrition in the rat. *Endocrinology.* 1999;140:4208-4213.

121 Garofano A, Czernichow P, Bréant B. Effect of ageing on beta-cell mass and function in rats malnourished during the perinatal period. *Diabetologia*. 1999;42:711-718.

122 Stoffers DA, Desai BM, DeLeon DD, Simmons RA. Neonatal exendin-4 prevents the development of diabetes in the intrauterine growth retarded rat. *Diabetes*. 2003;52:734-740.

123 Park JH, Stoffers DA, Nicholls RD, Simmons RA. Development of type 2 diabetes following intrauterine growth retardation in rats is associated with progressive epigenetic silencing of Pdx1. *J Clin Invest*. 2008;118:2316-2324.

124 Ham JN, Crutchlow MF, Desai BM, Simmons RA, Stoffers DA. Exendin-4 normalizes islet vascularity in intrauterine growth restricted rats: potential role of VEGF. *Pediatr Res*. 2009;66:42-46.

125 Thompson RF, Fazzari MJ, Niu H, Barzilai N, Simmons RA, Greally JM. Experimental intrauterine growth restriction induces alterations in DNA methylation and gene expression in pancreatic islets of rats. *J Biol Chem*. 2010;285:15111-15118.

126 Pinney SE, Jaeckle Santos LJ, Han Y, Stoffers DA, Simmons RA. Exendin-4 increases histone acetylase activity and reverses epigenetic modifications that silence Pdx1 in the intrauterine growth retarded rat. *Diabetologia*. 2011;54:2606-2614.

127 De Prins FA, Van Assche FA. Intrauterine growth retardation and development of endocrine pancreas in the experimental rat. *Biol Neonate*. 1982;41:16-21.

128 Cerf ME, Williams K, Nkomo XI, et al. Islet cell response in the neonatal rat after exposure to a high-fat diet during pregnancy. *Am J Physiol Regul Integr Comp Physiol*. 2005;288:R1122-R1128.

129 Cerf ME, Chapman CS, Muller CJ, Louw J. Gestational high-fat programming impairs insulin release and reduces Pdx-1 and glucokinase immunoreactivity in neonatal Wistar rats. *Metabolism*. 2009;58:1787-1792.

130 Reimer MK, Ahren B. Altered beta-cell distribution of pdx-1 and GLUT-2 after a short-term challenge with a high-fat diet in C57BL/6J mice. *Diabetes*. 2002;51(suppl 1):S138-143.

131 Foot VL, Richardson CC, Jefferson W, Taylor PD, Christie MR. Islets in early life are resistant to detrimental effects of a high-fat maternal diet: a study in rats. *Horm Metab Res*. 2010;42:923-929.

Development of this book was supported by funding from Sandoz

Chapter 18

Metabolic syndrome
Thomas Reinehr

Introduction

Children born small for gestational age (SGA) have an increased risk for metabolic syndrome, which is defined by a clustering of cardiovascular risk factors, and is also known as part of the 'deadly quartet' due to its association with heart attack, stroke, and atherosclerosis [1–3]. Studies reported an increased risk of cardiovascular disease (CVD) in adults when glucose intolerance, insulin resistance, (central) obesity, dyslipidemia, and hypertension group together [3–5]. Interestingly, this increased risk for metabolic syndrome is not caused by SGA status *per se* but to rapid weight gain in the first years of life [6,7]. Aside from children born SGA, children with lipodystrophia, and especially overweight and obese children and adolescents, demonstrate an increased risk for metabolic syndrome [6,7].

To screen for metabolic syndrome, the following diagnostic procedures should be performed in all overweight children, as well as children born SGA with rapid catch-up weight gain:

- blood pressure measurements;
- waist circumference measurements;
- fasting high-density lipoprotein (HDL), cholesterol, triglyceride and glucose levels; and
- an oral glucose tolerance test.

S. Zabransky (ed.), *Caring for Children Born Small for Gestational Age*,   243
DOI: 10.1007/978-1-908517-90-6_18, © Springer Healthcare 2013

Multiple definitions of the metabolic syndrome have been proposed for adults, and although they all generally agree on the essential components – glucose intolerance, (central) obesity, hypertension, and dyslipidemia – they can differ in the detail [8–10]. These definitions have been adapted to children and adolescents by different authors using widely varying criteria [7,11–13] leading to different estimates of the prevalence of the metabolic syndrome [12–14] (Table 18.1).

Proposed definitions of metabolic syndrome for children and adolescents				
Cook et al [15]	**Ferranti et al** [16]	**Viner et al** [17]	**Weiss et al** [7]	**IDF** [11]
				waist circumference ≥90th percentile *and*
≥3 of 5 of criteria below:	≥3 of 5 of criteria below:	≥3 of 4 of criteria below:	≥3 of 5 of criteria below:	≥2 of criteria below:
waist circumference ≥90 percentile	waist circumference ≥75 percentile	body mass index ≥95th percentile	body mass index >97th percentile	–
BP ≥90th percentile	BP ≥90th percentile	systolic BP ≥95th percentile	BP ≥95th percentile	systolic BP >30 mmHG *or* diastolic BP >85 mmHg
triglycerides ≥110 mg/dL	triglycerides ≥100 mg/dL		triglycerides >110 mg/dL	triglycerides >150 mg/dL
HDL-cholesterol ≤40 mg/dL	female: HDL ≤50 mg/dL male: HDL ≤45 mg/dL	1 of 3 of the following criteria: • triglycerides ≥150 mg/dL • HDL <35 mg/dL • total cholesterol ≥95th percentile	HDL cholesterol <40 mg/dL	HDL cholesterol <40 mg/dL
impaired fasting glucose	impaired fasting glucose	impaired fasting glucose or glucose tolerance	impaired glucose tolerance	impaired fasting glucose

Table 18.1 Proposed definitions of metabolic syndrome for children and adolescents. BP, blood pressure; HDL. high density lipoprotein; IDF, International Diabetes Federation; LDL, low density lipoprotein. Data taken from [7,11,15–17].

Cardinal factors

The pathogenesis of the metabolic syndrome is still not fully understood. Cardinal factors are insulin resistance and obesity, but also include ethnicity, genetic predisposition, inflammation, adipocytokines such as leptin, adiponectin, tumor necrosis factor alpha, and interleukin-6, as well as oxidative stress (Figure 18.1) [18]. Insulin resistance is suggested as a key component of metabolic syndrome [3] and interestingly, SGA status is associated with insulin resistance [6,7] (see Chapter 14).

Since insulin resistance is a cardinal factor of metabolic syndrome, it is not surprising that the risk for metabolic syndrome increases in puberty since this age range is associated with an insulin resistant status [13]. Furthermore, diseases associated with insulin resistance are more frequent in children with metabolic syndrome, such as polycystic ovarian syndrome (PCOS) and non-alcoholic fatty liver disease (NAFLD) [13]. While NAFLD is frequently asymptomatic, PCOS manifests with hirsutism and an irregular menstrual cycle [19]. Androgens and sex hormone-binding globulin are useful to diagnose PCOS, while

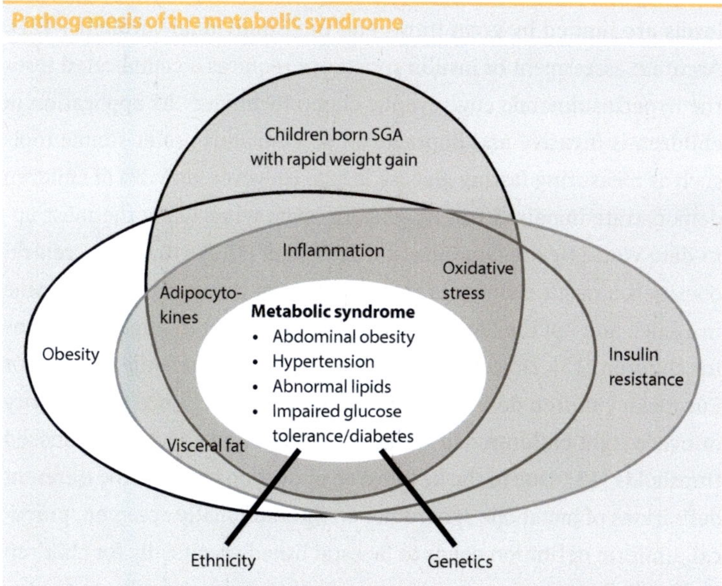

Figure 18.1 Pathogenesis of the metabolic syndrome. SGA, small for gestational age.

determination of transaminases and liver ultrasound should be performed to screen for NAFLD, which can be diagnosed only by liver biopsy [20]. In clinical practice, all children with metabolic syndrome should be screened for NAFLD and all pubertal girls with metabolic syndrome should be screened for PCOS.

Defining metabolic syndrome

Even if pediatricians 'diagnose' metabolic syndrome [13], in recent years, the definition of metabolic syndrome has continued to be debated, especially in children and adolescents [12,13]. In a study of obese children and adolescents, only 9% fulfilled all of the proposed definitions of metabolic syndrome [13], while the prevalence of metabolic syndrome had a wide range (6–39%) using the different proposed definitions. These findings point to a low degree of overlap between different definitions of metabolic syndrome.

One major problem is the determination of insulin resistance. Insulin levels without respect to glucose concentrations are not a good predictor of insulin resistance [21]. Furthermore, values of fasting insulin levels are limited by great intra- and inter-individual variability [21]. Accurate assessment of insulin resistance requires a complicated test - the hyperinsulinemic euglycyemic clamp technique. Its application in children is invasive and impractical, so clinicians prefer simple tools such as measuring fasting glucose levels. However, only 1% of children demonstrate impaired fasting glucose, even when using the most up-to-date World Health Organization definition [1]. Furthermore, central obesity is a major element in the definition of the metabolic syndrome in adults, and not the degree of overweight as used in some definitions for children [13]. However, waist circumference percentile cut-offs for European children do not seem to be very specific, since the majority of overweight children had waist circumferences above the proposed thresholds [13]. Due to the low degree of overlap between the different definitions of metabolic syndrome, an internationally accepted, practical, uniform definition needs to be established specifically for children and adolescents.

In order to attain the best definition of the metabolic syndrome, it would be ideal to study the impact of the different proposed definitions on clinical endpoints such as stroke, heart attack, or premature death. However, such longitudinal studies over decades are very difficult to perform. A measurement of early cardiovascular changes already detectable in childhood and adolescence, which has been shown to be predictive for later atherosclerotic diseases, would be an alternative, yet still practical, surrogate for such a clinical endpoint.

Measuring the intima-media thickness (IMT) of the common carotid artery, as a non-invasive marker for early atherosclerotic changes, has been reported to be reliable and predictive for development of later CVD [22–24]. A study in adults demonstrated that the prevalence of metabolic syndrome predicts IMT values [18]. Furthermore, in overweight children and adolescents, dyslipidemia, hypertension, and disturbed glucose metabolism were related to IMT [25,26]. Comparing different proposed definitions of metabolic syndrome, the best predictive value for increased IMT in children was achieved by the definition determined by Weiss and colleagues [7].

However, the entire concept of the metabolic syndrome is still controversial (at least in children) [13]. A major concern is the use of cut-off points for the various risk factors, thus implying that the values above the specified thresholds are associated with an excess risk. Yet the rationale for the different cut-off points has not yet been clearly delineated [12,13]. Moreover, the artificial dichotomization of continuous variables such as lipids, waist circumference, and blood pressure values seems debatable because dichotomization leads to an unnecessary loss of information [27]. This nonlinear relationship makes it all the more difficult and highlights the issue of how risk in the conglomeration of metabolic syndrome could be weighted more appropriately.

Finally, metabolic syndrome is based on the concept that the clustering of risk factors is predictive for CVD above and beyond the risks associated with its individual components [3,9,12–13]. However, this concept has not yet been tested empirically in childhood and adolescence. Analyzing the relationships between IMT and different definitions of metabolic syndrome, we have found no evidence of an increased risk beyond the sum of its components [14]. Furthermore, using the proposed cut-offs for these cardiovascular risk factors reduced the predictive value for increased IMT [14].

Indications for therapy

Indications for therapeutic procedures should be based on the estimation of the individual CVD risk factors, rather than on the dichotomous variable metabolic syndrome. Weight loss and increased physical activity are appropriate first-line approaches to reduce the related health risks associated with metabolic syndrome. For example, we have analyzed changes of weight status, two hour glucose levels from oral glucose tolerance tests (oGTT), fasting glucose, lipids, blood pressure, and the prevalence of metabolic syndrome in a one-year outpatient-lifestyle intervention that was based on physical activity, dietary counseling, and behavioral therapy in 288 obese children [28]. The data were compared to a study of 186 obese children without intervention with similar distributions of age, gender, and weight status. We found that the lifestyle intervention led to a significant weight decrease, while children without intervention demonstrated weight gain. Also, children in the lifestyle intervention group had a significant decrease of metabolic syndrome prevalence (from 19% to 9%) and an improvement of waist circumference, blood pressure, and two hour glucose values in the oGTT, in contrast to obese children without intervention [28] (Figure 18.2). The degree of weight loss was significantly associated with the amount of improvement of the components of the metabolic syndrome. Particularly, the children with a body mass index standard deviation score (BMI–SDS) reduction of >0.5 showed an improvement in all components associated with metabolic syndrome, as well as a decrease of IMT [28,29]. A reduction of 0.5 BMI–SDS is equal to body mass index reduction of 2 kg/m^2 (or a stable weight in the course of a year in growing children).

If lifestyle intervention does not work, pharmaceutical drugs should be used for treatment of cardiovascular risk factors. Hypertension should be treated (apart from restriction of sodium in the diet and stress management) with drug angiotensin inhibitors, calcium antagonists, or

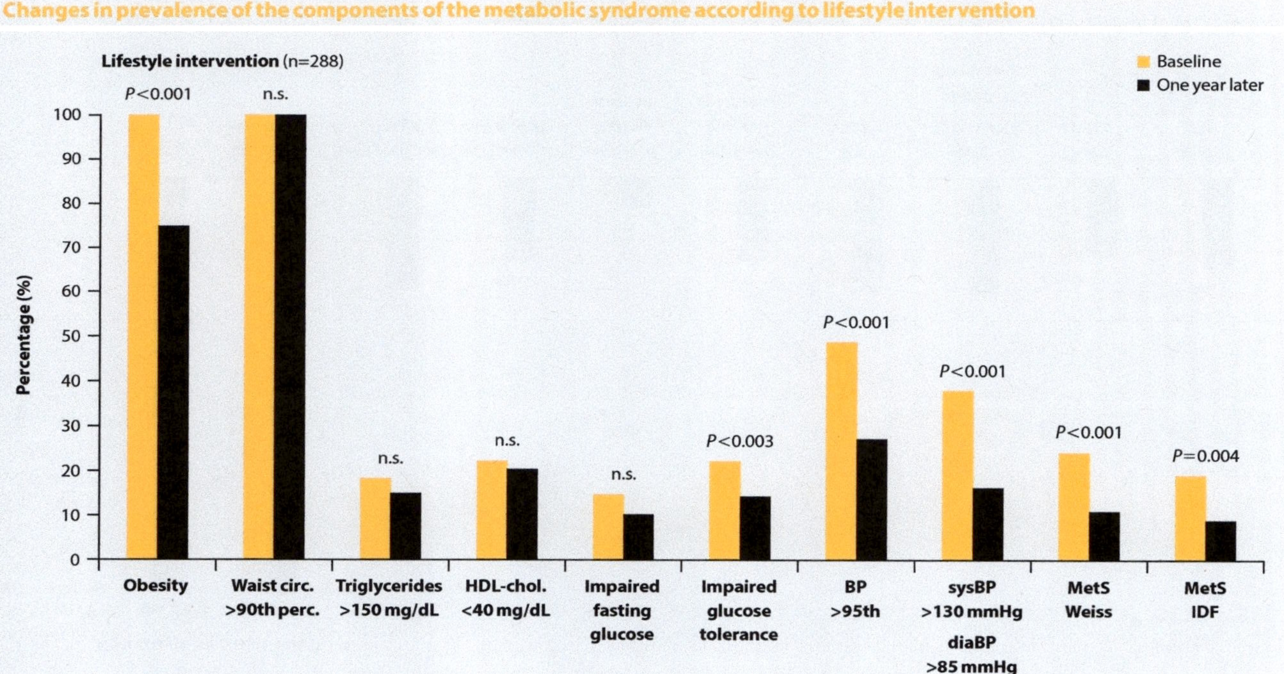

Figure 18.2 Changes in prevalence of the components of the metabolic syndrome according to lifestyle intervention (continues overleaf).

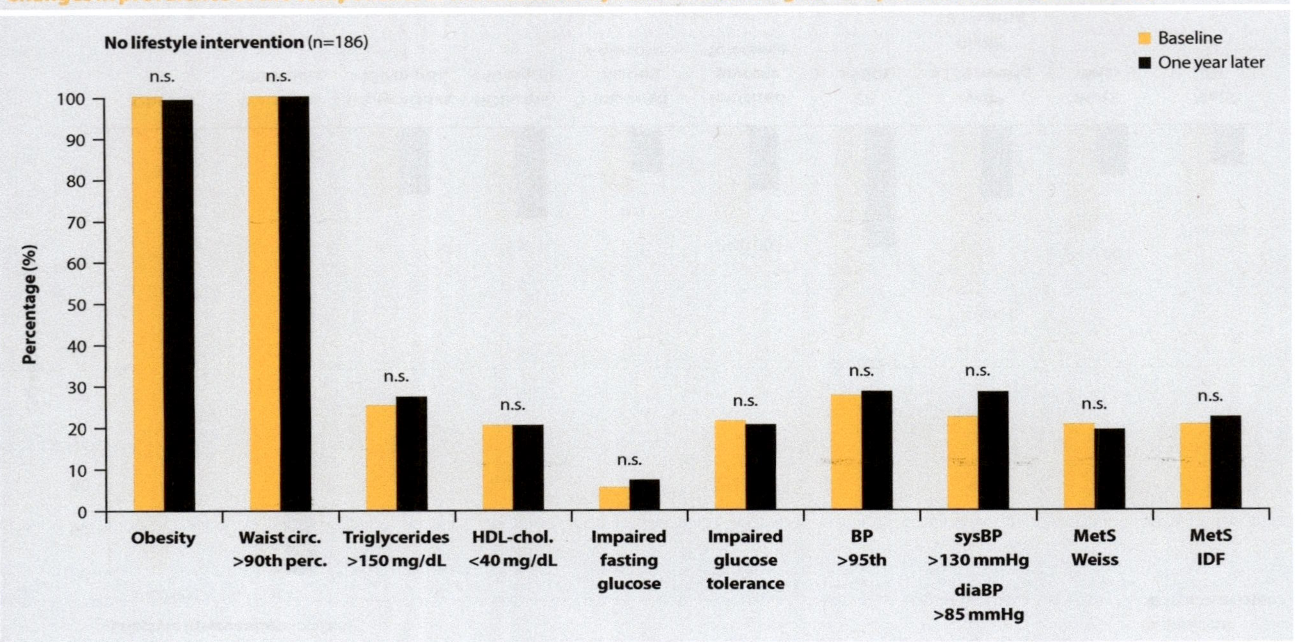

Figure 18.2 Changes in prevalence of the components of the metabolic syndrome according to lifestyle intervention (continued). BP, blood pressure; dias, diastolic; HDL, high-density lipoprotein; MetS, metabolic syndrome; perc, percentile; sys, systolic. Adapted with permission from Reinehr [26].

diuretics; beta blockers should not be used in obese patients, as they can reduce the basic metabolic rate [30].

Pharmaceutical intervention for dyslipidemia is seldom necessary in metabolic syndrome, as triglycerides are usually below 300 mg/dL. However, if triglycerides are above 350 mg/dL, fish oil, fibrates, or nicotinic acid are effective [30]. Since the major feature of dyslipidemia in metabolic syndrome is hypertriglyceridemia and low HDL cholesterol concentrations, increased low density lipoprotein cholesterol levels rarely occur.

Type 2 diabetes should be treated with metformin (if appropriate). However, the use of metformin in impaired glucose tolerance is remains controversial [31,32].

Conclusion

Children born SGA that experience rapid weight gain should be regularly screened for components of the metabolic syndrome. In these patients, first-line treatment for cardiovascular risk factors (eg, obesity, impaired glucose tolerance) should be lifestyle intervention.

References

1   l'Allemand D, Wiegand S, Reinehr T, et al. Cardiovascular risk in 26,008 European overweight children as established by a multicenter database. *Obesity (Silver Spring)*. 2008;16:1672-1679.
2   Ebbeling CB, Pawlak DB, Ludwig DS. Childhood obesity: public-health crisis, common sense cure. *Lancet*. 2002;360:473-482.
3   Reaven GM. Insulin resistance and compensatory hyperinsulinemia: role in hypertension, dyslipidemia, and coronary heart disease. *Am Heart J*. 1991;121:1283-1288.
4   Isomaa B, Almgren P, Tuomi T, et al. Cardiovascular morbidity and mortality associated with the metabolic syndrome. *Diabetes Care*. 2001;24:683-689.
5   Grundy SM. Obesity, metabolic syndrome, and coronary atherosclerosis. *Circulation*. 2002;105:2696-2698.
6   Kassi E, Pervanidou P, Kaltsas G, Chrousos G. Metabolic syndrome: definitions and controversies. *BMC Med*. 2011;9:48.
7   Weiss R, Dziura J, Burgert TS, et al. Obesity and the metabolic syndrome in children and adolescents. *N Engl J Med*. 2004;350:2362-2374.
8   Alberti KG, Zimmet P, Shaw J. Metabolic syndrome--a new world-wide definition. A Consensus Statement from the International Diabetes Federation. *Diabet Med*. 2006;23:469-480.
9   Eckel RH, Grundy SM, Zimmet PZ. The metabolic syndrome. *Lancet*. 2005;365:1415-1428.
10 Moebus S, Balijepalli C, Lösch C, et al. Age- and sex-specific prevalence and ten-year risk for cardiovascular disease of all 16 risk factor combinations of the metabolic syndrome - A cross-sectional study. *Cardiovasc Diabetol*. 2010;9:34.
11 Zimmet P, Alberti KG, Kaufman F, et al. The metabolic syndrome in children and adolescents - an IDF consensus report. *Pediatr Diabetes*. 2007;8:299-306.

12 Brambilla P, Lissau I, Flodmark CE, et al. Metabolic risk-factor clustering estimation in children: to draw a line across pediatric metabolic syndrome. *Int J Obes (Lond)*. 2007;31:591-600.

13 Reinehr T, de SG, Toschke AM, Andler W. Comparison of metabolic syndrome prevalence using eight different definitions: a critical approach. *Arch Dis Child*. 2007;92:1067-1072.

14 Reinehr T, Wunsch R, de Sousa G, Toschke AM. Relationship between metabolic syndrome definitions for children and adolescents and intima-media thickness. *Atherosclerosis*. 2008;199:193-200.

15 Cook S, Weitzman M, Auinger P, Nguyen M, Dietz WH. Prevalence of a metabolic syndrome phenotype in adolescents: findings from the third National Health and Nutrition Examination Survey, 1988-1994. *Arch Pediatr Adolesc Med*. 2003;157:821-827.

16 de Ferranti SD, Gauvreau K, Ludwig DS, Neufeld EJ, Newburger JW, Rifai N. Prevalence of the metabolic syndrome in American adolescents: findings from the Third National Health and Nutrition Examination Survey. *Circulation*. 2004;110:2494-2497.

17 Viner RM, Segal TY, Lichtarowicz-Krynska E, Hindmarsh P. Prevalence of the insulin resistance syndrome in obesity. *Arch Dis Child*. 2005;90:10-14.

18 Steinberger J, Daniels SR. Obesity, insulin resistance, diabetes, and cardiovascular risk in children: an American Heart Association scientific statement from the Atherosclerosis, Hypertension, and Obesity in the Young Committee (Council on Cardiovascular Disease in the Young) and the Diabetes Committee (Council on Nutrition, Physical Activity, and Metabolism). *Circulation*. 2003;107:1448-1453.

19 Lass N, Kleber M, Winkel K, Wunsch R, Reinehr T. Effect of lifestyle intervention on features of polycystic ovarian syndrome, metabolic syndrome, and intima-media thickness in obese adolescent girls. *J Clin Endocrinol Metab*. 2011;96:3533-3540.

20 Reinehr T, Schmidt C, Toschke AM, Andler W. Lifestyle intervention in obese children with =non-alcoholic fatty liver disease: 2-year follow-up study. *Arch Dis Child*. 2009;94:437-442.

21 Wallace TM, Matthews DR. The assessment of insulin resistance in man. *Diabet Med*. 2002;19:527-534.

22 Davis PH, Dawson JD, Riley WA, Lauer RM. Carotid intimal-medial thickness is related to cardiovascular risk factors measured from childhood through middle age: The Muscatine Study. *Circulation*. 2001;104:2815-2819.

23 Ahluwalia N, Drouet L, Ruidavets JB, et al. Metabolic syndrome is associated with markers of subclinical atherosclerosis in a French population-based sample. *Atherosclerosis*. 2006;186:345-353.

24 Lorenz MW, Markus HS, Bots ML, Rosvall M, Sitzer M. Prediction of clinical cardiovascular events with carotid intima-media thickness: a systematic review and meta-analysis. *Circulation*. 2007;115:459-467.

25 Meyer AA, Kundt G, Steiner M, Schuff-Werner P, Kienast W. Impaired flow-mediated vasodilation, carotid artery intima-media thickening, and elevated endothelial plasma markers in obese children: the impact of cardiovascular risk factors. *Pediatrics*. 2006;117:1560-1567.

26 Reinehr T, Kiess W, de Sousa G., Stoffel-Wagner B, Wunsch R. Intima media thickness in childhood obesity: relations to inflammatory marker, glucose metabolism, and blood pressure. *Metabolism*. 2006;55:113-118.

27 Royston P, Altman DG, Sauerbrei W. Dichotomizing continuous predictors in multiple regression: a bad idea. *Stat Med*. 2006;25:127-141.

28 Reinehr T, Kleber M, Toschke AM. Lifestyle intervention in obese children is associated with a decrease of the metabolic syndrome prevalence. *Atherosclerosis*. 2009;207:174-180.

29 Wunsch R, de Sousa G, Toschke AM, Reinehr T. Intima-media thickness in obese children before and after weight loss. *Pediatrics*. 2006;118:2334-2340.

30 Arbeitsgemeinschaft Adipositas im Kindes- und Jugendalter (AGA). www.aga.adipositas-gesellschaft.de/. Accessed February 20, 2013.

31 Meaney E, Vela A, Samaniego V, et al. Metformin, arterial function, intima-media thickness and nitroxidation in metabolic syndrome: the mefisto study. *Clin Exp Pharmacol Physiol*. 2008;35:895-903.

32 Wiegand S, l'Allemand D, Hüubel H, et al. Metformin and placebo therapy both improve weight management and fasting insulin in obese insulin-resistant adolescents: a prospective, placebo-controlled, randomized study. *Eur J Endocrinol*. 2010;163:585-592.

Development of this book was supported by funding from Sandoz

Chapter 19

Cardiovascular risks and diseases
Prakash M Kabbur, Nisha I Parikh

Introduction

During fetal development, body tissues and organ systems go through critical periods of development which coincide with rapid cell division [1]. This 'programming' is a process whereby a stimulus or insult during critical periods of development programs genetic and metabolic changes, resulting in life-long health outcomes [2]. Thus, programming in utero and in early-life can result in increased risks for developing cardiovascular disease (CVD), subclinical CVD, and ultimately overt cardiovascular events, including myocardial infarction and stroke [2]. From this, it is now becoming clear that being born small for gestational age (SGA) has implications for developing CVD that persist across the person's lifespan and may necessitate overlapping care provisions from several medical disciplines (Figure 19.1). Fetal programming is discussed in more detail in Chapter 11.

Primordial cardiovascular disease risk factor

Established nonbehavioral risk factors for CVD include hypertension, dyslipidemia, and diabetes mellitus [3]. Excess adiposity is considered a secondary risk factor for cardiovascular disease because it can influence the development and progression of hypertension, dyslipidemia, and diabetes mellitus [3]. Being born SGA can influence the trajectories of all of these CVD risk factors, and can thus be considered a primordial risk factor [4].

S. Zabransky (ed.), *Caring for Children Born Small for Gestational Age*,
DOI: 10.1007/978-1-908517-90-6_19, © Springer Healthcare 2013

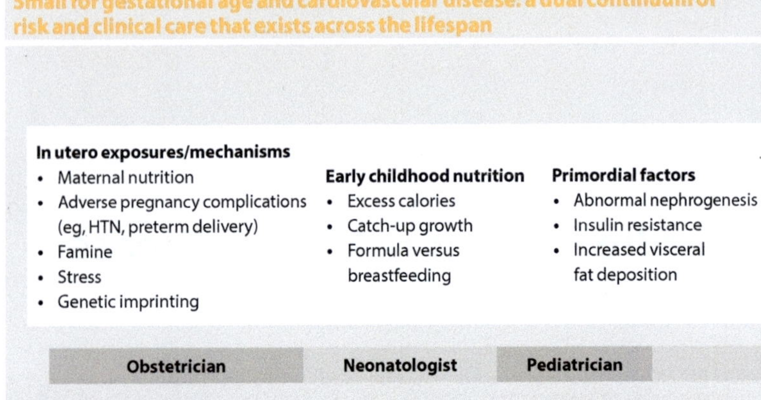

Figure 19.1 Small for gestational age and cardiovascular disease: a dual continuum of risk and clinical care that exists across the lifespan. CVD, cardiovascular disease; HTN, hypertension; IMT, intima-media thickness.

Accordingly, the importance of primordial disease prevention has been increasingly emphasized in scientific and public health communities [5] and mounting evidence supports the influence of early developmental influences such as being born SGA on CVD risk factor development.

Early nutrition imbalances that lead to babies being born SGA can affect blood pressure trajectories, cholesterol metabolism, insulin sensitivity, and a range of other metabolic, endocrine, and immune functions [6-8]. Human fetal adaptation to undernutrition is marked by an immediate catabolic response whereby the body begins to consume its own substrates to provide energy [9]. In utero, stressors can program hypertension through mechanisms which lead to a reduction in functional nephrons [10,11]. This paucity in the total number of nephrons can down-regulate the renin-angiotensin-aldosterone axis, leading to later renal dysfunction and hypertension [12]. A systematic meta-analysis of five high-quality studies of babies with low birth weight and preterm delivery demonstrated that these infants went on to have elevated blood pressure (3.8 mmHg; 95% CI, 2.6–5.0 mm Hg) later in childhood, adolescence, or adulthood [12].

It is widely accepted that growth-restricted infants lack skeletal muscle, which in turn decreases glucose uptake and causes insulin

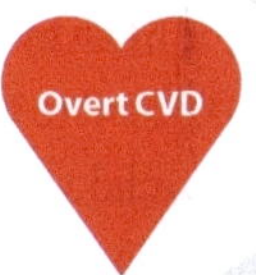

resistance [13,14]. Insulin resistance that develops early in life is associated with abnormal vascular development, leading to various metabolic problems and predisposition to hypertension [13]. Furthermore, early-life insulin resistance is also a risk factor for heart attack and congestive heart failure [14,15]. Studies have demonstrated associations between early growth restriction and postnatal accelerated growth with disproportionate fat mass accumulation and lack of skeletal muscle [14,16,17]. Furthermore, adults who were SGA at birth, of lower weight when compared to children not born SGA at 2 years of age, and who put on weight rapidly thereafter, were more prone to experience coronary events [17]. These data demonstrate that the rate of increase in body mass index (BMI) in childhood is more important than increase in BMI attained during any age in terms of the accompanying excess CVD risk [17].

Catch-up growth and cardiovascular disease

Low birth weight combined with rapid postnatal growth appears to be associated with later childhood and adult sequelae of hypertension, impaired glucose tolerance, and obesity [18]. Rapid growth after age 2 years may represent a particularly high-risk group for developing CVD risk factors and events [2]. As put forth by Barker, the adaptive responses to environmental insults during early life can be harmful above and beyond the initial insults [19,20] and it is important to note the impact of maternal undernutrition on young adults who were born SGA [21,22].

Observational studies conducted from regions affected by famine and war demonstrate the combined need for a healthy fetus, healthy mother, and a healthy postnatal course upon long-term health [23]. Individuals exposed to famine conditions (ie, lack of adequate nutrition) in utero were found to have a greater risk of impaired glucose tolerance, microalbuminuria, dyslipidemia, obesity, as well as three-fold increase in prevalence of coronary heart disease at age 50 [23].

Encouraging breastfeeding is of paramount importance, along with nutritional supplementation when deemed necessary, in order to maintain or minimize weight gain within recommended parameters [6,7]. Barker et al, in their Helsinki study of 13,345 men and women, showed that later coronary events were associated with low BMI at birth, at 2 years of age, and then with high BMI at 11 years of age, again indicating the coronary heart disease prediction not by body size at any particular age, but by the nature of childhood weight gain [2]. Given the dearth of randomized nutrition-focused studies evaluating multiple endpoints of catch-up growth (eg, cognitive health), it is difficult to provide clinical recommendations that focus solely on preventing the cardio-metabolic sequelae associated with aggressive catch-up growth. Nutrition during pregnancy is discussed in more detail in Chapter 3.

Subclinical cardiovascular disease

Markers of subclinical atherosclerosis reflect early-onset CVD and can predict incident CVD events. These include: brachial artery reactivity (a marker of endothelial function), arterial stiffness (a marker of vascular remodeling), and carotid intima-media thickness (IMT; a marker of atherosclerosis and vascular remodeling).

Metabolic syndrome

The metabolic syndrome consists of insulin resistance, hypertension, dyslipidemia, and adiposity, and predisposes to the development of CVD and diabetes in adults (see Chapter 18). Insulin resistance and dyslipidemia affect the endothelium and arterial wall which contributes to hypertension, CVD, and atherosclerosis [24,25]. Insulin is noted to have vasoactive and anticholinergic actions including direct actions on cellular and structural constituents of vascular wall [26,27]. Compared to normal birth weight infants, those with SGA showed a blunted vascular flow mediated dilation/endothelial function in childhood, adolescence, and adulthood [28–31].

Arterial stiffness

An important factor in regulation of blood pressure is wall stiffness of medium-to-large arteries [32]. Increased arterial stiffness in large arteries of children, adolescents, and adults who were born SGA is demonstrated through noninvasive methods such as pulse wave velocity measurement and pressure waveforms [33,34]. Arterial stiffness was measured by Ligi et al in very-low birth weight infants as early as fifth day of life using Doppler echocardiogram and pulse blood pressure measurements [35]. The association between SGA and arterial stiffness persisted until the 7th week of life [36]. Furthermore, coronary arteries and aortic root diameter are smaller and cardiac structure is altered in SGA infants [37].

Specific tissue biomarkers may mediate the association between arterial stiffness and hypertension. In particular, elastin deficiency plays a major role in the causation of stiffness of aorta and its major branches in growth-impaired fetuses [38]. The younger the gestational age, the lower the elastin content, as elastin accumulates in the late prenatal period.

Adiposity and atherogenic factors

Female infants born SGA are at risk for enlarged adipocytes, hyperinsulinemia, hypoadiponectinemia, faster bone maturation, and increased visceral and total adiposity in the absence of obesity [39] Compared to subcutaneous adipose depots, visceral adiposity is believed to have more deleterious cardiometabolic effects [39].

Infant size is related to endothelial dysfunction [40] through mechanisms of nutrition-mediated nitric oxide synthesis [41]. Thus, endothelial dysfunction in children and young adults born small may underlie the pathogenesis of adult atherosclerosis [31]. Greater IMT of the aorta, an early marker of atherosclerosis, was shown in late fetal life and in childhood among pregnancies associated with placental insufficiency and growth restricted newborns [42–45]. Higher blood pressure and fasting insulin were associated with higher IMT, and also increased risk for stroke [43]. Furthermore, thicker carotid IMT in relation to lumen size was seen in very-low birth weight infants as compared to term infants [43].

In the general population, serum lipid levels can be tracked over several years and childhood measurements may predict total cholesterol and low-density lipoprotein (LDL) cholesterol levels in adults [46,47]. When serum lipid levels were measured in children and young adults, they were demonstrated to be significantly associated with atherosclerotic changes in adulthood [48]. This particular finding was shown in 20-year-old adults who were born SGA [49]. Additionally, subjects with SGA had higher LDL and lower high-density lipoprotein (HDL) cholesterol levels when compared to non-SGA controls [50].

Conclusion

Being born SGA poses not only near-term harmful effects on growth and cognitive development early in life, but also increases the risk of developing CVD through several multifactorial mechanisms. SGA may predispose a patient to major non-behavioral CVD risk factors including hypertension, dyslipidemia, insulin resistance, and excess adiposity. The presence of these risk factors can in turn lead to subclinical atherosclerosis in childhood, adolescence, and early adulthood, and to overt CVD in adulthood. The recognition of being born SGA as a critical upstream mediator of several CVD pathways by health care providers across the lifespan continuum (eg, obstetricians, neonatologists, pediatricians, and internal medicine care providers) is critical to effectively addressing primordial, primary, and secondary CVD prevention.

References

1   Widdowson EM, McCance RA. A review: new thoughts on growth. *Pediatr Res.* 1975;9:154-156.
2   Barker DJ, Osmond C, Kajantie E, Eriksson JG. Growth and chronic disease: findings in the Helsinki Birth Cohort. *Ann Hum Biol.* 2009;36:445-458.
3   Centers for Disease Control and Prevention (CDC). "Heart Disease Risk Factors." CDC website. www.cdc.gov/heartdisease/risk_factors.htm. Accessed February 20, 2013.

4   Crispi F, Figueras F, Cruz-Lemini M, Bartrons J, Bijnens B, Gratacos E. Cardiovascular programming in children born small for gestational age and relationship with prenatal signs of severity. *Am J Obstet Gynecol.* 2012;207:e1-e9.

5   Pasternak RC, Abrams J, Greenland P, Smaha LA, Wilson PW, Houston-Miller N. 34th Bethesda Conference: Task force #1--Identification of coronary heart disease risk: is there a detection gap? *J Am Coll Cardiol.* 2003;41:1863-1874.

6   Lucas A. Programming by early nutrition in man. *Ciba Found Symp.* 1991;156:38-50.

7   Lucas A. Role of nutritional programming in determining adult morbidity. *Arch Dis Child.* 1994;71:288-290.

8   Lucas A. Programming by early nutrition: an experimental approach. *J Nutr.* 1998;128(2 suppl):401S-406S.

9   Harding JE, Johnston BM. Nutrition and fetal growth. *Reprod Fertil Dev.* 1995;7:539-547.

10   Wlodek ME, Westcott K, Siebel AL, Owens JA, Moritz KM. Growth restriction before or after birth reduces nephron number and increases blood pressure in male rats. *Kidney Int.* 2008;74:187-195.

11   Rueda-Clausen CF, Morton JS, Davidge ST. The early origins of cardiovascular health and disease: who, when, and how. *Semin Reprod Med.* 2011;29:197-210.

12   de Jong F, Monuteaux MC, van Elburg RM, Gillman MW, Belfort MB. Systematic review and meta-analysis of preterm birth and later systolic blood pressure. *Hypertension.* 2012;59:226-234.

13   Phillips DI. Insulin resistance as a programmed response to fetal undernutrition. *Diabetologia.* 1996;39:1119-1122.

14   Thompson JA, Regnault TR. In utero origins of adult insulin resistance and vascular dysfunction. *Semin Reprod Med.* 2011;29:211-224.

15   Contreras C, Sánchez A, Martínez P, et al. Insulin resistance in penile arteries from a rat model of metabolic syndrome. *Br J Pharmacol.* 2010;161:350-364.

16   Eriksson JG, Forsén T, Tuomilehto J, Jaddoe VW, Osmond C, Barker DJ. Effects of size at birth and childhood growth on the insulin resistance syndrome in elderly individuals. *Diabetologia.* 2002;45:342-348.

17   Barker DJ, Osmond C, Forsen TJ, Kajantie E, Eriksson JG. Trajectories of growth among children who have coronary events as adults. *N Eng J Med.* 2005;353:1802-1809.

18   Cameron N, Demerath EW. Critical periods in human growth and their relationship to diseases of aging. *Am J Phys Anthropol.* 2002;Suppl 35:159-184.

19   Barker DJ. In utero programming of chronic disease. *Clin Sci (Lond).* 1998;95:115-128.

20   Barker DJ. The fetal and infant origins of adult disease. *BMJ.* 1990;301:1111.

21   Barker DJ. Fetal nutrition and cardiovascular disease in later life. *Br Med Bull.* 1997;53:96-108.

22   Barker DJ. The origins of the developmental origins theory. *J Intern Med.* 2007;261:412-417.

23   Painter RC, de Rooij SR, Hutten BA, et al. Reduced intima media thickness in adults after prenatal exposure to the Dutch famine. *Atheroscleorosis.* 2007;193:421-427.

24   Celermajer DS, Sorensen KE, Bull C, Robinson J, Deanfield JE. Endothelium-dependent dilation in the systemic arteries of asymptomatic subjects relates to coronary risk factors and their interaction. *J Am Coll Cardiol.* 1994;24:1468-1474.

25   Verma S, Anderson TJ. Fundamentals of endothelial function for the clinical cardiologist. *Circulation.* 2002;105:546-549.

26   Dimmeler S, Fleming I, Fisslthaler B, Hermann C, Busse R, Zeiher AM. Activation of nitric oxide synthase in endothelial cells by Akt-dependent phosphorylation. *Nature.* 1999;399:601-605.

27   Montagnani M, Golovchenko I, Kim I, et al. Inhibition of phosphatidylinositol 3-kinase enhances mitogenic actions of insulin in endothelial cells. *J Biol Chem.* 2002;277:1794-1799.

28   Leeson CP, Whincup PH, Cook DG, et al. Flow-mediated dilation in 9- to 11-year-old children: the influence of intrauterine and childhood factors. *Circulation.* 1997;96:2233-2238.

29   Goodfellow J, Bellamy MF, Gorman ST, et al. Endothelial function is impaired in fit young adults of low birth weight. *Cardiovasc Res.* 1998;40:600-606.

30 Martin H, Hu J, Gennser G, Norman M. Impaired endothelial function and increased carotid stiffness in 9-year-old children with low birthweight. *Circulation*. 2000;102:2739-2744.

31 Leeson CP, Kattenhorn M, Morley R, Lucas A, Deanfield JE. Impact of low birth weight and cardiovascular risk factors on endothelial function in early adult life. *Circulation*. 2001;103:1264-1268.

32 Cecelja M, Chowienczyk P. Role of arterial stiffness in cardiovascular disease. *J R Soc Med Cardio*. 2012;1:411.

33 Lurbe E, Torro MI, Carvajal E, Alvarez V, Redón J. Birth weight impacts on wave reflections in children and adolescents. *Hypertension*. 2003;41:646-650.

34 Oren A, Vos LE, Bos WJ, et al. Gestational age and birth weight in relation to aortic stiffness in healthy young adults: two separate mechanisms? *Am J Hypertens*. 2003;16:76-79.

35 Ligi I, Grandvuillemin I, Andres V, Dignat-George F, Simeoni U. Low birth weight infants and the developmental programming of hypertension: a focus on vascular factors. *Semin Perinatol*. 2010;34:188-192.

36 Tauzin L, Rossi P, Giusano B, et al. Characteristics of arterial stiffness in very low birth weight premature infants. *Pediatr Res*. 2006;60:592-596.

37 Jiang B, Godfrey KM, Martyn CN, Gale CR. Birth weight and cardiac structure in children. *Pediatrics*. 2006;117:e257-e261.

38 Martyn CN, Greenwald SE. Impaired synthesis of elastin in walls of aorta and large conduit arteries during early development as an initiating event in pathogenesis of systemic hypertension. *Lancet*. 1997;350:953-955.

39 Ibáñez L, Lopez-Bermejo A, Diaz M, de Zegher F. Catch-up growth in girls born small for gestational age precedes childhood progression to high adiposity. *Fertil Steril*. 2011;96:220-223.

40 Touwslager RN, Houben AJ, Gielen M, et al. Endothelial vasodilatation in newborns is related to body size and maternal hypertension. *J Hypertens*. 2012;30:124-131.

41 Franco Mdo C, Arruda RM, Dantas AP, et al. Intrauterine undernutrition: expression and activity of the endothelial nitric oxide synthase in male and female adult offspring. *Cardiovasc Res*. 2002;56:145-153.

42 Oren A, Vos LE, Uiterwaal CS, Gorissen WH, Grobbee DE, Bots ML. Birth weight and carotid intima-media thickness: new perspectives from the atherosclerosis risk in young adults (ARYA) study. *Ann Epidemiol*. 2004;14:8-16.

43 Koklu E, Kurtoglu S, Akcakus M, et al. Increased aortic intima-media thickness is related to lipid profile in newborns with intrauterine growth restriction. *Horm Res*. 2006;65:269-275.

44 Koklu E, Ozturk MA, Kurtoglu S, Akcakus M, Yikilmaz A, Gunes T. Aortic intima-media thickness, serum IGF-I, IGFBP-3, and leptin levels in intrauterine growth-restricted newborns of healthy mothers. *Pediatr Res*. 2007;62:704-709.

45 Cosmi E, Visentin S, Fanelli T, Mautone AJ, Zanardo V. Aortic intima media thickness in fetuses and children with intrauterine growth restriction. *Obstet Gynecol*. 2009;114:1109-1114.

46 Lauer RM, Lee J, Clarke WR. Factors affecting the relationship between childhood and adult cholesterol levels: the Muscatine Study. *Pediatrics*. 1988;82:309-318.

47 Webber LS, Srinivasan SR, Wattigney WA, Berenson GS. Tracking of serum lipids and lipoproteins from childhood to adulthood. The Bogalusa Heart Study. *Am J Epidemiol*. 1991;133:884-899.

48 Berenson GS, Srinivasan SR, Bao W, Newman WP 3rd, Tracy RE, Wattigney WA. Association between multiple cardiovascular risk factors and atherosclerosis in children and young adults. The Bogalusa Heart Study. *N Eng J Med*. 1998;338:1650-1656.

49 Salonen M, Tenhola S, Laitinen T, et al. Tracking serum lipid levels and the association of cholesterol concentrations, blood pressure and cigarette smoking with carotid artery intima-media thickness in young adults born small for gestational age. *Circ J*. 2010;74:2419-2425.

Development of this book was supported by funding from Sandoz

Chapter 20

Ophthalmological findings and visual function disorders

Barbara Käsmann-Kellner

Introduction

The wide-ranging sequelae of premature birth on morphology and function of the visual system are now well known following the discovery of an inverse relationship between prevalence of retinopathy of prematurity (ROP) and critical birth weight [1]. Parallel to the continuing decrease in critical and life-threatening birth weight, many papers have described the general and ocular outcomes in premature children, as more children survived despite their low birth weight [2–5].

The ocular and visual consequences of starting life as a child small for gestational age (SGA) – born prematurely or full-term – have not been widely described in ophthalmological literature. Particular attention should therefore be paid to children who have been delivered on due day, but who are born SGA. Generally, these children usually are not given ophthalmological screening examinations during the first weeks of their lives, in contrast to premature children. For example, in Germany, in general, no ophthalmological or visual attention is given to children born SGA until the third year of life, when a pediatrician (not an ophthalmologist) performs an eye screening and vision test in the mandatory preventive medical check-up. If the pediatrician notices any vision deficit or visual acuity asymmetry, it is only then that an ophthalmologist becomes involved. If this is not the case in infancy, the child may well live up to 6 or 7 years

S. Zabransky (ed.), *Caring for Children Born Small for Gestational Age*,   263
DOI: 10.1007/978-1-908517-90-6_20, © Springer Healthcare 2013

of age before visual deficits become evident. Thus, there are still a number of children whose visual deficit is only noticed when they enter school and undergo a school entry health exam.

Children born SGA at term may show morphological and functional abnormalities of the visual system, which may be present at birth or may develop during childhood years [6,7]. The pathological ocular and central findings can affect any structure of the eye and any quality of vision (eg, visual function, visual field, binocularity, strabismus, visual perception) [7].

The visual system forms nearly one-third of the telencephalon volume and the visual pathways connect many other neural structures on their way from the frontal to the occipital cortex and into the associative higher areas. Concerning ocular anatomy, the development of the retinal vessels is of particular interest, as this is the origin of pathological development in retinopathy of prematurity (ROP). Unlike with brain and cortical structures, one can examine retinal vessels in vivo, thus, as in ROP, being able to draw inferences to other critical vessel development sites, such as kidneys, gastrointestinal tract, and any neuronal structures.

Altered retinal vascular architecture

Retinal vascular structure changes in relation to the retinal locus. For example, at the vascular and non-functional center of the retina (the optic nerve head); the vessels are completely different from those in the retinal periphery [8]. Just as the retinal neural dendrites thin away in the periphery, the capillary net of the retinal vessels changes accordingly [8]. At the posterior pole, retinal vessels are surrounded by a dense and thick network of perivascular mesenchymal capillaries [8]. At the equator, this capillary net is already considerably thinner. In the peripheral retinal area that merges into the ora serrata, the capillary extensions are barely detectable [8].

Both in prematurity (very evident with the risk of development of ROP), as well in infants born SGA, it has been postulated that critical alimentary shortage and malnutrition before birth leads to permanent changes in some physiological and metabolic variables which are essential for normal vessel development [9,10]. It has been demonstrated that children born SGA, both in utero and postpartum, exhibit reduced levels of insulin-like growth factor (IGF-I), which in turn activates vascular endothelial growth factor leading to increased endothelial cell proliferation and survival [9]. Thus, IGF-I has a direct influence on retinal angiogenesis. In children born SGA, a reduced retinal vascularization has been found, apparent by a reduced number of retinal vessel branchings in the periphery [9]. Thus, not only retinal vascularization, but also the shape and morphology of the optic nerve head, can be affected in preterm and children born SGA.

Exemplary work on retinal vessel development and optic nerve head anomalies in children born SGA has been performed in recent years by using digital image analysis [11–14]. The researchers elucidated certain distinct differences in ocular and visual system changes between different etiological groups, such as SGA with prematurity, SGA due to fetal exposition to alcohol or nicotine, and SGA in septo-optic dysplasia (de Morsier syndrome, often accompanied by low levels of growth hormone). Table 20.1 gives a summary of the results from the aforementioned studies examining children with varying underlying causes of malnutrition.

Figure 20.1 and Figure 20.2 show the results of one of the most important papers written by Helstrom and colleagues, who first described the retinal findings in SGA in a standardized way, supplying standardized photographic evaluations to underline their findings.

In Figure 20.2, both for subjects with IUGR and children born SGA, the number of vessel branchings were more often significantly below the median of normal infants [15]. The altered development of retinal vascular and neural structures under malnutrition conditions occurred in utero and directly after birth. However, these tissues are definitely not the only vascular and neural structures in the growing human which are affected by malnourishment leading to a child being born SGA.

Figure 20.3 shows the retinal vascular pattern in children of nearly the same age who received an evaluation of their strabismus. Here, besides the atypical branching, the paleness of the optic nerve head in SGA is clearly evident.

Figure 20.4 shows the difference between adult persons (one born AGA and other born SGA), both in their early twenties, with reduced adult retinal vascularization [16]. The images demonstrate that these differences persist beyond childhood.

Literature survey: Alterations of the optic nerve head and retinal vessels in small for gestational age		
Etiology of malnutrition	**Optic nerve head**	**Retinal vessels**
Controls: 100 healthy non-preterm and non-SGA adolescents	Reference group for the digital image analysis of the subgroups examined	
Premature children without PVL	Normal	Less ramifications
Premature children with PVL	Larger cup-disc relation	Less branching
Small for gestational age (SGA)	Small neuroretinal rim of the optic nerve head Optic nerve head small	Lower number of retinal vessels
Fetal ethanol syndrome	Small optic nerve head	Arteries and veins show tortuositas
Formerly IUGR; age upon examination=18 years	Small neuroretinal rim of the optic nerve head, correlating to the extend of SGA It still is unclear whether the individual neurons show less volume or if there is a reduced number of dendrites	Significantly less retinal vessels and less vessel branching; this correlates to the extent of SGA
Septo-optic dysplasia (de Morsier Syndrome)	Extremely small and dysplastic optic nerve head and optic nerve	Tortuositas only of the venous vessels
Isolated growth hormone deficiency	Optic nerve head may be smaller	Lower numbers of retinal branchings
Laron-Syndrome	Optic nerve head may be smaller	Lower numbers of retinal branching

Table 20.1 Literature survey: Alterations of the optic nerve head and retinal vessels in small for gestational age. IUGR, intrauterine growth restriction; PVL, periventricular leukomalacia. Data compiled from [11–14].

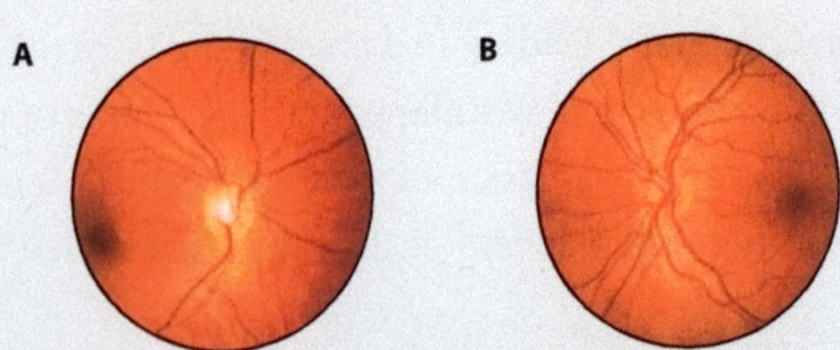

Figure 20.1 Typical SGA findings as compared to normal findings in ophthalmoscopy. A, Reduced retinal vascularization in an 18-year-old woman with a birth weight SGA and fetal aortic BFC III; B, Normal vascularization in an 18-year-old woman with a normal birth weight and normal fetal aortic BFC. BFC, blood flow class. Reproduced with permission from Hellström et al [15].

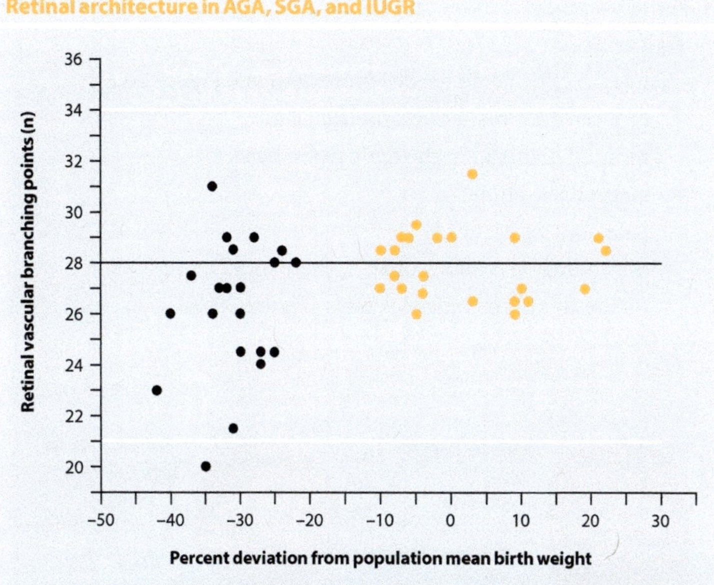

Figure 20.2 Retinal architecture in AGA, SGA, and IUGR. Number of retinal vascular branching points in test subjects with IUGR (n=21; orange dots), in subjects with SGA (n=23; black dots) and a healthy control group (AGA; not represented). Solid line: median of vessel branchings depending on the birth weight in AGA infants; dotted lines: maximum and minimum of vessel branchings in AGA. Black dots: SGA; orange dots: IUGR. AGA, average for gestational age; IUGR, intrauterine growth restriction; SGA, small for gestational age. Reproduced with permission from Hellström et al [15].

Other ophthalmological sequelae

The following is an abbreviated list and discussion of other possible consequences of IUGR and being born SGA on the eyes and visual system. Many of them may have a negative impact on the visual function of the child, which can cause life-long impairment. These include:

- changes to ocular morphology;
- lanugo (fine downy hair) of the eyelids (Figure 20.5);
- persistent tunica vasculosa lentis;
  - fine vessels from the stroma to the anterior lens surface
  - severe maturation disorders
  - slow decline in visual function
  - lens opacification (cataracta subcapsularis anterior)

- retinal vascular architecture (Table 20.1; Figure 20.2, Figure 20.3; Figure 20.4);
- changes to optic nerve head (Figure 20.3 and Figure 20.6);
  - reduced and smaller neuroretinal rim
  - reduced diameter of the optic nerve head
  - larger excavation
  - pale optic nerve head
  - depending on etiology of SGA, there may be prominent tortuositas of the retinal vessels (Figure 20.6).

Retinal vascular pattern and optic nerve head findings in children born AGA and SGA

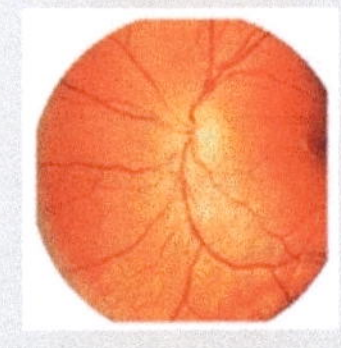

Female, 10 years

AGA
- ONH vital
- Normal branching numbers of retinal vessels

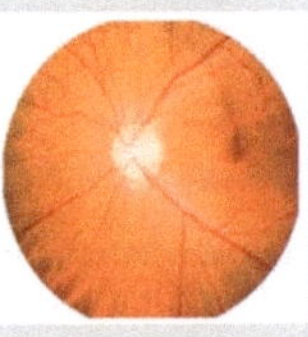

Female, 11 years

SGA
- ONH pale
- Less branchings of retinal vessels

Figure 20.3 Retinal vascular pattern and optic nerve head findings in children born AGA and SGA. AGA, appropriate for gestational age; ONH, optic nerve head; SGA, small for gestational age.

Differences in AGA and SGA adult retinal vascularization

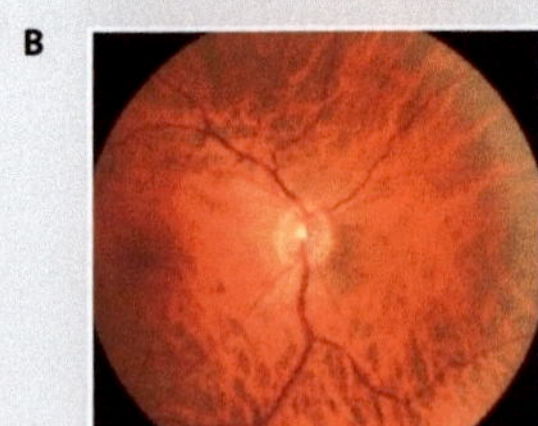

A — Female patient, AGA, 25 years of age, normal branching of retinal vessels; best to be seen in inferior retina

B — Female patient, SGA, 27 years of age, clearly reduced branching of retinal vessels, including atypical branching of the inferior veins; best seen in the lower part of the retina

Figure 20.4 Differences in AGA and SGA adult retinal vascularization. AGA, appropriate for gestational age; SGA, small for gestational age. Reproduced with permission from Kistner et al [16].

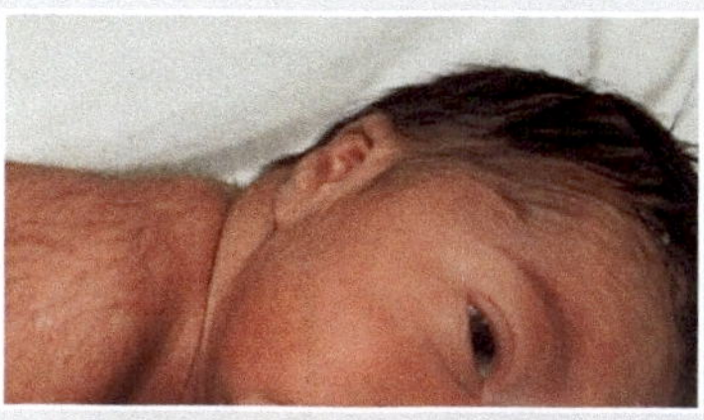

Figure 20.5 Marked lanugo above brows and on forehead and shoulders.

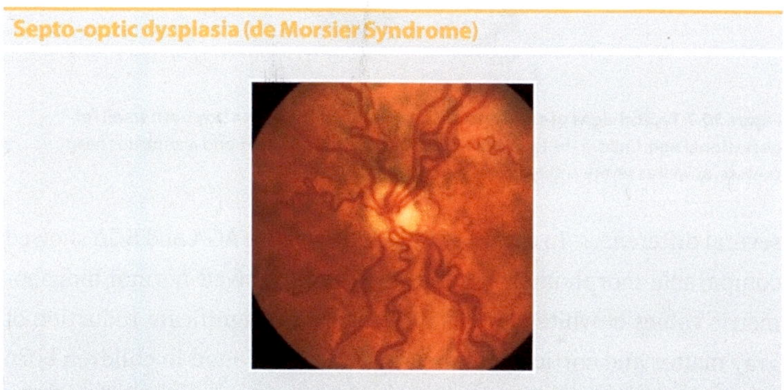

Figure 20.6 Septo-optic dysplasia (de Morsier Syndrome). Optic nerve head dysplasia, paleness especially of the temporal part of the optic nerve head, massively torted veins and arteries.

Refraction

Children born SGA are, on average, slightly more hyperopic than an AGA control group and, when compared to former preterm infants, myopia was more frequent than in children born SGA [13,17].

Ocular alignment and ocular motility

Early childhood strabismus syndrome (congenital esotropia) is found in children born SGA more frequently (Figure 20.7), but the difference when compared with children born AGA is not significant [18].

Postchiasmatic visual pathway and visual cortex

Cerebral morphometry in children born SGA and AGA and in children born with a very low birth weight (VLBW) has been found to have

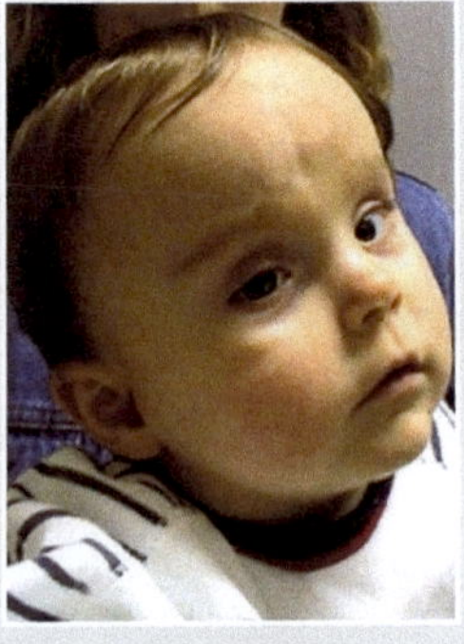

Figure 20.7 Typical signs of early onset strabismus syndrome in a boy born small for gestational age. Child in the figure exhibits esotropia, cross fixation, and anomalous head posture, as well as severe amblyopia of the right eye.

several differences. In a 2011 study, children born AGA and SGA showed comparable morphometric values and both showed normal morphometric values of white matter [19]. However, a significant reduction of gray matter and cortical white matter was only found in children born with a VLBW [14,20]. A slight enlargement of the anterior horn of the ventricular system was also only seen in VLBW, as is a distinct narrowing of the corpus callosum [20]; no significant differences were found between children born AGA and SGA [19].

Functional impairments

Development of visual acuity

In children born SGA and low-risk premature infants, there is no significant difference in the development of the grating acuity within the first 2 years of life as compared to children born AGA [3]. However, in a study of 4-year-old children born SGA, there was significantly worse detection acuity as compared to children born AGA [3]. Additionally, children born SGA show more recognition problems when viewing far away objects as compared to children born AGA [3] (Figure 20.8).

As previously noted, strabismus (in which the eyes are not properly aligned with each other) is often seen in children born SGA and is a

Evaluating grating acuity in preverbal children using LEA grating paddles

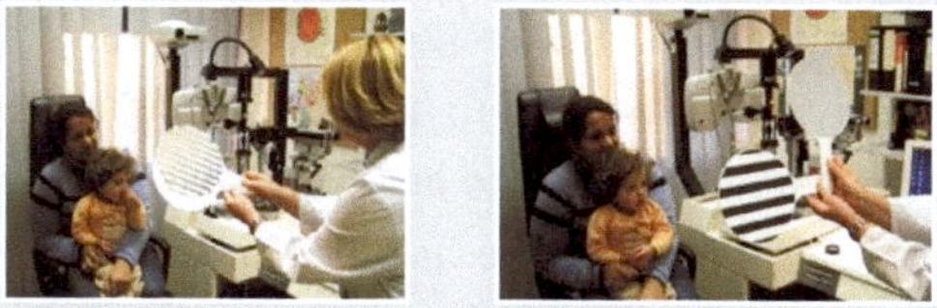

Figure 20.8 Evaluating grating acuity in preverbal children using LEA grating paddles.

condition that carries an increased risk of amblyopia (or 'lazy eye') and stereopsis, a lack of binocular depth perception [16,18,21].

Development of the visual fields

In children born SGA and low-risk premature infants there is no evidence of significant differences in the development of the peripheral visual field borders in the first 2 years of life when compared to children born AGA [21]. In formerly premature babies, there was a very slight, but significantly faster, development of the upper half of the visual field [22]. Even at the age of 4 years, there were no significant differences between children born AGA and SGA concerning visual fields [3].

Visual field lesions and defects. In IUGR and children born SGA, when compared to AGA controls, more relative scotomas were found in the computer-aided perimetry of the central 30 [21]. These findings, however, do not apply to another technique of visual field examination, the so-called frequency-doubling perimetry [21].

Color vision. Children born SGA were not found to have a greater risk of color vision deficiencies when compared to a control group [23].

Contrast sensitivity. There are no known differences in contrast sensitivity between children born SGA and AGA [16].

Disorders of fixation gaze deviations. Conditions associated with SGA/IUGR include:

- deficient slow eye movements;
- difficulties performing saccades;
- reading deficits (in childhood);
- gaze deviations (rare compared to premature children).

Visual perception disorders

Pronounced visual perception deficits can be present in normal or near-normal cognition and intelligence [24]. Typically, the child displays inconsistent behavior and appears to have normal sight, while at other times, the same child can appear to be severely visually handicapped. Visual perception disorders could be classified into the following groups:

- recognition;
- orientation;
- depth perception;
- spatial detection;
- motion perception;
- simultaneous vision;
- combination of the above.

An example of a visual perception disorder can be seen in Figure 20.9.

Major visual pathways

The area of the visual pathway where motion is perceived is called the dorsal (or "where") pathway. This area is often affected in premature or SGA-related brain damage [25]. If a lesion in this pathway is present, the child may have impaired visually-guided motor activity, especially concerning the legs, and impaired saccades and deficits of fixational changes [25,26]. These perception deficits are often combined with bilateral lower visual field defects.

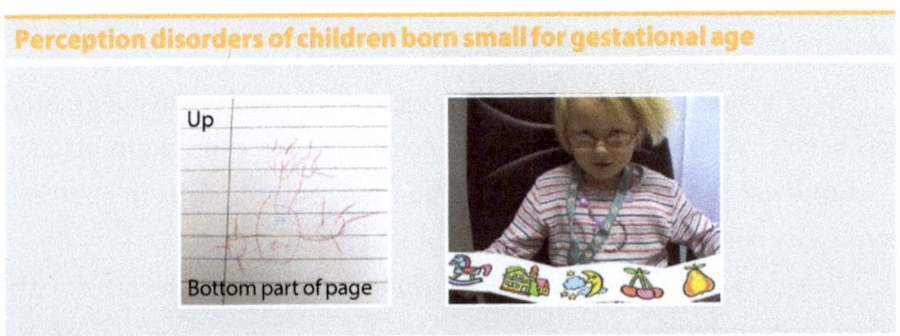

Figure 20.9 Perception disorders of children born small for gestational age. These disorders can include reading and drawing upside down. They are often transient but may be early indicators of severe perceptual deficits.

Another large visual pathway is the so-called ventral (or "what") pathway. Lesions in this area lead to deficits in shape recognition, figure-ground problems, and problems of facial recognition [27,28]. For example, maps may be hard to read and understand.

Children born SGA who were admitted to a medical department for the visually-impaired were found to present with a higher degree of central visual perception disorders [22]. Visual impairment due to morphological damage to the eye (eg, retinopathy of prematurity, optic atrophy) were significantly less frequent than the damage to the higher visual pathway and consequential perceptual disorders [23,29,30].

Table 20.2 gives a summarized overview on the different impacts of prematurity and being born SGA have on the visual system and on visual perception. Although some of the deficits are comparable, there are clear differences between premature children and children born SGA concerning some morphological aspects and the degree of perceptual deficits.

Conclusion

Children born SGA should be subjected to the same routine ophthalmo-logical and orthoptic screening examinations as those that are performed in premature children, as it has been established that being born SGA can yield multiple morphological and functional disorders to the eye and the higher visual centers. Only standardized orthoptic and ophthalmological examinations during the first six years of life can detect any SGA-related changes in early childhood and can induce treatment.

A suitable time for a first eye and vision exam would be the fourth month of life for all full-term children born SGA; children born SGA who have additionally been born prematurely should be first examined 4 months after the expected delivery date. In the long-term, children born SGA should be seen by an ophthalmologist and an orthoptist on a regular basis, as ocular and functional deficits may not become apparent during infancy, and, just as in preterm infants, may only become evident in school age. This espe-cially applicable to perception deficits, which often become evident around the sixth year of life when a child starts learning how to read and write.

Survey of the morphological and functional findings in premature children and in children born small for gestational age without prematurity

	Prematurity and visual system
	Morphology of the eye
First weeks of life	• Persistent tunica vasculosa lentis • Cataract • Glaucoma • Retinopathy of prematurity Stage I to V • Retinal detachment
First year of life	• Ectopic macula • Residual retinal scar formation (Stage I to V retinal scar formation following ROP, phthisis and atrophia bulbi) • High refractive anomalies (especially myopia) • Late-onset cataract • Late-onset glaucoma
First to fifth year of life	• Elevated risk of retinal detachment especially in myopic children • Progression of myopia • Astigmatism • Late-onset cataract • Late-onset glaucoma • Slow improvements of central visual acuity may occur up to the 6th year of life

School age, youth and adult	• Direct correlation exists between degree of ocular pathology and central visual acuity
	• Children with **any** form of former ROP always show a higher frequency of late ocular complications such as:
	  – Retinal detachment
	  – Cataract, glaucoma
	  – Phthisis/atrophia bulbi

Clinical pearls	• Mandatory yearly exams in multiply handicapped children include:
	  – Ophthalmoscopy
	  – Intraocular pressure
	  – Retinoscopy
	  – Refraction
	• No multiply handicapped child may be subjected to missing corrective glasses or to omitting necessary medication just because the ophthalmologist does not manage the child's examination
	• Lack of treatment means lack of early supportive measurements and lack of developmental possibilities

Table 20.1 Survey of the morphological and functional findings in premature children and in children born small for gestational age without prematurity (continues overleaf).

Optic nerve head

- Ascending or descending optic atrophy due to retinal and/or cerebral lesions
- Glaucomatous optic nerve cupping and atrophy

- Optic atrophy
  - Of cerebral origin
  - Of retinal origin
  - Glaucomatous
  - Mixed
- Important: in optic atrophy the optic nerve head shows no swelling in elevated cerebrospinal pressure!

- See above
- In the case of non-diagnosed late-onset glaucoma progression of optic nerve atrophy occurs in spite of seemingly unaltered cerebral and ocular findings
- Regular measurements of intraocular pressure mandatory

- See above
- Regular VEP-monitoring might help to distinguish the different forms of optic atrophy and might be a help to diagnose progression of optic atrophy
- Severe optic atrophy and low vision often prevents the diagnosis of concurrent perception deficits

- Description of the cup-disc-relation should start during ROP-screening during the first weeks of life
- Documentation of CDR at every exam facilitates the diagnosis of late-onset glaucoma
- If in doubt: perform an exam under general anaesthesia
- Regular VEPs help to monitor the course of optic atrophy of any kind and is the only way to document glaucoma treatment, as the children usually are not able to perform visual field exams

Optic pathways, visual

- Cerebral hemorrhages
- Periventricular leukomalacia (PVL)
- Hydrocephalus
- No/little fixation
- Gaze deviations

- Delayed visual maturation (DVM)
- DD: Central visual impairment (CVI)
- Gaze deviations
- Nystagmus
- Strabismus

- CVI, nystagmus
- Strabismus, gaze deviations
- Visual performance depends on the location and on the degree of sustained cerebral hemorrhage and on the extent of PVL
- Visual field defects
- Perceptual deficits become apparent

- No direct correlation between the degree of morphological cerebral changes and amount of visual and perceptual deficits
- Visual perception deficits may be on the **sensory** side (visual field, color perception, face recognition, movement detextion) or on the **motor** side (gaze deviations, no stereopsis)

- Keep in mind that visual perception is transferred into the brain via two ways
- **"Where"-pathway:** detection of movement, orientation (dorsal pathway)
- **"What"-pathway:** object and face recognition, figure-grund-discrimination, colour discrimination (ventral pathway)
- Perceptual deficits can arise in only one or both sectors of visual signal transmission and the two pathways should therefore be tested separately

Survey of the morphological and functional findings in premature children and in children born small for gestational age without prematurity (continued)

	SGA and visual system
	Morphology of the eye
First weeks of life	• Morphology depends on the cause for IUGR and SGA • Lanugo, persistent tunica vasculosa lentis • Cataract (anteriorly) • Reduced number of retinal vessels • Reduced number of vessel branchings • Tortuous arteries and veins (FES, SOD)
First year of life	• Macula hypoplasia or dysplasia • Refractive anomalies: hyperopia much more often than in premature children • Retinal vessels: see above
First to fifth year of life	• Retinal vessels: see above (less ramifications, occasionally tortuous) • Moderate to high hyperopia and astigmatism
School age, youth and adult	• Significantly less retinal vessels and less vessel branching • The amount of vessel rarefication correlates to the extend of IUGR and SGA • Macular differentiation often lacks foveolar reflex characteristics

Clinical pearls	• Mandatory yearly exams in SGA children include:
	  • Ophthalmoscopy
	  • Intraocular pressure
	  • Retinoscopy
	  • Refraction
	• Lack of diagnosis of treatable findings such as hyperopia, strabismus, amblyopia means lack of early supportive measurements and lack of developmental possibilities
	• If there are discrepancies between (good) central visual acuity and poor visual performace → exclude perception deficits!

Table 20.1 Survey of the morphological and functional findings in premature children and in children born small for gestational age without prematurity (continued).

Optic nerve head	**Optic pathways**
• Morphology depends on the cause of IUGR and SGA	• Damage of the optic pathways depends mainly on the underlying cause of SGA and may be normal or severely pathological
• Small neuroretinal rim of the optic nerve	• Delayed onset of fixation
• Optic nerve head small	• Gaze deviations more frequent than in AGA
• Larger CDR in children with additional PVL	
• Extreme optic hypoplasia/dysplasia in septo-optic dysplasia (SOD-Syndrome)	
• Optic nerve head often pale and small	• Visual development up to 2 years comparable to AGA children
• Optic atrophy has to be ruled out (VEP)	• Moderate delayed visual maturation may occur during the first 6 months
• Enlarged CDR	• Strabismus more frequent than in AGA
• Up to now, glaucoma has not been identified as a complication of IUGR and nonsyndromatic SGA	• Nystagmus rare
• Morphology depends on the cause for IUGR and SGA	• Detection and recognition acuity are significantly lower than in AGA children
• Small neuroretinal rim of the optic nerve head	• Early strabismus syndrome and no stereopsis is frequent
• Optic nerve head small	• Perceptual deficits may become apparent even if no cerebral pathologies can be detected (less often than in prematurity, but more often than in AGA)
• No differences in visual field examinations up to the age of 4 between SGA and AGA	
• Small neuroretinal rim of the optic nerve head, correlating to the extend of SGA	• Distinctly more visual perception deficits than in AGA children
• It still is unclear whether the individual neurons show less volume or if there is a reduced number of dendrites	• Perceptual deficits may exist in children of normal intelligence
• Relative scotomata are more frequent in SGA than in AGA children	• Perceptual deficits can often not clearly be correlated to the 2 visual pathways
	• Colour discrimination normal
	• Contrast sensitivity comparable to AGA
• In small and pale optic nerve heads always think of the possibility of septo-optic dysplasia!	• SGA children often show marked differences between good recognition acuity and visual performance!
• Neuroimaging necessary	• Rule out perceptual deficits and visual field defects
• Endocrine exam should be performed	• If perceptual vision deficits are present, they are less clearly associated to just one of the two transmission pathways and less often accompanied by visible cerebral defects than is the case in former premature children
• In small and pale and/or dysplastic optic discs regular VEPs should be performed every one or two years	
• The smaller the optic nerve head is, the more probable visual field defects are → visual field exams should be performed even if SOD could be excluded	

References

1   Chalam KV, Lin S, Murthy RK, Brar VS, Gupta SK, Radhakrishan R. Evaluation of modified reniopathy of prematurity screening guidelines using birth weight as the sole inclusion criteria. *Middle East Afr J Opthalmol.* 2011;18:214-219.

2   Dutton G, Ballantyne J, Boyd G, et al. Cortical visual dysfunction in children: a clinical study. *Eye (Lond).* 1996;10:302-309.

3   Getz L, Dobson V, Luna B. Development of grating acuity, letter acuity, and visual fields in small-for-gestational-age preterm infants. *Early Hum Dev.* 1994;40:59-71.

4   Jacobson L, Hård AL, Svensson E, Flodmark O, Hellström A. Optic disc morphology may reveal timing of insult in children with periventricular leucomalacia and/or periventricular haemorrhage. *B J Ophthalmol.* 2003;87:1345-1349.

5   Martinussen M, Fischl B, Larsson HB, et al. Cerebral cortex thickness in 15-year-old adolescents with low birth weight measured by an automated MRI-based method. *Brain.* 2005;128:2588-2596.

6   Goyen T-A, Lui K, Woods R. Visual-motor, visual-perceptual, and fine motor outcomes in very-low-birthweight children at 5 years. *Dev Med Child Neurol.* 1998;40:76-81.

7   O'Connor AR, Stephenson TJ, Johnson A, et al. Long-term ophalmic outcome of low birth weight children with and without retinopathy of prematurity. *Pediatrics.* 2002;1:12-18.

8   Anand-Apte B, Hollyfield JG. Developmental anatomy of the retinal and chorodial vasculature. Elsevier Direct. www.elsevierdirect.com/brochures/eyes/PDFs/Developmental-Anatomy-Retinoid-Chorodial-Vasculature.pdf. Accessed February 20, 2013.

9   Hellström A, Ley D, Hansen-Pupp I, et al. New insights into development of retinopathy of prematurity – importance of early weight gain. *Acta Paediatr.* 2009;99:502-508.

10 Hellström A, Carlsson B, Niklasson A, et al. IGF-I is critical for normal vascularisation of the human retina. *J Clin Endocrin Metab.* 2000;87:3413-3416.

11 Hård AL, Aring E, Hellström A. Subnormal visual perception in school-aged ex-preterm patients in a paediatric eye clinic. *Eye (Lond).* 2004;18:628-634.

12 Hellström A, Hård AL, Svensson E, Niklasson A. Ocular fundus abnormalities in children born before 29 weeks of gestation: a population-based study. *Eye (Lond).* 2000;14:324-329.

13 Hellström A, Svensson E, Carlsson B, Niklasson A, Albertsson-Wikland, K. Reduced retinal vascularization in children with growth hormone deficiency. *J Clin Endocrinol Metab.* 1999;84:795-798.

14 Hellström A, Wiklund LM, Svensson E, Albertsson-Wikland K, Stromland K. Optic nerve hypoplasia with isolated tortuosity of the retinal veins: a marker of endocrinopathy. *Arch Ophthalmol.* 1999;117:880-884.

15 Hellström A, Dahlgren J, Marsál K, Ley D. Abnormal retinal vascular morphology in young adults following intrauterine growth restriction. *Pediatrics.* 2004;113:e77-e80.

16 Kistner A, Jacobson L, Jacobson SH, Svensson E, Hellström A. Low gestational age associated with abnormal retinal vascularization and increased blood pressure in adult women. *Pediatric Res.* 2002;51:675-680.

17 Denne C, Käsmann-Kellner B, Ruprecht KW. [Prevalence of optic atrophy and associated ocular and system diseases in a department of paediatric opthamology]. *Klin Monbl Augenheilkd.* 2003;220:767-773.

18 O'Connor AR, Stepenson TJ, Johnson A, Tobin MJ, Ratib S, Fielder AR. Strabismus in children of birth weight less than 1707g. *Arch Opthalmol.* 2002;767-773.

19 De Bie HM, Oostrom KJ, Boersma M, et al. Global and regional differences in brain anatomy of young children born small for gestational age. *PLoS One.* 2011;6:e24116.

20 Inder TE, Warfield SK, Wang H, Hüppi PS, Volpe JJ. Abnormal cerebral structure is present at term in premature infants. *Pediatrics.* 2005;115:286-294.

21 Lindqvist S, Vik T, Indredavik MS, Brubakk AM. Visual acuity, contrast sensitivity, peripheral vision and refraction in low birthweight teenagers. *Acta Ophthalmol Scand.* 2007;85:157-164.

22 Martin, L, Ley D, Marsal K, Hellström A. Visual function in young adults following intrauterine growth retardation. *J Pediatr Ophthalmol Strabismus*. 2004;41:212-218.

23 Hellström A, Wiklund L, Svensson E. The clinical and morphologic spectrum of optic nerve hypoplasia. *J AAPOS*. 1999;3:212-220.

24 Torrioli MG, Frisone MF, Bonvin L, et al. Perceptual-motor, visual and cognitive ability in very low birthweight preschool children without neonatal ultrasound abnormalities. *Brain Dev*. 2000;22:163-168.

25 Jakobson LS, Frisk V, Knight RM, Downie ALS, Whyte H. The relationship between periventricular brain injury and deficits in visual processing among extremely-low-birthweight (<1000g) children. *J Pediatr Psych*. 2001;26:503-512.

26 Jongmans M, Mercuri E, Henderson S, de Vries L, Sonksen P, Dubowitz L. Visual function of prematurely born children with and without perceptual motor difficulties. *Early Hum Dev*. 1996;45:73-82.

27 Rosander K, Nystrom P, Gredeback G, von Hofsten C. Cortical processing of visual motion in young infants. *Vision Res*. 2007;47:1614:1623.

28 Strand-Brodd K, Ewald U, Grönqvist H. Development of smooth eye pursuit eye movements in very preterm infants: 1. General aspects. *Acta Paediatr*. 2011;100:983-991.

29 Skranes JS, Martinussen M, Smevik O, et al. Cerebral MRI findings in very-low- birth-weight and small-for-gestational-age children at 15 years of age. Pediatric Radiol. 2005;35:758–765.

30 Käsmann-Kellner B, Heine M, Pfau B, Singer A, Ruprecht KW. Screening for amblyopia, strabismus and refractive abnormalities in 1,030 kindergarten children. *Klin Monbl Augenheilkd*.1998;213:166-173.

Development of this book was supported by funding from Sandoz

Chapter 21

Auditory function disorders
Philipp S van de Weyer and Peter K Plinkert

Introduction

Hearing loss is one of the most common human sensory disabilities and both children and adults can be affected. For example, in Germany approximately 15 million people (or 18.5% of the population) have experienced hearing loss to some degree [1]. Additionally, approximately 2–3 out of every 1000 newborns are born with congenital deafness [2]. Risk factors for developing congenital hearing loss include multiple pregnancies, intrauterine infections, hyperbilirubinemia, and being born small for gestational age (SGA) [2].

Auditory development

The auditory system can be divided anatomically into: the middle ear, inner ear, and the central auditory pathway (Figure 21.1).

After conversion of sound waves into mechanical motion through the middle ear, a nerve signal is generated by the hair cells of the inner ear and the resulting nerve signal causes stimulation of the auditory cortex. The central auditory pathway develops over approximately 15 years and it appears that cognitive development is closely linked to an adequate auditory stimulation of the central nervous system (CNS) [3,4]. Electrical signals of the CNS (eg, auditory evoked potentials) indicate neural information processing, while abnormal event related potentials in the neonatal period are associated with later deficiencies in language-processing skills [5].

S. Zabransky (ed.), *Caring for Children Born Small for Gestational Age*, DOI: 10.1007/978-1-908517-90-6_21, © Springer Healthcare 2013

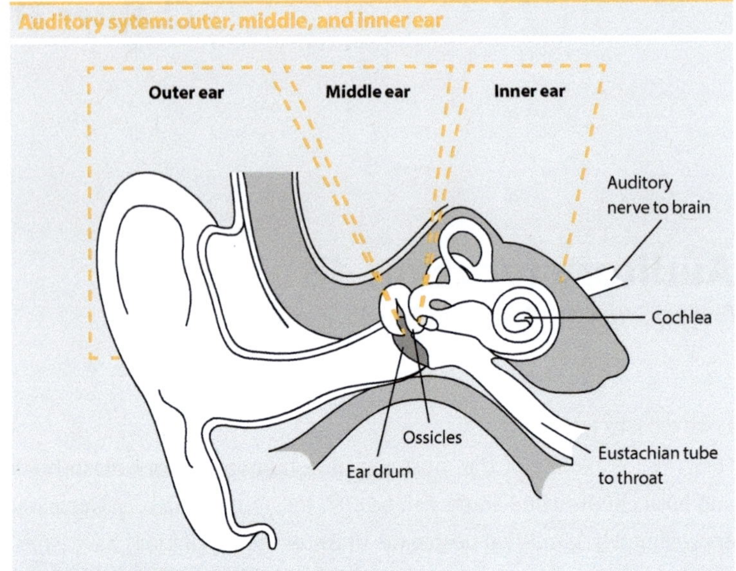

Figure 21.1 Auditory sytem: outer, middle, and inner ear.

Auditory dysfunction in children born small for gestational age

Increased rates of deformity or functional impairment of the middle ear have not yet been described for children born SGA. However, in the area of the central auditory pathway, subtle differences have now been recognized and may be related to intrauterine growth restriction and head growth [6]. Also, it has been found that from the second trimester of development, the fetal brain is able to discriminate auditory information. [7]. After birth, it is possible to measure its capacity non-invasively by monitoring auditory evoked potentials [8,9]. Additionally, the running time of more centrally-generated waves (III and V) in children born SGA are significantly extended [3,6]. This is visible directly after birth, develops over the first year, and cannot be reserved. Thus, children born SGA may have hearing difficulties throughout life [10,11].

Diagnosing and treating auditory disorders in children born small for gestational age

Early detection of hearing loss is essential, especially for infants and young children. During the sensitive phase of speech development, adequate hearing is necessary to ensure the development of the child's verbal and listening skills. Otherwise, speech delays, learning difficulties, and other associated limitations of social and intellectual development can occur.

For children born SGA, a complete diagnostic determination of location and presence of hearing loss is essential. The first hearing test should be performed immediately after birth in the hospital, or shortly after at another appropriately-equipped facility. In cases where irregularities are detected, a diagnostic confirmation should be undertaken in a pediatric audiology or an ear-nose-throat department that is especially equipped for further investigation and assessment.

References

1   Zahnert T. The differential diagnosis of hearing loss. *Dtsch Arztebl Int.* 2011;108:433-443.
2   Neumann K, Gross M, Bottcher P, Euler HA, Spormann-Lagodzinski M, Polzer M. Effectiveness and efficiency of a universal newborn hearing screening in Germany. *Folia Phoniatr Logop.* 2006;58:440-455.
3   Fellman V, Kushnerenko E, Mikkola K, Ceponiene R, Leipala J, Naatanen R. Atypical auditory event-related potentials in preterm infants during the first year of life: a possible sign of cognitive dysfunction? *Pediatr Res.* 2004;56:291-297.
4   Eldredge L, Salamy A. Functional auditory development in preterm and full term infants. *Early Hum Dev.* 1996;45:215-228.
5   Molfese DL. Predicting dyslexia at 8 years of age using neonatal brain response. *Brain Lang.* 2000;72:238-245.
6   Jiang ZD, Brosi DM, Wang J, Wilkinson AR. Brainstem auditory-evoked responses to different rates of clicks in small-for-gestational age preterm infants at term. *Acta Paediatr.* 2004;93:76-81.
7   Draganova R, Eswaran H, Murphy P, Huotilainen M, Lowery C, Preissl H. Sound frequency change detection in fetuses and newborns, a magnetoencephalographic study. *Neuroimage.* 2005;28:354-361.
8   Näätänen R. *Attention and Brain Function.* Hillsdale, NJ: Lawrence Erlbaum; 1992:102-200.
9   Cheour M, Leppänen PH, Kraus N. Mismatch negativity (MMN) as a tool for investigating auditory discrimination and sensory memory in infants and children. *Clin Neurophysiol.* 2000;111:4-16.
10 Monset-Couchard M, de Bethmann O, Relier JP. Long term outcome of small versus appropriate size for gestational age co-twins/triplets. *Arch Dis Child Fetal Neonatal Ed.* 2004;89:F310-F314.
11 Viggedal G, Carlsson G, Hugdahl K. Language asymmetry and auditory attention in young adulthood after being born small-for-gestational age or with cardio-pulmonary resuscitation at birth. *Child Neuropsychol.* 2004;10:195-200.

Development of this book was supported by funding from Sandoz

Chapter 22

Neurological, neurocognitive, and behavioral aspects

Fritz Haverkamp

Introduction

Being born small for gestational age (SGA) is associated with increased neonatal morbidity and mortality [1]. Additionally, children born SGA are at increased risk for other chronic health conditions such as cardiovascular disease and diabetes mellitus later in life [1]. Thus, it is important to address key health issues and methods for providing the necessary care for children born SGA.

When compared with chronic diseases in general, neonatal survival rates of very-low birthweight infants has improved considerably in the last two decades, mostly due to improved prenatal and perinatal care [2]. Also, especially during the last 10 years, research into clinical care for the neurocognitive, emotional, and behavioral effects of being born SGA has increased [3–5]. However, many times it is not until a child starts school (ie, the first setting that requires complex social, emotional, and cognitive skills outside of the home) that deficits in vulnerable developmental areas related to being born SGA are recognized and diagnosed [6,7].

In this chapter, the available empirical evidence for neurocognitive impairment in children born SGA will be discussed, and the importance of early detection to prevent potential developmental delays will be highlighted. As prematurity is an independent risk factor, studies will be classified in accordance to gestational age either in full-term or in preterm children.

S. Zabransky (ed.), *Caring for Children Born Small for Gestational Age*,
DOI: 10.1007/978-1-908517-90-6_22, © Springer Healthcare 2013

Neurological and visuosensory handicaps

In very preterm infants (gestational age of 22–32 weeks) born SGA, the prevalence of neurodevelopmental handicap, including cerebral palsy, microcephaly, mental retardation, blindness, and deafness is double the rate reported in infants born average for gestational age (AGA) [8]. The etiology of neurodevelopmental morbidity, including cerebral paresis, remains unclear but is thought to be multifactorial. In the past, neurodevelopmental morbidity was attributed to hypoxia and/or ischemia associated with perinatal asphyxia [9]. However, only a small proportion of children who are neurologically impaired have evidence of acute perinatal stress [10]. There is increasing evidence that intrauterine or early postnatal inflammation or placental insufficiency due to a different etiology may play a role in the development of cerebral paresis and other neurological handicaps in SGA [11–13].

Intelligence, neurocognitive domains, and learning

Intelligence refers to neuropsychological functions such as visual and auditory perception, abstract reasoning, and cognitive processing. It is essential for learning and is often evaluated as a person's intelligence quotient (IQ). While there is evidence that general IQ is lower in individuals born SGA, irrespective if the infant was born preterm or on time, it never exceeds 1 standard deviation (<15 IQ points) [14]. It is also widely accepted that the mean IQ in children born SGA in most studies still remained in the average range of the normal population (85–115 IQ points) [11,15–19].

In individuals born SGA, a higher prevalence for a specific delay or disorder in each of the developmental cognitive and motor domains such as speech, language, visual-spatial perception and processing, verbal and non-verbal memory, attention, executive functions (such as planning), and developmental motor coordination disorder have also been identified [20,21]. Additionally, there have been studies showing higher rates (up to 55%) of learning disabilities, such as reading and writing disability, dyscalculia [6,15,20,22].

Behavioral and emotional problems

In addition to the neurosensory and cognitive deficits, many studies [2,12,17,23] have found a correlation between prematurity and IUGR/very low birth weight (VLBP) and later emotional and behavioral problems and mental health disorders, with up to 25% of study participants being affected. A wide range of symptoms either with externalizing or internalizing psychiatric disorders (eg, attention deficit hyperactivity disorder, aggressive and delinquent behavior, low self esteem, withdrawal, anxiety, poor social skills, depression) have been reported. Compared to individuals born AGA, the prevalence of these disorders is three times as great [2,12,17,23].

These emotional and behavioral problems or disorders generally become apparent or even more pronounced upon school enrollment [22,23]. It is thought that this is because, for most children, school acts as the first setting that requires complex social skills, such in coping with children of different ages and genders, and finding ways of relating to peers [23]. For psychological and educational surveillance of children born SGA in a clinical care setting, it is important to consider clinical precursors of emotional behavioral disorders (some of which may already present at preschool age) [17,24].

SGA-related risk factors

The overall likelihood of an individual born SGA developing neurocognitive, behavioral, and/or emotions problems is result of a complex interaction between several specifically SGA-related and non SGA-related factors and processes. Furthermore postnatal catch-up growth of both the body and head can follow various patterns [11]. In literature specific to predicting SGA-related neurocognitive, emotional and social outcomes, study parameters often refer to:

- the point of time of IUGR and weight retardation occurred;
- head growth pattern.

Further key players in determining outcome are perinatal complications (eg, prematurity) [11].

Onset and severity of intrauterine and postnatal growth retardation

If IUGR is already present at the 26th week of gestation, the affected children will have a higher risk of developing psychomotor problems, as compared to those demonstrating a later onset of growth restriction [25]. The same is true for the onset and severity of weight retardation. Thus, the earlier the onset, and the more severe it is, the greater the neurodevelopmental risk [17].

Prenatal and postnatal microcephaly

An optimal intrauterine environment is essential for brain development. The neurocognitive prognosis in SGA is dependent on the coexistence of accompanying microcephaly [26]. There is evidence that SGA is associated with reduced brain volume, though it is unclear if this is caused by a reduction of cerebral gray matter or cerebral white matter volume [27,28].

If a microcephaly is present at birth and persists beyond the second year of life, the patient has a greater likelihood of developing neurocognitive deficits [29]. Another high risk group is children with congenital microcephaly who have catch up head circumference growth that places them into normal head circumference range [29]. In case of a normal head circumference at birth (but growth that decreases postnatally), the risk for disturbed psychomotor development also increases [6]. Children with a normal head circumference at birth and postnatally have the best prognosis for healthy psychomotor development [29]. However even in this subgroup, children born SGA show more subtle deficits, especially in language development (eg, spelling) [29].

Determining an overall risk of children born SGA (which comprises IUGR, low birth weight, prematurity, and microcephaly) developing a neurological disorder remains controversial in literature [30].

General risk factors

Postnatal health and socioeconomic status

In general, children born SGA are similarly affected by the same deleterious (and protective) influencing factors and processes as other children. Therefore postnatal health, parental care, environmental, educational, and psychological co-influences are very important determinants in neurological, neurocognitive, and behavioral outcomes [31].

It has been repeatedly shown that parents with lower levels of education and below average income are more likely to have children born SGA [32]. Therefore, offspring born SGA are more likely to live in unfavorable conditions for good health and education [32]. This alone may be responsible for the higher occurrence of emotional and social problems later in life, as well as for specific developmental delays (eg, language development) and learning disabilities. Conversely, in general, children born SGA from families with a high socioeconomic status have a better neurodevelopmental prognosis and postnatal catch-up growth. This is thought to be due to differences in educational resources, as well as better environmental conditions [29,33].

Postnatal nutrition

Cooke and Foulder-Hughes found in a study of 280 preterm babies and 210 full-term children that impaired postnatal growth (length, weight, head) did not seem to be exclusively determined from the intrauterine clinical course, but was also influenced by parental postnatal feeding and care [13]. Similarly, McCowan et al provided evidence that children who were not fed with breast milk during the first 3 months of their life had lower psychomotor development index scores (odds ratio=3.5; 95% CI, 1.2–10.1) regardless of birth weight [34]. However, a recent study did not confirm this hypothesis. In fact, in children born SGA, catch-up growth was not found to be associated with an increase of cognitive functioning [35].

Socioeconomic status

IUGR and being born SGA has been associated with indicators of socioeconomic status, as well as physical environment [36]. This issue is an important health concern, due to the increasing body of evidence that suggests adverse health processes or events that occur very early in life (or indeed, in vitro) can lead to diseases in childhood and later in life [24,36]. In this manner, socioeconomic status is an important indicator, as it can generally act as a measure of access to health care, empowerment, level of stress and violence, and likelihood of exposure to negative environmental factors [33]. Living under restricted life conditions (eg, low income, high crime neighborhood, exposure to pollution, etc) has often problematic consequences [24,37,38]. Among others, they are at greater risk of obtaining a lower level of education and have lower literacy rates, resulting in inferior academic participation, as compared to children born to undeprived parents [38].

A biopsychosocial model of psychomotor development

In the face of the confounding SGA-related and non-SGA related risk factors, the challenge is to identify and differentiate the direct effects of being born SGA on neurological, neurocognitive, and behavioral outcomes. In general, it has been recognized that the greatest risks exist for those children born SGA that had early onset IUGR, microcephaly, and have minimal postnatal catch-up growth, especially beyond the second year of life [1,38]. Careful and comprehensive surveillance and care (especially for children from lower socioeconomic backgrounds) from the beginning of life is crucial. This can be provided through optimal postnatal nutrition, supporting strong mother-child bonding and interaction, and promoting an adequate psychological and educational atmosphere. In Figure 22.1, an advancement of an earlier biopsychosocial model of psychomotor development for SGA is demonstrated [8].

If clinical symptoms such as neurological disturbances (eg, microcephaly) or other developmental problems (eg, feeding and sleeping problems), are present and/or the parental background is at higher risk for impairing a child's development, the respective child and family should be offered early intervention. Again, because lower social status is overrepresented in this subgroup of children, children born SGA should be considered for educational and psychological intervention and implementation of interdisciplinary care settings, which may include the assignment of a social worker.

Biopsychosocial inclusive diagnostic and care processes in children born small for gestational age

Body funtction and structure

- short stature
- expressive language disorders
- fine and gross motor coordination disorders

Activities

- self-help group
- play and sports activities
- special education

Personal/ environmental factors

- self-esteem
- intelligence
- familial empowerment
- parental relationship status
- familial income

Health system

- pediatric endocrinologist
- neuropediatrican
- logopedic

Education system

- inclusive pedagogic intervention with healthy and affected subjects
- patient and family education

Social welfare system

- social and clinical worker
- supporting familial competencies
- financial support

Participation

Activation of social inclusion

Figure 22.1 Biopsychosocial inclusive diagnostic and care processes in children born small for gestational age.

References

1   Clayton PE; Cianfarani S, Czernichow, Johannsson G, Rapaport R, Rogol A Management of the child born small for Gestational age through to adulthood: a consensus statement of the International Societies of Pediatric Endocrinology and the Growth Hormone Research Society. *J Clin Endocrinol Met*. 2007;92:804-810.

2   Hayes B, Sharif F. Behavioural and emotional outcome of very low birth weight infants -- literature review. *J Matern Fetal Neonatal Med*. 2009;22:849-856.

3   Hack M, Wilson-Costello D, Friedman H, Taylor GH, Schluchter M, Fanaroff AA. Neurodevelopment and predictors of outcomes of children with birth weights of less than 1000 g:1992–1995. *Arch Pediatr Adolesc Med*. 2000;154:725-731.

4   Hille ET, den Ouden AL, Saigal S, et al. Behavioral problems in children who weigh 1000 g or less at birth in four countries. *Lancet*. 2001;357:1641-1643.

5   Anderson P, Doyle LW, Victorian Infant Collaborative Study Group. Neurobehavioral outcomes of school-age children born extremely low birth weight or very preterm in the 1990s. *JAMA*. 2003;289:3264-3272.

6   Strauss RS. Adult functional outcome of those born small for gestational age: twenty-six-year follow-up of the 1970 British Birth Cohort. *JAMA*. 2000;283:625-632.

7   Reijneveld SA, de Kleine MJ, van Baar AL, et al. Behavioural and emotional problems in very preterm and very low birthweight infants at age 5 years. *Arch Dis Child Fetal Neonatal Ed*. 2006;91:F423-F428.

8   Haverkamp F, Haverkamp-Krois A, Kavsek M. Intelligenz, Teilleistungsstörungen, und Schulleistungen. In: Zabranky S, ed. *SGA-Syndrom. Risiken für die Entwicklung des Nervensystems.*, Saarbrücken: CONTE-Verlag; 2006:123-130.

9   Volpe JJ. Hypoxic-ischemic encephalopathy: Clinical aspects In, *Neurology of the Newborn*. Philadelphia: WB Saunders; 2000. 331-396.

10 Blair E, Stanley FJ. Intrapartum asphyxia: a rare cause of cerebral palsy. *J Pediatr*. 1988;112:515.

11 De Bie HM, Oostrom KJ, Boersma M,et al. Global and regional differences in brain anatomy of young children born small for gestational age. *PLoS ONE*. 2011;6:e24116.

12 De Bie HM, Oostrom KJ, Delemarre-van de Waal HA. Brain development, intelligence and cognitive outcome in children born small for gestational age. *Horm Res Paediatr*. 2010;73:6-14.

13 Cooke RW, Foulder-Hughes L. Growth impairment in the very preterm and cognitive and motor performance at 7 years. *Arch Dis Child*. 2003;88:482-487.

14 van Pareren YK, Duivenvoorden HJ, Slijper FS, Koot HM, Hokken-Koelega AC. Intelligence and psychosocial functioning during long-term growth hormone therapy in children born small for gestational age. *J Clin Endocrinol Metab*. 2004;89:5295-5302.

15 Haverkamp F, Rünger M, Haverkamp-Krois A. Small for gestational age – Neurologische und kognitive Entwicklungsperspektiven. In: Zabranky S, ed. *SGA-Syndrom-Ursacehn und Folge*n. Malburg: Jonas Verlag; 2003:124-128.

16 Hollo O, Rautava P, Korhonen T, Helenius H, Kero P, Sillanpää M. Academic achievement of small-for-gestational-age children at age 10 years. *Arch Pediatr Adolesc Med*. 2002;156:179-187.

17 Koller H, Lawson K, Rose SA, Wallace I, McCarton C. Patterns of cognitive development in very low birth weight children during the first six years of life. *Pediatrics*. 1997;99:383-389.

18 Morsing E, Asard M, Ley D, Stjernqvist K, Marsál K. Cognitive function after intrauterine growth restriction and very preterm birth. *Pediatrics*. 2011;127:e874-e882.

19 Scherjon S, Briët J, Oosting H, Kok J. The discrepancy between maturation of visual-evoked potentials and cognitive outcome at five years in very preterm infants with and without hemodynamic signs of fetal brain-sparing. *Pediatrics*. 2000;105:385-391.

20 Guellec I, Lapillonne A, Renolleau S, et al. Neurologic outcomes at school age in very preterm infants born to severe or mild growth restriction. *Pediatrics*. 2011;127:e883-e891.

21 Sommerfelt K, Sonnander K, Skranes J, et al. Neuropsychologic and motor function in small-for-gestation preschoolers. *Pediatr Neurol*. 2002;26:186-191.

22 Calame A, Fawer CL, Claeys V, Arrazola L, Ducret S, Jaunin L. Neurodevelopmental outcome and school performance of very-low-birth-weight infants at 8 years of age. *Eur J Pediatr.* 1986;145:461-466.

23 Elgen I, Sommerfelt K. Low birthweight children: coping in school? *Acta Paediatr.* 2002;91:939-945.

24 Grady SC, Enander H. Geographic analysis of low birthweight and infant mortality in Michigan using automated zoning methodology. *Int J Health Geogr.* 2009;8:10.

25 Villar, Smeriglio V, Martorell R, Brown CH, Klein RE. Heterogenous growth and mental development of intrauterine growth-retarded infants during the first 3 years of life. *Pediatrics.* 1984;74:783-791.

26 Hille ET, Dorrepaal C, Perenboom R, Gravenhorst JB, Brand R, Verloove-Vanhorick SP; for the Dutch POPS-19 Collaborative Study Group. Social lifestyle, risk-taking behavior, and psychopathology in young adults born very preterm or with a very low birthweight. *J Pediatr.* 2008;152:793-800.

27 Tolsa CB, Zimine S, Warfield SK, et al. Early alteration of structural and functional brain development in premature infants born with intrauterine growth restriction. *Pediatr Res.* 2004;56:132-138.

28 Martinussen M, Flanders DW, Fischl B, et al. Segmental brain volumes and cognitive and perceptual correlates in 15-year-old adolescents with low birth weight. *J Pediatr.* 2009;155:848-853.

29 Frisk V, Amsel R, Whyte HE. The importance of head growth patterns in predicting the cognitive abilities and literacy skills of small-for-gestational-age children. *Dev Neuropsychol.* 2002;22:565-593.

30 Gutbrod T, Wolke D, Soehne B, Ohrt B, Riegel K. Effects of gestation and birth weight in the growth and development of very low birthweight and small for gestational age infants: a matched group comparison. *Arch Dis Child Fetal Neonatal Ed.* 2000;82:F208-F214.

31 DeFries JC, Johnson RC, Kuse AR, et al. Familial resemblance for specific cognitive abilities. *Behav Genet.* 1979;9:23-43.

32 Zeka A, Melly SJ, Schwartz J. The effects of socioeconomic status and indices of physical environment on reduced birth weight and preterm births in Eastern Massachusetts. *Environ Health.* 2008;7:60.

33 Koeppen-Schomerus G, Eley TC, Wolke D, Gringras P, Plomin R. The interaction of prematurity with genetic and environmental influences on cognitive development in twins. *J Pediatr.* 2000;137:527-533.

34 McCowan LM, Pryor J, Harding JE. Perinatal predictors of neurodevelopmental outcome in small-for-gestational-age children at 18 months of age. *Am J Obstet Gynecol.* 2002;186:1069-1075.

35 Beyerlein A, Ness AR, Streuling I, Hadders-Algra M, von Kries R. Early rapid growth: no association with later cognitive functions in children born not small for gestational age. *Am J Clin Nutr.* 2010;92:585-593.

36 Zelkowitz P, Feeley N, Shrier I, et al. The Cues and Care Trial: a randomized controlled trial of an intervention to reduce maternal anxiety and improve developmental outcomes in very low birthweight infants. *BMC Pediatr.* 2008;8:38.

37 Smedler AC, Faxelius G, Bremme K, Lagerstrom M. Psychological development in children born with very low birth weight after severe intrauterine growth retardation: a 10-year follow-up study. *Acta Paediatr.* 1992;81:197-203.

38 Haverkamp F. Gesundheit und soziale lebenslage: herausforderung für eine inklusive gesundheitsversorgung. In: Huster EU, Boeckh, J, Mogge-Grotjahn H, eds. *Handbuch Armut und soziale Ausgrenzung.* Hessen: Springer Fachmedien Wiesbaden; 2012:365-382.

Development of this book was supported by funding from Sandoz

Chapter 23

Prevention and long-term care
Siegfried Zabransky

Introduction

Primary prevention of children being born small for gestational age (SGA) and intrauterine growth restriction (IUGR) should target the main etiology and mechanisms, which in developed countries are smoking, alcohol, infection, and preeclampsia as major causes of decreased placental flow [1]. In light of the topics discussed in this book, the following preventative measures should be taken:

- no alcohol, smoking, or ingesting other toxic substances (eg, illegal drugs) during pregnancy and breastfeeding periods;
- regular surveillance of body weight, blood pressure, urine analyses, control of fetal growth;
- adequate quantity and quality of nutrition with sufficient intake of vitamins and trace elements; and
- hygienic precautions in order to prevent infections.

Upon examination of clinical and experimental data, overnutrition during neonatal life and in infancy should be regarded as a primary cause of deleterious long-term outcomes in children born SGA and/or with IUGR [2]. Avoidance of early overnutrition can be most effectively realized by breastfeeding. Breastfeeding for at least 6 months should be recommended wherever possible and promoted, not only with respect to the short-term benefits (eg, adequate nutrition, greater immunity to infection), but also long-term benefits such as decreased risk of high blood pressure and obesity [3,4].

S. Zabransky (ed.), *Caring for Children Born Small for Gestational Age*, 295
DOI: 10.1007/978-1-908517-90-6_23, © Springer Healthcare 2013

There should be regular documentation of body length, head circumference, and weight. If there is no catch up growth during the first 2 years, a physician should check for an indication for growth hormone therapy [5].

References

1   Bull J, Mulvihill C, Quigley R. Prevention of low birth weight: assessing the effectiveness of smoking cessation and nutritional interventions. Evidence briefing. Health Development Agency (NICE UK).
    www.nice.org.uk/niceMedia/documents/low_birth_weight_evidence_briefing.pdf. Accessed February 20, 2013.
2   Barker DJP, Eriksson JG, Forsén T, OsmondC. Fetal origins of adult disease: strength of effects and biological basis. *Int J Epidemiol*. 2002;31:1235-1239.
3   World Health Organization (WHO). Global strategy for infant and young child feeding. The optimal duration of exclusive breastfeeding. WHO website.
    apps.who.int/gb/archive/pdf_files/WHA54/ea54id4.pdf. Accessed February 20, 2013.
4   World Health Organization (WHO). Optimal feeding of low birthweight infants in low-and middle-income countries 2011. WHO website.
    www.who.int/maternal_child_adolescent/documents/9789241548366.pdf.
    Accessed February 20, 2013.
5   National Institute for Clinical Excellence (NICE). Guidance on use of human growth hormone (somatropin) in children with growth failure. Technology Appraisal Guidance No. 42. London, UK; NICE. www.guidance.nice.org.uk/TA42. Accessed February 20, 2013.

Development of this book was supported by funding from Sandoz

Chapter 24

Considerations for future research

Jörg Dötsch, Miguel A Alejandre Alcázar, Sarah Appel,
Ruth Kuschewski, Eva Nüsken, Kai Nüsken, Eva Rother

Future research

The study fields of investigating children born small for gestational age (SGA) and developmental origins of health and disease (DOHaD) have been closely linked in the past few decades, leading to new perspectives in both areas and increased understanding of functional adaptations during fetal life and childhood that may predict future course of health and disease.

In what ways can the field further develop? Are there opportunities for future research? Will researchers be able to develop treatment and prevention studies that are affordable for health systems that are under constant financial pressure? In this short chapter, a personal approach to these questions will be offered. These considerations are based on personal perspectives in the field.

Approaches for further experimental research

Experimental studies should focus on the examination of underlying molecular mechanisms. The discovery of such mechanisms will provide the opportunity to explain concepts of DOHaD and help to develop effective preventive and therapeutic strategies. Because IUGR has no uniform etiology, approaches on different levels need to be made to clarify the underlying mechanisms that determine individual and population-based

S. Zabransky (ed.), *Caring for Children Born Small for Gestational Age*, 297
DOI: 10.1007/978-1-908517-90-6_24, © Springer Healthcare 2013

risks for poor health and development. These levels include continuation of basic research and evaluation of follow-up programs for continuous control of somatic and neurologic development in later infancy and adulthood and improvement of medical care during pregnancy and around birth.

Additionally, the role of epigenetic pathways should be explored with regard to the underlying mechanisms and should not stop at looking for methylation patterns only. Hypothesis generation methods (eg, arrays, metabolomics) might help initiate a mechanistic approach. Longitudinal data needs to be generated to further elucidate developmental kinetics in the effects of programming factors and systematic experimental approaches are needed to determine the vulnerable time windows for each relevant compromising factor (eg, fetal growth restriction).

Aims for further clinical research

The broad variety of underlying causes for being born SGA must be carefully considered when recruiting study populations. An in-depth characterization of all study participants should start as early as implantation to determine whether or not fetal programming may have taken place. Human studies should aim to identify clinical parameters and biomarkers that can serve as targets for interventional and experimental approaches. Translational approaches, building a bridge between clinical observations and molecular mechanisms, will ultimately help to move the field of perinatal programming towards a providing greater scientific impact.

Interventional studies

Interventional studies should be focused and based on molecular mechanisms that have been identified in experimental approaches. Interdisciplinary approaches involving obstetricians, pediatricians, and midwives are needed to implement comprehensive preventive and interventional strategies.

The goals for future research of medical care during pregnancy and around birth may include the following: early detection of maternal risks that lead to asymmetric and symmetric growth retardation; using the best method to monitor maternal and fetal health; developing protective obstetric practices; determining the optimal time and mode of delivery, using a multidisciplinary approach; taking precautions against the heightened neonatal morbidities of growth-restricted infants, especially the risk of hypoglycemia; and putting together treatment strategies for the infant that involve specialized care from a pediatric endocrinologist and/or neurologist.

Another goal for future studies should be to contribute to an area of research that is well-recognized among other research fields, not for its spectacular theories, but for its profound research methods.

Development of this book was supported by funding from Sandoz

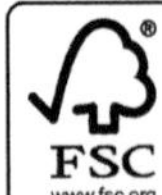

If you have any concerns about our products,
you can contact us on
ProductSafety@springernature.com

In case Publisher is established outside the EU,
the EU authorized representative is:
Springer Nature Customer Service Center GmbH
Europaplatz 3, 69115 Heidelberg, Germany

Printed by Libri Plureos GmbH
in Hamburg, Germany